Functional
VISION

Functional
VISION

A Practitioner's
Guide to
Evaluation and
Intervention

Amanda Hall Lueck, Editor

AFB PRESS

American Foundation for the Blind

Printed in the United States of America

Library of Congress Cataloging-in-Publication Data

Functional vision : a practitioner's guide to evaluation and intervention
/ Amanda Hall Lueck, editor.
    p. ; cm.
Includes bibliographical references and index.
ISBN 978-0-89128-871-8 (alk. paper)
1. Low vision. 2. Vision disorders.
[DNLM: 1. Vision Disorders—diagnosis. 2. Vision
Disorders—therapy. WW 140 F9786 2004] I. Lueck, Amanda Hall, 1949–
  RE91.F87 2004
  617.7—dc22

                      2003059589

Dedication

Working with individuals with low vision is a challenging and rewarding experience. The field of low vision is changing rapidly, with new
advances occurring all the time in our basic understanding of visual
conditions, training effects, and new technological applications. Yet at
the heart of this process are people: the people who have low vision
and the people who facilitate the multifaceted aspects of low vision care.
This book is dedicated to all of them.

—A. H. L.

Contents

PART 3: INTERVENTION METHODS

Acknowledgments

I would like to thank all the contributors for their dedication to the preparation of this manuscript. A special thanks is extended to our editor at AFB Press, Natalie Hilzen, for her insights, persistence, and care. Without her constant support, this book would not have come to fruition. Ellen Bilofsky's thoughtful and careful preparation of the final manuscript was especially appreciated. Barbara Chernow was a positive force in bringing the book through the final production phase.

A number of people informally reviewed chapters or sections of chapters. The contributors and I would like to thank Lee Berdinski, Harvey Clark, Dennis Brooks, August Colenbrander, Helen Dornbusch, Jamie Dote-Kwan, and Penny Rosenbloom. A very special thanks to Ian Bailey for his patient explanations and advice.

And, for their encouragement and love during the many long days (and nights) devoted to this project, I thank my husband, Scott, and my daughter, Tasha Ariana.

Foreword

This book deals with the education and rehabilitation needs of people with visual impairments. Its goal is to help professionals from the fields of education, rehabilitation, and health care gain a better understanding of methods used to evaluate and work with functional vision as they provide services for their clients with low vision. The rehabilitation and education services that are appropriate for a person with low vision depend primarily on that individual's functional vision. The educator or rehabilitation specialist is faced with the question of what visual capabilities can be used or enhanced to enable or facilitate the client's performance of functional tasks in daily life. What visual abilities and skills have been retained by the individual who has a partial loss of vision? Can his or her performance of tasks and participation in the activities of normal daily life be enhanced, or optimized, through maximizing the use of vision by means of devices, environmental modifications, and the teaching of different visual behaviors? Alternatively, would it be preferable to use some nonvisual strategies and devices to enable or facilitate the performance of tasks for which vision would normally be used? Service providers must have a good understanding of the functional vision capabilities of the person with visual impairments when decisions are being made about treatments and interventions and the plans and strategies for their implementation.

Success in the provision of education and rehabilitative care and assistance therefore depends to a large extent on collaborations. The professionals involved may come from ranks of the medical, educational, or rehabilitation communities. Family members, friends, colleagues, and other nonprofessionals often play crucially important roles in this process. The relative importance of the different participants and their interactions with each other can vary enormously from one client or student to the next. For a given individual, the nature and the magnitude of support that is necessary or appropriate will vary from task to task and from day to day.

There has long been a need for a structured framework for the practical and rational assessment of functional vision and a logical and systematic approach to intervention methods that focus on functional vision abilities. *Functional Vision* begins with an outline of visual functions related to functional vision, and it describes the optical devices that are used to assist in the performance of visual tasks. It goes on to describe methods for the practical assessment of functional vision. From a platform of the practitioner's understanding of functional vision abilities, the book describes methods of intervention that the practitioner may use. Emphasis is given to developing structured intervention programs, built on sequences aimed at developing selected skills and accomplishing the performance of selected tasks. The book provides a blueprint for education and rehabilitation practitioners, giving them a rational approach to understanding, analyzing and working with functional vision for the benefit of their students and clients with low vision.

Functional Vision is a most welcome and highly important contribution to the literature and to the field. The title appropriately promises guidance to its primary audience—practitioners in the field of low vision rehabilitation and education. The book, however, is more than a manual of practical advice and recommendations. From a scholarly and scientifically sound foundation, it has built a logical structure for the evaluation of functional vision and the development of intervention strategies and programs. It serves as a valuable resource informing all participants about the roles, procedures, and intervention options of others. Its more direct impact will come from the guidance and frameworks that it gives to professionals for improving and expanding their assessment methods and their intervention procedures and strategies. *Functional Vision* is a welcome addition to low vision literature and practice, providing education and rehabilitation practitioners, experts and neophytes alike, with a new and more fundamentally rational approach to understanding, analyzing, and working with functional vision for the benefit of their students and clients with low vision.

Ian L. Bailey
Professor of Optometry and Vision Science
School of Optometry
University of California, Berkeley

About the Contributors

Amanda Hall Lueck, Ph.D., is Associate Professor and Coordinator, Program in Visual Impairments, at San Francisco State University. A teacher of visually impaired students, she was a Fulbright Professor in Katmandu, Nepal, and has also taught and consulted in India, Nairobi, Cyprus, and Sri Lanka. She is chair-elect and past president of the Northern California Chapter of the Association for Education and Rehabilitation of the Blind and Visually Impaired and received their 2002 Education Award. Dr. Lueck has published widely in the area of low vision and reading, and is a coauthor of *Developmental Guidelines for Infants with Visual Impairment: A Manual for Early Intervention* as well as of the *Bailey-Hall Cereal Test for the Measurement of Visual Acuity in Children* and the *U.C. Berkeley Preferential Looking Test.*

Aries Arditi, Ph.D., is a senior fellow at the Arlene R. Gordon Research Institute at the Lighthouse International in New York City.

Lori Cassells, M.A., is a certified orientation and mobility instructor at the California School for the Blind, Fremont.

Robert Dister, O.D., J.D., is Associate Clinical Professor, School of Optometry, at the University of California, Berkeley. A fellow of the American Academy of Optometry, he has coauthored journal articles and book chapters, made numerous conference presentations, and conducted research in the areas of low vision, contact lenses, and legal issues in optometry.

Roanne Flom, O.D., is Associate Professor of Clinical Optometry, School of Optometry, and Chief, Vision Rehabilitation Service, at Ohio State University in Columbus. A fellow of the American Academy of Optometry and diplomate in its Low Vision section, she has made numerous presentations on low vision and written journal articles and a book chapter on low vision management.

Gregory Goodrich, Ph.D., is Supervisory Research Psychologist, Psychology Service and Western Blind Rehabilitation Center, Veterans Affairs Health Care System in Palo Alto, California. He is coauthor of *Low Vision—The Reference* (now in its third edition) and contributor of numerous book chapters and journal articles on low vision rehabilitation as well as its history. Goodrich is president-elect and former treasurer of the Association for Education and Rehabilitation of the Blind and Visually Impaired and received its 2002 Division VII (Low Vision) Award for Outstanding Contributions to the Division.

Robert Greer, O.D., is Associate Clinical Professor, School of Optometry, at the University of California, Berkeley. A fellow of the American Academy of Optometry and a diplomate in its Low Vision section, he has coauthored a number of articles on low vision and received several teaching awards.

Gunilla Haegerstrom-Portnoy, O.D., Ph.D., is Associate Dean for Academic Affairs and Professor of Optometry and Vision Science, at the School of Optometry, University of California, Berkeley. She has authored and coauthored many papers and book chapters and made numerous presentations on vision, low vision, and optometry.

Toni Heinze, Ed.D., is Associate Professor, Department of Teaching and Learning, at Northern Illinois University in Dekalb and a psychologist. She contributed the chapter on "Comprehensive Assessment" in *Foundations of Education, Vol. II: Instructional Strategies for Teaching Children and Youths with Visual Impairments.*

Jillian King, M.A., is a speech and learning pathologist for Placer Nevada Special Education Local Plan Area in Auburn, CA.

Deborah Tierney Kreuzer, M.A., is Director of Education at the California School for the Blind in Fremont.

Patricia Morgan, M.Ed., is a teacher for the visually impaired at the Marin County Office of Education in San Rafael, California. She is a coauthor of the Visual Functioning Assessment Tool (VFAT).

Ike Presley, M.Ed., is National Program Associate, National Literacy Center, American Foundation for the Blind in Atlanta.

R. D. Quillman, M.A., is Blind Rehabilitation Specialist (Low Vision), Southeastern Blind Rehabilitation Center, at the Veterans Affairs Medical Center in Birmingham, Alabama. A certified low vision therapist and orientation and mobility specialist, he is the author the *Low Vision Training Manual* and coauthor of the *Study Guide for the Low Vision Therapist Certification Examination.* Quillman is president-elect of the Alabama chapter of the Association for Education and Rehabilitation of the Blind and Visually Impaired and past chair of Division VII (Low Vision) of the national association and has received several professional awards for his contributions in low vision.

Janice Smith, Ph.D., is a low vision specialist at the Arizona State Schools for the Deaf and Blind in Tucson. A certified low vision therapist, Smith has written on the topic of students with low vision.

Irene Topor, Ph.D., is Adjunct Associate Professor, Vision Specialization Program, at the University of Arizona in Tucson; Allied Health Professional with the Children's Rehabilitative Services of the State of Arizona; and consultant to the Arizona Division of Developmental Disabilities. A certified low vision therapist and teacher of students with visual impairments, she has written several book chapters on functional vision assessment of infants and children and visual impairment among Native Americans. Topor received the 2001 Margaret Bluhm Worker of the Year Award from the Arizona chapter of the Association for Education and Rehabilitation of the Blind and Visually Impaired.

Introduction

AMANDA HALL LUECK

The practice of low vision education and rehabilitation has advanced rapidly since Natalie Barraga completed her landmark study (1964) verifying the effectiveness of vision intervention for children with visual impairments. This work marked the end of the "sight saving" era in the schools, in which the use of sight was discouraged in the belief that limiting its use would in fact preserve it. It heralded the beginning of the promotion of methods to encourage and enhance the use of vision by persons with visual impairments. Various intervention methods were developed subsequently to foster the use of vision skills and abilities by persons with visual impairments.

LOW VISION EVALUATION AND INTERVENTION IN PERSPECTIVE

In the 1970s and 1980s, many intervention approaches in education to promote the use of functional vision centered around the performance of isolated visual skills not related to critical activities, such as following a penlight in a dimly lit room (Lundervald, Lewin, & Irvin, 1987). This approach was most often used with very young children and students with visual and multiple impairments. Some exceptions to this general approach were available for academically oriented schoolchildren, such as a program to increase visual efficiency in skills related to reading (Barraga & Morris, 1978–80). Current methodologies have evolved to emphasize the complete infusion of vision instruction and other compensatory techniques into functional tasks completed in the home, school, work, or community environments for all individuals with low vision (Corn & Koenig, 1996; Goetz & Gee, 1987; Lueck, Dornbusch, & Hart, 1999).

Along with systematic instruction to improve vision skills and abilities, other intervention methods have been developed to support the performance of tasks of daily living for adults and children as well as work-related tasks for adults. Instruction to enhance overall task performance now takes into account the complex interplay of visual factors, additional sensory skills, environmental conditions, and use of assistive and adaptive devices. These comprehensive instructional programs are derived from an assessment of a person's overall capabilities and the various demands of his of her daily life. Assessment in low vision has received increased attention in recent years from medical, education, and re-habilitation professionals. This has resulted in the steady development of formal and informal methods to evaluate different aspects of the visual functioning of individuals with low vision (Goodrich & Sowell, 1996).

FRAMEWORK FOR THIS BOOK

This book is meant to be a primary reference tool for professionals who have a basic knowledge of visual impairments from educational or rehabilitation per-spectives. However, it contains important information of use to anyone engaged in work related to low vision rehabilitation and the delivery of low vision services. It contains detailed and practical information about various steps associated with the functional vision evaluation and instruction process. As an outgrowth of the editor's earlier work, which organized low vision intervention practices into a cohesive plan for research and service delivery (Hall & Bailey, 1989; Lueck, 1997), this volume considers various ways to deliver instruction to promote the use of vision in activities in the school, home, work, or community.

The original approach has been expanded and updated in order to present a systematic and integrated approach to functional vision evaluation and instruc-tion, in which evaluation findings are linked to the creation of meaningful and effective instructional programs for persons with low vision. Emphasis is placed on instruction to promote visual functioning within usual activities of daily life, including educational, vocational, and leisure pursuits. References are provided throughout the text for readers who wish to delve more deeply into current prac-tices about general evaluation and instruction topics specific to early childhood education, students with multiple impairments, programming for school age stu-dents, vocational training for adults, and special concerns regarding elderly per-sons. The book is organized into three sections: Overview of Low Vision Care, Evaluation of Functional Vision, and Intervention Methods.

Part 1: Overview of Low Vision Care

This section provides a brief introduction to low vision services and some key definitions used in this book. The role of professionals and consumers in the com-prehensive process of low vision care is reviewed. Collaborative methods that can be used by professionals and consumers are examined that can promote independence and improved quality of life for individuals with low vision. Visual functions such as acuity, contrast, and visual fields affected by common eye con-ditions are analyzed along with a description of ways in which a reduction in these capacities can affect an individual's performance. Information on basic optical principles related to frequently prescribed low vision optical devices is also presented in this section.

Part 2: Evaluation of Functional Vision

The first chapter in this section, Chapter 4, presents an overview of critical elements in the low vision evaluation process that apply to persons of all ages. Chapters 5 and 6 address specific assessment methodologies. Specific practices involving tasks with less complex cognitive, motor, and language requirements for the assessment of young children with visual impairments as well as some individuals with visual and multiple disabilities are presented first. This is followed by a chapter detailing assessment methods that can be used with both older children and adults. According to a report from the National Research Council (2002), most school age children at least 6 years of age and older can be evaluated using standard adult tests of visual acuity and contrast sensitivity and shorter versions of adult methods for testing visual fields. Chapter 6 presents these and other methods.

Part 3: Intervention Methods

A model for training vision functioning for individuals with low vision of all ages is introduced. Methods to modify environments to accommodate persons with various visual impairments are furnished, and methods to infuse intervention programs into strategic life tasks are elucidated. The design and development of instructional programs for young children as well as children with severe cognitive impairments in home and school settings are discussed in Chapter 8. Children in school require different instructional methods from those presented for young children and children with multiple disabilities, and these approaches are presented in Chapter 9. Intervention approaches for adults, including elderly individuals, are discussed in the final chapter.

COLLABORATION AND FAMILY INVOLVEMENT

With their varied backgrounds, the book's contributors reflect the cross-disciplinary nature of services for persons with low vision. This book stresses the need for collaboration and cooperation across all medical, education, rehabilitation, and social service disciplines to serve persons with low vision effectively. It also emphasizes the need to involve individuals who have low vision and their families throughout the evaluation and instruction process to determine meaningful and realistic educational, vocational, and rehabilitation goals and to implement instructional plans. Only through carefully coordinated teamwork can successful outcomes be achieved for persons served by comprehensive low vision care.

REFERENCES

Barraga, N. C. (1964). *Increased visual behavior in low vision children*. New York: American Foundation for the Blind.

Barraga, N. C., & Morris, J. E. (1978–80). *Program to develop efficiency in visual functioning.* Louisville, KY: American Printing House for the Blind.

Lundervald, D., Lewin, L., & Irwin, L. (1987). Rehabilitation of visual impairments: A critical review. *Clinical Psychology Review, 7,* 169–185.

Corn, A. L., & Koenig, A. J. (1996). *Foundations of low vision: Clinical and functional perspectives.* New York: AFB Press.

Goetz, L., & Gee, K. (1987). Functional vision programming: A model for teaching visual behavior in natural contexts. In L. Goetz, D. Guess, & K. Stremmel-Campbell (Eds.), *Innovative program design for individuals with dual sensory impairments.* Baltimore, MD: Paul Brookes.

Goodrich, G. L., & Sowell, V. M. (1996). Low vision: A history. In A. L. Corn & A. J. Koenig (Eds.), *Foundations of low vision: Clinical and functional perspectives.* New York: AFB Press.

Hall, A., & Bailey, I. L., (1989). A model for training vision functioning. *Journal of Visual Impairment & Blindness. 83,* 390–396.

Lueck, A. H. (1997). Education and rehabilitation specialists in the comprehensive low vision care process. *Journal of Visual Impairment & Blindness, 91,* 423–434.

Lueck, A. H., Dornbusch, H., & Hart, J. (1999). An exploratory study to investigate the effects of training on the vision functioning of young children with cortical visual impairment. *Journal of Visual Impairment & Blindness, 93,* 778–793.

National Research Council (2002). *Visual impairments: Determining eligibility for social security benefits.* Washington, DC: National Academy Press.

Part 1

OVERVIEW OF LOW VISION CARE

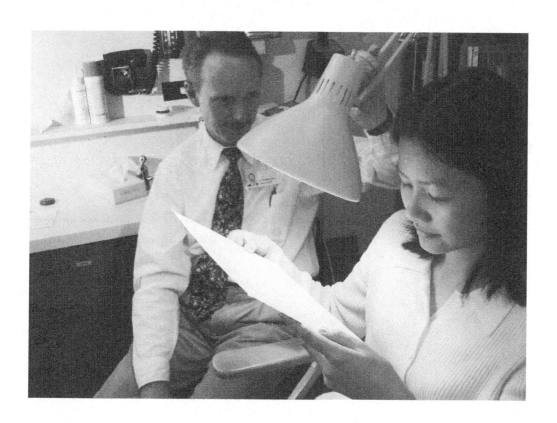

Comprehensive Low Vision Care

AMANDA HALL LUECK

There are numerous definitions of low vision, each organized around one or more of the following factors: loss of organ function, degree of available vision, and participation in life tasks (see, e.g., Corn & Koenig 1996; Colenbrander, 1997). In keeping with this book's emphasis on functional vision—the application of available vision skills and behaviors in various activities of daily life—the definition of low vision adopted here stresses a person's ability to use vision in learning and performing critical and meaningful tasks (Bailey & Hall, 1990; Lueck, Chen, & Kekells, 1997):

> Low vision is defined as a vision loss that is severe enough to impede an individual's ability to learn or perform usual tasks of daily life, given that individual's level of maturity and cultural environment, but still allows some functionally useful visual discrimination. Low vision cannot be corrected to normal by regular eyeglasses or contact lenses and covers a range from mild to severe vision loss but excludes full loss of functional vision. The majority of persons who are legally blind are included within the category of low vision.

GOALS OF LOW VISION CARE

Low vision care is a coordinated and collaborative system of discrete services designed to maximize independence and quality of life for individuals with low vision. Services may include vision evaluation and eye care, provision of assistive devices, instruction to promote the use of vision or alternative sensory strategies in life tasks, training to promote safe and efficient travel, and psychosocial services for individuals with low vision and their families.

Low vision care professionals promote strategies that will maximize effective use of vision in tasks that both promote independent functioning and are deemed to be important by each person with low vision and his or her family. For example, a recent high school graduate with low vision may want to find employment in the computer industry. Both the graduate and the team of professionals must work together along with the graduate's family, to identify and implement realistic steps to reach this goal. It is essential that service providers, consumers, and their families understand and agree upon the steps toward reaching this goal and work together to achieve it.

Goals of Professionals

To understand the goal of low vision care from the vantage point of service providers, it is necessary to have a clear understanding of the distinctions among visual impairment, activity limitation, and participation restriction in order to see how health, education, rehabilitative, and social services fit conceptually into the broad picture of comprehensive low vision care. The *International Classification of Functioning, Disability, and Health* defines these as follows:

1. *Visual impairment* results from problems in body function or structure such as a significant deviation or loss.

2. A difficulty in performing activities of daily life due to a visual impairment is classified as an *activity limitation.*

3. An activity limitation becomes a *participation restriction* when the inability to perform a specific activity creates problems for an individual in becoming involved in broader life situations. (Colenbrander, 1977; World Health Assembly, 1980; World Health Organization, 2001)

Based on these definitions, comprehensive low vision care has been conceptualized as any treatment or assistance to individuals with low vision that prevents their visual impairment from becoming an activity limitation or a participation restriction. Low vision care includes:

1. Restoring function by enhancing impaired vision (that is, through medical and optometric intervention)

2. Teaching strategies to compensate for impaired vision

3. Accessing a full range of education/rehabilitation supports and services (Massof et al., 1995)

According to these definitions, when it is not possible to prevent impairments from becoming activity limitations or participation restrictions solely through restoration of function by medical or optometric interventions, health care, education, and rehabilitation practitioners are mobilized to teach compensatory strategies or, along with social service professionals, to provide a full range of educational and rehabilitative support and services. Although a full range of services is a part of comprehensive low vision care, this book will focus on teaching strategies that compensate for impaired vision; such strategies can be facilitated by health care, rehabilitation, and education professionals.

Goals of Consumers

From the viewpoint of consumers—patients and their families—low vision care must generate positive outcomes. These outcomes must be meaningful, and this "meaning" can best be determined by consumers themselves. Outcomes address issues related to independence and quality of life. To facilitate this process, low vision care must involve the following:

1. The education of consumers so that they are aware of the range of possible outcomes and the steps required to reach them (Lund & Dietrichson, 2000)
2. A determination of meaningful and critical outcomes, with consumers playing a major role
3. The identification and implementation of instructional strategies and activities leading to identified outcomes
4. An assessment that focuses on the achievement of desired outcomes

Outcomes of Low Vision Care

An overall goal for low vision care should combine the needs of consumers with the capabilities of service providers. It entails continued communication between consumers and service providers so that goals and objectives can be revised to reflect an individual's changing needs and perceptions over time.

The ultimate goal of low vision care is to optimize outcomes determined by consumers that increase self-perceived independence and quality of life. Any system of education, rehabilitation, health, or social service must empower consumers to achieve those outcomes, with professionals facilitating the process by encouraging consumer competence in selecting meaningful and critical outcomes that may change over time and implementing activities that lead to the successful achievement of those outcomes.

The need for rehabilitation programs to demonstrate positive service outcomes for their clients has resulted in projects to define and categorize measurable and meaningful areas of change that also reflect those clients' wishes (Crews, 2000). This has also led to efforts to develop standardized instruments to evaluate outcomes of vision rehabilitation for adults with low vision that can eventually be readily incorporated into rehabilitation programs (e.g., Stelmack, et al., 2000; De L'Aune, Welsh, & Williams, 2000; Massof, 2003).

LOW VISION SERVICE DELIVERY OPTIONS

The growing need for coordinated low vision services resulting from demographic trends, such as the aging of the population, and social trends, such as the recognized importance of early intervention, has resulted in the creation of varied service and funding models. Low vision service delivery systems can vary greatly in their philosophical base, organization, level of service, as well as degree of interactive planning and implementation across disciplines. Service delivery paradigms of programs committed to low vision care are dependent on the resources, organizational scheme of sponsoring programs or agencies (including their funding base), the range of services available in a single setting, the degree and quality of interaction among the professionals involved, and extent of referral to external or internal resources. Services can be rendered in such diverse settings as general or teaching hospitals, teaching clinics in optometry schools, rehabilitation agencies, educational agencies, or private low vision practices of specialists in ophthalmology or optometry (Massof & Lidoff, 2001).

COLLABORATIVE TEAMS

To meet the need for client-centered services, low vision practitioners have adopted methods by which professionals in the specialties of health, educational, rehabilitative, and social services work as teams to implement collaborative comprehensive care (Maino, 2000; Mehr & Fried; 1975; Wilkinson, Stewart, & Trantham, 2000).

Teams may be defined as multidisciplinary, interdisciplinary, or transdisciplinary. In multidisciplinary teams, various specialists work individually with a person and communicate very little among themselves. In interdisciplinary teams, specialists work individually with clients or students, but there is communication among the specialists. In transdisciplinary teams, specialists work jointly to plan and implement assessment and instruction for an individual, often with designated professionals or family members serving as the primary implementers of activities (Smith & Levack, 1996). In practice, true transdisciplinary teaming may be rare. In early childhood special education programs, for example, multidisciplinary teams primarily conduct assessments and interdisciplinary teams primarily conduct interventions (Chen & Dote-Kwan, 1998). The nature of teams in low vision care, which include the individual with low vision and family members, is determined by such factors as the members' field of expertise, the team's organizational structure, the location of service delivery, the quality and quantity of interaction among team members, and the role of individual members.

Composition

Team members come from a variety of disciplines, and the composition of the low vision care team depends upon the needs of the individual and the services available within a given system. Members can include ophthalmologists, physicians from other specialties, nurses, optometrists, rehabilitation teachers, vocational counselors, teachers of students who are visually impaired, orientation and mobility (O&M) specialists, social workers, low vision therapists, occupational therapists, physical therapists, and psychologists, among others. The most important team members are individuals with low vision and their families.

Organizational Structure

Some teams are made up of members who all work within the same organization, while other teams may have members from different organizations. For example, a rehabilitation agency may have on its staff all the team members required to meet the needs of a particular client, including an eye care practitioner, social worker, rehabilitation teacher, assistive technology specialist, and O&M instructor. In another case, an ophthalmology practice may employ several team members required to provide comprehensive low vision care for a particular person (e.g., ophthalmologist, optometrist, occupational therapist), but some patients may be referred to additional team members from several other organizations (teacher of visually impaired students, O&M specialist, school psychologist, genetic counselor) to ensure that the patient receives comprehensive services. Teaming across organizational boundaries can be particularly important in working with individuals with low vision, whose individual needs can vary greatly.

Clinical or Applied Service Settings

Some teams will work entirely in clinical settings, while others may work extensively in practical settings such as the home, community, or workplace, depending on the needs of the individuals being served and the services available in a particular organization or agency. For example, a special unit from an agency may go into nursing homes to perform vision screening, low vision evaluations, and functional vision evaluations, as well as to develop and implement compensatory strategies. That same agency may have an in-house low vision clinic that provides low vision evaluations for other clients, along with rehabilitation teachers who perform functional vision evaluations in the home and provide training in special computer software programs at the agency site.

Quality and Quantity of Team Interaction

Teams have been described in terms of the type and extent of collaborative interaction among their members. In the provision of low vision care, such interaction may be affected by the composition of the team and its organizational structure. For example, teams composed of a few specialists working closely together within one organization may be able to work together more collaboratively than teams consisting of many diverse specialists from different organizations.

In addition, some members of a team may work more closely together than others, based on the individual client's needs. Team interactions may relate to the following tasks:

➤ Determining the most appropriate assessment procedures to implement

➤ Implementing assessment procedures (e.g., rather than having every team member conduct observational assessments, one or two team members may carry out these assessments in the natural setting to address issues of interest identified by the entire team)

➤ Determining low vision care goals and objectives

➤ Determining the most appropriate intervention procedures

➤ Implementing intervention procedures (e.g., having one or two team members, possibly a family member, implement interventions recommended by several members of the team)

➤ Evaluating the effectiveness of services provided

Teams can vary along a continuum of collaboration, from those with many specialists, each working separately, with little communication among team members to those with specialists working jointly to plan and implement assessment, intervention, and service evaluation procedures.

Roles of Team Members

Team coordination and the roles of individual team members can vary significantly depending on how closely a team works together, the organizational structure of the team, and the degree to which team members collaborate on various procedures. For example, in a highly interactive team, a rehabilitation teacher may complete an initial interview with a new client while the optometrist who will be conducting the low vision evaluation and the O&M instructor listens and takes notes, adding comments and asking questions at the end. In another team, the rehabilitation specialist, optometrist, and O&M instructor may each conduct separate interviews. The degree of input required from team members can vary, depending on the needs of individuals with low vision and their families. Recent trends in rehabilitation care advocate that consumers play a large role in determining goals and evaluating outcomes (Lund & Dietrichson, 2000).

Collaboration as Best Practice

Collaborative models for comprehensive low vision care have been deemed best practice for many years to promote strong and effective service delivery (Jose, 1983). Sinclair et al. (2000) have found a number of advantages and disadvantages of team members working in an interdisciplinary low vision care program.

Advantages for patients include more holistic care, fewer appointments required, and the ability to upgrade low vision devices in the patient's home. They found the following direct benefits for team members: increased respect among professionals, avenues for interchange of ideas and skills, opportunities for joint professional development, and diminished isolation. Disadvantages identified in the study included unclear role definition resulting in unnecessary overlap or underutilization of services by team members, and lack of coordination with existing community services (in this study, low vision optometric services).

Another study examining collaboration among professional groups in low vision care in the United Kingdom concluded that involving a variety of professional groups on the low vision team resulted in more extensive services and cooperation among professionals and agencies (Ryan et al., 2000). This research group also noted that a user-centered orientation was critical for success. More research is needed to determine the most effective methods to promote efficient and effective collaboration among low vision care team members within the wide range of available service settings.

Practitioners on the Low Vision Team

This book focuses on the evaluation of and interventions for functional vision in low vision care. Service providers on the low vision team who most often participate in this process are listed by primary discipline, and according to which part of the evaluation and care they provide, in Table 1.1. In health care settings, these professionals most often include ophthalmologists, optometrists, occupational therapists and low vision therapists. (In some instances, nurses or certified ophthalmic medical assistants may participate in the assessment of visual functions and the dispensing of low vision devices and training in their use.) In educational settings, the team can include teachers of students with visual impairments and O&M instructors. In the process of rehabilitation, the team can include rehabilitation teachers, O&M instructors, and low vision therapists. The precise role of a particular individual in the process depends on the nature of the low vision care team. For purposes of discussion in this book, the terms practitioners, professionals, or service providers will be used to indicate people who are appropriately trained to implement functional vision evaluation and intervention activities for individuals with low vision. National certification standards that include professional competencies in functional vision evaluation and intervention (for low vision therapists) have been developed to ensure appropriate services to persons with low vision (Watson, Quillman, Flax, & Gerritson, 1999).

OVERVIEW OF THE COMPREHENSIVE LOW VISION CARE PROCESS

A discussion of low vision evaluation and instructional strategies requires a description of how these two activities fit within the broader area of comprehensive

TABLE 1.1

Common Service Providers:
Low Vision Evaluation and Instruction

SPECIALIST	GENERAL EYE EXAMINATION	LOW VISION EXAMINATION	FUNCTIONAL VISION EVALUATION	FUNCTIONAL VISION INSTRUCTION
Low vision therapist			X	X
Occupational therapist with training in low vision			X	X
Ophthalmologist	X			
Ophthalmologist specializing in low vision		X	X	X
Optometrist	X			
Optometrist specializing in low vision		X	X	X
O&M instructor			X	X
Rehabilitation teacher for people who are visually impaired			X	X
Teacher of students who are visually impaired			X	X

low vision care. Figure 1.1 summarizes the comprehensive low vision care process.

To understand the different components in this process, it is important to clarify the differences between *visual functions* and *functional vision*. According to Colenbrander (2002), examinations of visual functions describe how the *eye* and the visual system function; they involve measures of functional changes at the organ level. Visual functions (such as visual acuity or visual field) are often measured quantitatively, are usually measured for each eye separately, test threshold performance, have precise categories, and evaluate a single variable at a time. Tests of visual functions are usually performed in a static environment.

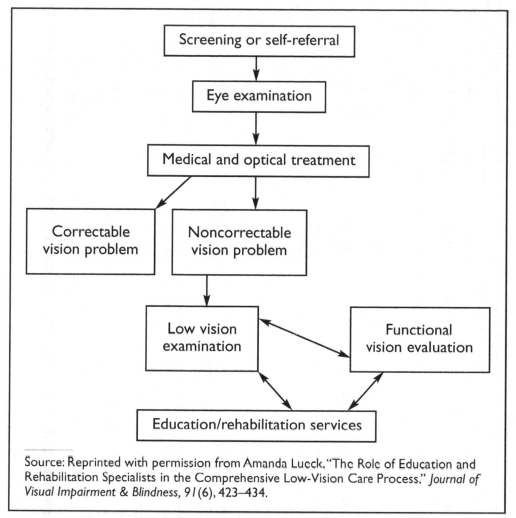

Source: Reprinted with permission from Amanda Lueck, "The Role of Education and Rehabilitation Specialists in the Comprehensive Low-Vision Care Process," *Journal of Visual Impairment & Blindness, 91*(6), 423–434.

Figure 1.1. Comprehensive low vision care process.

By contrast, functional vision describes how the *person* functions and involves measures of a person's visual skills and abilities as applied to the performance of the usual tasks of daily life, such as reading. Functional vision is often described qualitatively (although some quantitative measures are available for some tasks such as reading). It is measured binocularly to replicate the individual's visual performance in the real world, and examines suprathreshold (i.e., above threshold) performance so that a person's comfort level for an activity is identified. An evaluation of functional vision involves categories that are less precise than measures of visual functions, and often is affected by multiple variables at one time. Functional vision evaluations are usually performed in dynamic environments.

Table 1.2 presents the types of assessments that are commonly performed in each of the different types of vision evaluations: a basic eye examination, a low

TABLE 1.2

Common Assessment Activities in Different Types of Vision Evaluations

TYPE OF EVALUATION	THE EYE			VISUAL FUNCTIONS						FUNCTIONAL VISION
	OCULAR HEALTH	REFRACTIVE ERROR	VISUAL ACUITIES	VISUAL FIELD	CONTRAST SENSITIVITY	RESPONSE TO LIGHT[a]	COLOR VISION	OCULO-MOTOR FUNCTION	ACCOM-MODATION	USE OF VISION IN FUNC-TIONAL TASKS
Basic Eye Examination	usually	usually	usually	usually	sometimes	sometimes	sometimes	usually	usually	infrequently
Low Vision Examination	only if indicated for eye health check or to check recent vision change	often modified techniques; alternative instrumentation	often modified techniques; alternative instrumentation	often modified techniques; alternative instrumentation	often modified techniques; alternative instrumentation	Special procedures	often modified techniques; alternative instrumentation	usually	often modified techniques	frequently
Functional Vision Evaluation			observation of behavior during replication of tests done within basic or low vision examination	observation of behavior during replication of tests done within basic or low vision examination	observation of behavior during replication of tests done within basic or low vision examination	observation of changes in behavior & performance in different lighting conditions	observation of behavior during replication of tests done within basic or low vision examination			observation of behavior & performance while completing various functional tasks

[a] Assessment of response to light: (1) variation of visual function at different lighting levels; (2) glare disability (or veiling glare); (3) glare discomfort; an adverse consequence of extraneous light within the visual environment; and (4) light adaptation; the gradual change in the ability to see when going from one light level to another.

vision examination, and a functional vision examination. The table also indicates whether the assessments focus mainly on the visual functions of the eye or on functional vision, as does the discussion of each type of examination that follows.

Basic Eye Examination

When a person notices decreased visual functioning or when decreased visual performance is noted during a routine screening procedure, an eye examination is warranted. A basic eye examination, performed by an ophthalmologist or optometrist, focuses primarily on ocular health and the need for eyeglasses, gathering information about ocular history, refractive error, accommodation, visual fields, distance and near acuities, coordinated use of both eyes, and ocular motility in this process. Based on the findings from this eye examination, identified vision problems are treated by the appropriate eye care specialist with surgery, medication, or corrective lenses. Correctable refractive errors are treated with spectacles or contact lenses. Health concerns are addressed through medication or surgery. For most people, their vision concerns can be corrected at this phase.

If an individual's vision problem is not correctable with surgery, medication, or corrective lenses, he or she enters the comprehensive low vision care process. At this point, the person can be referred for a low vision evaluation and for education and rehabilitation services.

Comprehensive Low Vision Evaluation

A comprehensive low vision examination, performed by an optometrist or ophthalmologist, investigates many of the same factors as a basic eye examination, but it may involve the use of different techniques that provide more precise results for individuals with low vision (Mehr & Fried, 1975; Cole & Rosenthal, 1996). The same or additional critical visual functions are examined in detail, along with aspects of functional vision, in order to accomplish the following:

1. Prescribe appropriate correction for refractive errors and accommodation anomalies

2. Prescribe low vision optical devices (e.g., magnifiers, and telescopes) and adaptive devices (e.g., large-print checks, and reading stands)

3. Determine appropriate environmental modifications to optimize visual functioning (e.g., recommending best lighting for reading at school or for cooking at home)

4. Determine specific visual interventions to optimize visual functioning (e.g., using visual field information to determine the best method for teaching eccentric viewing)

5. Provide information that individuals with low vision, their families, and practitioners, can use to determine the individual's entitlement to expanded services (e.g., education or rehabilitation services) and optimal use of these services.

Important components of the low vision examinations include conveying vision information clearly and compassionately to patients and their families; providing appropriate referral to additional services; and interacting with other medical, education, rehabilitation, or social services professionals. This creates a coordinated effort to optimize comprehensive care. An important service of the low vision ophthalmologist or optometrist is the prescription of conventional or low vision optical devices. Some ophthalmologists or optometrists perform detailed assessments of functional vision within the clinical setting. Some may also teach individuals to maximize their visual functioning, particularly related to the use of optical devices. Others may not have the time or resources to implement and monitor training procedures or environmental modifications. Working with a team of professionals who can integrate low vision evaluation recommendations into intervention programs is a practical solution to these variations in practice.

Functional Vision Evaluation

The functional vision evaluation differs from the basic eye examination and the low vision evaluation in that it primarily assesses how the individual applies his or her vision in real-life tasks or environments outside the clinical setting. A functional vision evaluation sets the stage for education and rehabilitation services, providing direction for the use of methods to promote the use of vision in tasks of daily living, vocational pursuits for older children and adults, and educational programming for students. It can, ideally, be conducted in the person's home, school, or work environment. It is also performed in specialized settings set up for this purpose by educators, rehabilitation specialists, or allied health personnel. Some functional vision assessment procedures may be completed by medical or rehabilitation personnel as part of a low vision evaluation. Therefore there may be some overlap among functional assessments performed during the low vision evaluation and those performed during the functional vision evaluation.

The functional vision evaluation may repeat assessments of visual functions and functional tasks (such as reading), but the purpose of these assessments may be different. For example, a near vision word reading test administered during a low vision evaluation may be used to determine the type of magnification device to be prescribed. That same information will be combined with other pertinent information in a functional vision evaluation to help determine appropriate reading instruction methods.

Performance differences noted in the low vision clinical setting and education or rehabilitation settings may also provide information that is valuable in determining the appropriate intervention. A functional vision evaluation often includes the use of formal tests, but it also involves observation of an individual's visual functioning in typical surroundings as well as an analysis of the person's environment to determine visual demands and accommodation requirements.

It is recommended that the functional vision evaluation be conducted after the individual has undergone an initial low vision evaluation, although it is often helpful for education and rehabilitation personnel to perform some preliminary observations of functional vision prior to the low vision evaluation. This is done so that current performance levels can be clearly presented to the ophthalmologist or optometrist during the low vision evaluation. One reason to wait until the low vision evaluation is performed before conducting a functional vision evaluation is that refractive status (level or extent of refractive errors and accommodation anomalies) may be determined and corrected through conventional optical devices during the low vision evaluation. The resulting improvement in vision might radically alter the individual's performance on functional vision assessments, which, in turn, could affect the type of interventions recommended.

Education and Rehabilitation Services

Information obtained from the initial eye examination, the low vision examination, and the functional vision evaluation is used in the determination of eligibility for and extent of education or rehabilitation services required. This information is also the basis of a profile of visual skills and behaviors that will be used in determining necessary compensatory strategies to promote an individual's vision use for functional tasks in their school, workplace, home, and community settings.

Educational and rehabilitation services for individuals with low vision range from programs for infants and toddlers to school programs to programs for adults in the workforce to community programs for elderly persons. They can include instruction and support in daily living, O&M, and academic and preacademic skills as well as psychological, medical, and vocational counseling. These services most often involve individuals' families to promote maximum outcomes (Lewis & Allman, 2000; Silverstone, 2000). More complete descriptions of services available are provided elsewhere (Holbrook & Koenig, 2000; Orr, 1992; Ponchilla & Ponchilla, 1996).

Referral within the Low Vision Care System

In the comprehensive low vision care process, individuals need to return for low vision examinations or functional vision evaluations, based on medical recommendations for follow-up care, changes in the status of their vision, or changes in life circumstances. For example:

An eye care specialist has recommended that an elderly person with diabetic retinopathy return for low vision examinations on a regular basis. In the course of a routine examination, a marked decrease in visual acuity is noted in conjunction with the patient's report that many household tasks are becoming difficult to perform. The specialist prescribes a handheld magnifier for the individual to read such items as mail, can labels, and grocery receipts. In addition, the patient is referred to a rehabilitation specialist for another functional vision evaluation to make any necessary revisions to intervention priorities and strategies that address the patient's daily living needs.

In another example, an office worker with ocular albinism who has changed to a new job that requires more extensive use of computer and telecommunications equipment might ask for assistance from a rehabilitation counselor. The counselor could then recommend another low vision examination as well as a functional vision evaluation to determine the optimal equipment for this individual in the new work setting.

Informing Consumers about Available Services

When all segments of the low vision care system work as a network, it can meet clients' complex needs using the talents and skills of a variety of professionals who can share information and coordinate efforts for maximum effectiveness. Individuals with low vision need to be informed of the array of services available to them, how these fit together, and how best to use them. Service providers must be alert to the multiple needs of their clients and be ready to accommodate their changing needs. Low vision optical devices may be sufficient for some individuals with less severe vision problems, but most individuals can also benefit from becoming knowledgeable consumers. Knowing that there are services, products, and support groups available to them may help to shorten the period of adjustment to vision loss and encourage people to continue their everyday activities with necessary modifications (Weisse, 1991). Practitioners can provide information about the following:

➤ The organization and capabilities of relevant health, rehabilitation, and education services

➤ Low vision services available to a particular person and family based on local availability, the individual's age, eligibility for service, or other variables

➤ Suppliers of low vision adaptive devices

➤ Consumer organizations

➤ Professional organizations

➤ Financial assistance and government entitlement programs

ADDRESSING CONSUMERS' CONCERNS

Issues of acceptance, self-worth, family dynamics, and interpersonal relations arise for individuals with low vision and their families throughout the comprehensive low vision care process (Fitzmaurice, Osborne, & Kendig, 2000; Reinhardt & D'Allura, 2000; Warnke, 1991). Changes in the health care system in the United States, brought about, in part, by the disability rights movement, are encouraging more active roles for consumers in the direction and evaluation of care (Kizer, 2001; Rhoades, McFarland & Knights, 1995; Shapiro, 1993). Providing education and training to increase consumer competence in decision-making and involvement has proven successful in rehabilitation care (Patterson & Marks, 1992).

Professionals can assist by taking the role of support person, information provider, and referral agent for patients. These functions cannot be separated from the functional vision assessment and instruction process since adjustment issues related to vision loss affect intervention programs and their outcomes, and consumer education is critical to the success of education or rehabilitation programs (Lang, 2000; Ringering & Amaral, 2000). Finally, involving the individual's family in the low vision care process in ways appropriate to a person's age and life situation can be critical to successful low vision intervention and care (Lang, 2000; Ringering & Amaral, 2000). Because of their importance, consumer issues that can be addressed by professionals who provide functional vision assessment and interventions are discussed briefly in the following section.

Supporting Interactions with Medical Professionals

Many individuals with low vision and their families feel overwhelmed, anxious, and confused about information provided to them during a low vision examination. Often a person undergoes a low vision evaluation in the hope that normal or near-normal visual function can be restored; that expectation cannot always be met. Parents of young children, especially those who have multiple disabilities, can be emotionally drained from their experiences with numerous medical personnel and may not absorb all that is occurring in the whirlwind of services, treatments, and specialists. Even though medical staff demonstrate a high degree of care and concern, additional support may be needed to explain eye conditions and their ramifications in comprehensible terms to individuals and their families. Service providers can provide assistance by repeating these explanations in a nonthreatening environment over time.

Facilitating Acceptance of Visual Impairment

The diagnosis of permanent and irreversible vision loss affects families deeply. Reactions to vision loss are varied and intense (Tuttle & Tuttle, 1996). Understanding the complex maze of health, education, or rehabilitation opportunities is usually the last thing on people's minds when they learn that they have permanent and irreversible vision loss. Individuals with low vision and their families are thinking about why this change has happened to them; how it will affect their lives and those of their loved ones; how they will pay the bills; and what will happen to them. Parents are wondering if their child will be able to work or get married; who will take care of their child when they die; how they will successfully raise a child with a disability (Warnke, 1991). These are all important concerns related to survival and loss. Few families are able to think about the comprehensive low vision care process or how to work sucessfully with professionals.

The process of accepting this diagnosis for persons with acquired and congenital visual impairments continues throughout their lives, although the milestones along the way will be different for each (Tuttle & Tuttle, 1996). Some are able to jump the initial, highly personal hurdles and meet the demands of adjusting to vision loss without professional assistance or with the assistance of family and friends. Others may require additional professional support to gain a degree of composure to begin thinking about the concept of rehabilitation or education for their specific situation.

What each person brings to the acceptance process varies with his or her temperament, life experiences, and existing systems of support. Professionals must learn about each individual's unique attitudes, needs, and wants while being sensitive to contributing factors from the individual's cultural background (Millian, 2000; Schultz & Chao, 2000). The eye care professional (usually the ophthalmologist and, occasionally, the optometrist) is most frequently the first person to inform an individual of the diagnosis of visual impairment. Regardless of what might be termed a professional's bedside manner, such statements as "You are legally blind, " "Your vision is impaired," "You will never see normally again," or "You are blind" hit patients and their families hard no matter how well or with how much kindness they are delivered. Some individuals with low vision and their families may have an inkling of what they will hear, but no one wants to hear the finality of those words. Individuals and their families are busy coping with and learning about the medical realities that must be understood and faced. Professionals are in a position to ease this process and set the stage for building effective consumer-professional relationships. Werner (2000, p. 675), an optometrist, offers some general guidelines to help professionals ease the impact on an individual of first learning of a visual impairment:

➤ Be clear and brief.

➤ Keep it simple, with no jargon.

➤ Offer hope, but do not lie.

➤ Allow time for reaction.

➤ Respond to reactions but do not argue.

➤ Solicit and answer questions.

➤ Provide a follow-up plan.

➤ Summarize to be certain there is understanding.

➤ Assure that you are available should questions arise.

Facilitating Successful Referrals

Most adults do not use rehabilitation services immediately after being diagnosed with low vision, unless they are referred immediately by their ophthalmologist or optometrist (Greenblatt, 1991). In many instances, even when individuals are given referral information, some are not ready to accept additional services until they have had time to digest and accept the news of their diagnosis. Sometimes, general information and support are the initial services accepted. Many very young children are not referred early enough to education services that can be crucial to their optimal development. Many with less severe visual impairments or those with disabilities in addition to visual impairments are not identified until well into their elementary school years (Trief & Morse, 1987). Adults of working age may be more persistent, and therefore more successful, in their efforts to secure services than elderly persons (Greenblatt, 1991). For many elderly individuals and their families, vision loss is seen as a part of the aging process that must be accepted as conclusive and final and, for that reason, additional services are not sought (Yeadon, 1984). The elderly visually impaired population in long-term care facilities all too often receive minimal low vision services, and initial vision screening and eye examinations may also be limited (Duffy & Beliveau Tobey, 1991).

Service providers in the initial phases of the low vision care process can help to promote comprehensive low vision care by providing information about low vision services and resources themselves or by providing and monitoring timely referrals to appropriate information and referral sources (Weisse, 1991). At some points, consumers may require assistance from professionals to sort out the wealth of information available. Information on available low vision services can be overwhelming to people who are just learning of the extent of their vision loss or to those with multiple disabilities who are medically fragile.

Encouraging Involvement in the Rehabilitation Process

New models of rehabilitation place more responsibility on consumers in directing and assessing their care (Kizer, 2001). Service providers can facilitate this process by encouraging individuals with low vision to ask for assistance when appropriate, to make informed choices about their low vision care, to determine their rehabilitation or education goals, and to assess the success of service outcomes (Reed, Fried, & Rhoades, 1995). This involves providing information to individuals with low vision and their families in a timely manner, listening to consumer needs and designing low vision care plans to meet those needs, being responsive to an individual's cultural background, and supporting the consumer in making independent decisions.

CONCLUSION

The comprehensive low vision care process involves a complex array of services and a variety of professionals who need to work with each other, and in concert with consumers and their families, to maximize outcomes for persons with low vision. It is up to professionals in the low vision care process to create medical, educational, and rehabilitation environments that enable all consumers to achieve a level of independence and competence required to promote this process. It is crucial that persons with low vision and their families have the amount of support appropriate to their individual situations to negotiate these systems well. Functional vision evaluation and instruction are part of this process. Professionals must understand the role of evaluation and instruction in low vision care and make provisions to accommodate consumer input in providing functional evaluation and intervention for individuals of all ages. As consumers participate in different aspects of low vision evaluation and instruction, they need to be active participants who can understand the many factors involved and services available.

REFERENCES

Bailey, I. L., & Hall, A. P. (1990). *Visual impairment: An overview*. New York: American Foundation for the Blind.

Chen, D., & Dote-Kwan, J. (1998). Early intervention services for young children who have visual impairments with other disabilities and their families. In S. Z. Sacks & R. K. Silberman (Eds.), *Educating students who have visual impairments with other disabilities* (pp. 303–334). Baltimore, MD: Paul H. Brookes.

Cole, R. G., & Rosenthal, B. P. (1996). Remediation and management of low vision. New York: Mosby.

Colenbrander, A. (1977). Dimensions of visual performance. *Transactions of the American Academy of Ophthalmology and Otolaryngology, 83*, 332-337.

Colenbrander, A. (2002, August). Visual standards: Aspects and ranges of vision loss with emphasis on population surveys. Report for the International Council of Ophthalmology, 29th International Congress of Ophthalmology, Sydney, Australia.

Corn, A. L., & Koenig, A. J. (1996). Perspectives on low vision. In Corn & Koenig (Eds.), *Foundations of low vision: Clinical and functional perspectives* (pp. 3–25). New York: AFB Press.

Crews, J. E. (2000). The evolution of public policies and services for older people who are visually impaired. In B. Silvertone, M. A. Lang, B. P. Rosenthal, & E. F. Faye (Eds.), *The Lighthouse handbook on vision impairment and vision rehabilitation. Vol. 2. Vision rehabilitation.* (p. 1287–1300). New York: Oxford University Press.

De L'Aune, W. R., Welsh, R. L., & Williams, M. D. (2000). Outcome assessment of the rehabilitation of the visually impaired: A national project in the United States. In C. Stuen, A. Arditi, A. Horowitz, M. A. Lang, B. Rosenthal, & K. Seidman (Eds.), *Vision rehabilitation: Assessment, intervention, & outcomes* (pp. 771–773). Lisse, Netherlands: Swets & Zeitlinger.

Duffy, M. A., & Beliveau-Tobey, M. (1991). Providing services to visually impaired elders in long term care facilities: A multidisciplinary approach. In S. Greenblatt (Ed.), *Meeting the needs of people with low vision: A multidisciplinary perspective* (pp. 93–107). Lexington, MA: Resources for Rehabilitation.

Fitzmaurice, K,, Osborne, D., & Kendig, H. (2000). The impact of sight loss on older persons living in the community. In C. Stuen, A. Arditi, A. Horowitz, M. A. Lang, B. Rosenthal, & K. Seidman (Eds.), *Vision rehabilitation: Assessment, intervention, and outcomes* (pp. 659–671). Lisse, Netherlands: Swets & Zeitlinger.

Goetz, L., & Gee, K. (1987). Functional vision programming: A model for teaching visual behavior in natural contexts. In Goetz, D. Guess, & K. Stremmel-Campbell (Eds.), *Innovative program design for individuals with dual sensory impairments* (pp. 77–97). Baltimore, MD: Paul Brookes.

Greenblatt, S. (1991). What people with vision loss need to know. In S. Greenblatt (Ed.), *Meeting the needs of people with low vision: A multidisciplinary perspective* (pp. 7–20). Lexington, MA: Resources for Rehabilitation.

Holbrook, M. C., & Koenig, A. J. (Eds.). (2000). *Foundations of education: Vol. 1. History and theory of teaching children and youths with visual impairments.* (2nd ed.). New York: AFB Press.

Jose, R. T. (1983). The low vision rehabilitation service. In R. Jose (Ed.), *Understanding low vision* (pp. 61–71). New York: American Foundation for the Blind.

Kizer, K. W. (2001). Establishing health care performance standards in an era of consumerism. *Journal of the American Medical Association, 286,* 1213–1217.

Lang, M. A. (2000). The role of psychosocial factors in adaptation to vision impairment and habilitation outcomes for children and youth. In B. Silverstone, M. A. Lang, B. P. Rosenthal, & E. F. Faye. (Eds.), *The Lighthouse handbook on vision impairment and vision rehabilitation: Vol. 2. Vision rehabilitation* (pp. 1011–1028). New York: Oxford University Press.

Lewis, S., & Allman, C.B. (2000). Educational programming. In M. C. Holbrook & A. J. Koenig (Eds.), *Foundations of education: Vol. 1. History and theory of teaching children and youths with visual impairments* (2nd ed., pp. 218–259). New York: AFB Press.

Lueck, A. H., Chen, D., & Kekelis, L. S., (1997). *Developmental guidelines for infants with visual impairment: A manual for early intervention.* Louisville, KY: American Printing House for the Blind.

Lund, R., & Dietrichson, J., (2000). Rehabilitation of people with visual impairments and quality of life. In C. Stuen, A. Arditi, A. Horowitz, M. A. Lang,

B. Rosenthal, & K. Seidman (Eds.), *Vision rehabilitation: Assessment, intervention, & outcomes* (pp. 780–786). Lisse, Netherlands: Swets & Zeitlinger.

Maino, J.M (2000, August). *Low vision as a subset of medical rehabilitation.* Paper presented at Issues in Blindness Conference, Kansas City, MO.

Massof, R. W. (2003, February). *Functional evaluation and measuring functional outcomes for visually impaired elderly.* Paper presented at Vision Loss in the 21st Century, Los Angeles, CA.

Massof, R. W., Dagnelie, G., Deremeik, J. T., DeRose, J. L., Alibhai, S. S., & Glasner, N. M. (1995). Low vision rehabilitation in the U.S. health care system. *Journal of Vision Rehabilitation, 9,* 3–25.

Massof, R. W., & Lidoff, L. (Eds.). (2001). *Issues in low vision rehabilitation: Service delivery, policy, and funding.* New York: AFB Press.

Mehr, E. B., & Freid, A. N. (1975). *Low vision care.* Chicago: Professional Press.

Millian, M. (2000). Multicultural issues. In M. C. Holbrook & A. J. Koenig (Eds.), *Foundations of education: Vol. 1. History and theory of teaching children and youths with visual impairments* (2nd ed., pp 197–217). New York: AFB Press.

Orr, A. L. (Ed.). (1992). *Vision and aging: Crossroads to service delivery.* New York: American Foundation for the Blind.

Patterson, J. B., & Marks, C. (1992). The client as customer: Achieving service quality and customer satisfaction in rehabilitation. *Journal of Rehabilitation, 58,* 16-21.

Ponchilla, P. E., & Ponchilla, S. V. (Eds.) (1996) *Foundations of rehabilitation teaching with persons who are blind or visually impaired.* New York: AFB Press.

Reed, B. J., Fried, J. H., & Rhoades, B. J. (1995). Empowerment and assistive technology: The local resource team model. *Journal of Rehabilitation. 61,* 30–35.

Reinhardt, J. P., & D'Allura, T. (2000). Social support and adjustment to vision impairment across the life span. In B. Silverstone, M. A. Lang, B.P. Rosenthal, & E. F. Faye. (Eds.), *The Lighthouse handbook on vision impairment and vision rehabilitation: Vol. 2. Vision rehabilitation* (pp. 1049–1068). New York: Oxford University Press.

Rhoades, D. R., McFarland, K. F., & Knights, P. G. (1996). Evolution of consumerism in rehabilitation counseling: A theoretical perspective. *Journal of Rehabilitation, 62,* 26–29.

Ringering, L., & Amaral, P. (2000). The role of psychosocial factors in adaptation to vision impairment and rehabilitation outcomes for adults and older adults. In B. Silverstone, M. A. Lang, B. P. Rosenthal, & E. F. Faye. (Eds.), *The Lighthouse handbook on vision impairment and vision rehabilitation: Vol. 2. Vision rehabilitation* (pp. 1029–1048). New York: Oxford University Press.

Ryan, B., Culham, L. E., Hill, A. R., Jackson, A. J., Jones, B., Bird, A. C., & Bunce, C. (2000). Multi-disciplinary low vision services in the United Kingdom. In C. Stuen, A. Arditi, A. Horowitz, M. A. Lang, B. Rosenthal, & K. Seidman (Eds.), *Vision rehabilitation: Assessment, intervention, and outcomes* (pp. 542–545). Lisse, Netherlands: Swets & Zeitlinger.

Schultz, L., & Chao, R. (2000). Cultural/ethnic sensitivity in vision rehabilitation. In C. Stuen, A. Arditi, A. Horowitz, M. A. Lang, B. Rosenthal, & K. Seidman (Eds.), *Vision rehabilitation: Assessment, intervention, and outcomes* (pp. 677–681). Lisse, Netherlands: Swets & Zeitlinger.

Shapiro, J.P. (1993). *No pity: People with disabilities forging a new civil rights movement.* New York: Three Rivers Press.

Silverstone, B. (2000). Aging, vision rehabilitation, and the family. In J. E. Crews & F. J. Whittington (Eds.), *Vision loss in an aging society: A multidisciplinary perspective.* (pp. 155–180). New York: AFB Press.

Sinclair, A., Grimsley, A. Horobin, J., Inchley, J., MacDonald, M., Park, J., Paterson, H., & Suttie, A. (2000). The interdiscipinary approach to low vision services—how does it work in practice? In C. Stuen, A. Arditi, A. Horowitz, M. A. Lang, B. Rosenthal, & K. Seidman (Eds.), *Vision rehabilitation: Assessment, intervention, and outcomes* (pp. 546–549). Lisse, Netherlands: Swets & Zeitlinger.

Smith, M., & Levack, N. (1996). Teaching students with visual and multiple impairments: A resource guide. Austin: Texas School for the Blind and Visually Impalred.

Stelmack, J., Szlyk, J., Joslin, C., Swetland, B. A., & Myers (2000). Pilot study: Use of the NEI VFQ-25 to measure outcomes of low vision rehabilitation services in the Department of Veterans Affairs. In C. Stuen, A. Arditi, A. Horowitz, M. A. Lang, B. Rosenthal, & K. Seidman (Eds.) *Vision rehabilitation: Assessment, intervention, and outcomes* (pp. 774–776). Lisse, Netherlands: Swets & Zeitlinger.

Trief, E., & Morse, A. R. (1987). An overview of preschool vision screening. *Journal of Visual Impairment & Blindness,* 81, 197–200.

Tuttle, D. W., & Tuttle, N. R. (1996). *Self-esteem and adjusting with blindness: The process of responding to life's demands.* Springfield, IL: Charles C. Thomas.

Warnke, (1991). The role of the family in the adjustment to blindness or visual impairment. In S. Greenblatt (Ed.), *Meeting the needs of people with low vision: A multidisciplinary perspective* (pp. 37–45). Lexington, MA: Resources for Rehabilitation.

Watson, G., Quillman, D., Flax, M., & Gerritson, B. (1999). Development of low vision certification standards. *Journal of Visual Impairment & Blindness,* 93, 451–456.

Weisse, F. A. (1991). Information and referral services for people with low vision. In S. Greenblatt (Ed.), *Meeting the needs of people with low vision: A multidisciplinary perspective* (pp. 21–36). Lexington, MA: Resources for Rehabilitation.

Werner, D. L. (2000). Honesty versus cultural differences in the presentation of bad news to low vision patients. In C. Stuen, A. Arditi, A. Horowitz, M. A. Lang, B. Rosenthal, & K. Seidman (Eds.), *Vision rehabilitation: Assessment, intervention, and outcomes* (pp. 774–776). Lisse, Netherlands: Swets & Zeitlinger.

Wilkinson, M. E., Stewart, I., & Trantham, C. S., (2000). The Iowa model for pediatric low vision services. *Journal of Visual Impairment & Blindness,* 94, 446–452.

World Health Assembly (1980). *International classification of impairments, disabilities, and handicaps: A manual of classification relating to the consequences of disease.* Geneva: World Health Organization.

Yeadon, A. (1987). The informal care group: Problem or potential? *Journal of Visual Impairment & Blindness, 78,* 149–154.

World Health Organization. (2001). *International classification of functioning, disability, and health.* Geneva: World Health Organization.

2

Visual Functions as Components of Functional Vision

ROANNE FLOM

F unctional vision, as explained in Chapter 1, refers to an individual's ability to use his or her vision in the everyday tasks of real life, such as reading, doing housework, getting around independently from place to place, or enjoying a television program. An individual's ability to see and function visually is determined largely by the relative contributions of a number of underlying components of vision. The combined effect of these factors on visual functioning is similar to the ways in which the quality of the picture on a television screen is determined by underlying factors such as the resolution of the monitor, the size of the screen, the contrast created, the color accuracy, and the overall brightness. A variety of terms have been used to refer to these components of vision, but this book will use the term *visual function* (as discussed in Chapter 1) or sometimes *visual capacity.* The authors have attempted to reserve the term *visual abilities* or *capabilities* for visual performance in real-world situations.

Certain specific visual functions seem to explain many variations in visual performance across the spectrum of visual impairment. Understanding which visual functions are most affected by an individual's visual impairment, as well as the nature and severity of those effects for the given individual, can provide powerful insights into how that person sees. With such knowledge, practitioners can identify aspects of behavior affected by vision loss, better focus rehabilitation and assessment efforts, anticipate problems, and empathize with the frustrations the individual experiences.

VISUAL FUNCTIONS

This chapter focuses on the seven visual functions that are considered most important in adequately understanding the spectrum of visual functioning among those with impaired vision:

1. visual acuity

2. visual field

3. contrast sensitivity

4. light sensitivity

5. color discrimination

6. oculomotor control

7. accommodation

These variables are typically considered during eye examinations and are also included in assessments of functional vision.

The first three visual functions—visual acuity, visual field, and contrast sensitivity—warrant the greatest attention, since deficits in these areas usually have the greatest influence on the ability to perform important tasks. Indeed, visual acuity and visual field have been considered so important that their evaluation is a part of nearly every vision examination and their measurement is the basis of most definitions of visual impairment. In recent years, contrast sensitivity has emerged as an important additional test of basic visual functioning.

Light sensitivity and color discrimination warrant discussion since severe impairment of these abilities can be caused by certain vision conditions and may require specific interventions.

Impairments of oculomotor control can lead to abnormalities of eye movements and eye alignment that are common in persons with many serious eye conditions. How these often conspicuous abnormalities influence or, more importantly, do not influence visual functioning is particularly relevant to an understanding of the visual functioning of persons with congenital visual impairments or brain injuries.

Accommodation (or internal focusing) warrants attention because adults gradually lose this accommodative ability. This capacity is particularly important for young people with reduced vision who must hold reading materials close to their faces in order to see the print clearly.

Data from tests of these seven visual functions can be compiled to create what we might call a profile of visual functioning for any given individual. This type of profile can explain much about how a vision deficit may affect an individual's ability to perform tasks in daily life and which strategies may be most effective in enhancing his or her functioning. Some examples are presented at the end of this chapter.

Before detailing the individual components of visual functioning, the chapter will review the roles of age and diagnosis in creating this profile of visual functioning. Then the strengths and weaknesses of clinical vision testing will be addressed in explaining how vision affects an individual's ability to function in complex and varied environments. Each of the seven visual functions evaluated in developing a profile of visual impairment is then discussed extensively. A final section reviews special considerations when brain damage is the cause of an individual's visual impairment.

ROLES OF AGE AND DIAGNOSIS

Age

Age is an important variable in understanding vision. Although it is natural for very young children to still be developing their visual functions, it is typical for adults and older adults to be losing certain of them. During a person's fifth decade, the decline in natural focusing abilities for reading becomes noticeable for most fully sighted persons. In later decades, a decline in pupil size and increased clouding of the lens within the eye are associated with dimming of vision, increased sensitivity to glare, and other subtle changes. Advancing age is also associated with greater likelihood of certain eye conditions, such as cataract, macular degeneration, glaucoma, and diabetic retinopathy.

Diagnosis

Simply knowing the cause of a person's visual impairment helps to identify which of his or her visual functions are more likely to be affected. The table presented in the Appendix of this book describes 23 of the more common causes of visual impairment and, for each, indicates generalizations about how specific visual functions are most likely to be affected. Some visual disorders have their greatest impact on only a few of visual functions, while others affect nearly all aspects of vision. Such varied patterns result from differences in which parts of the eye and the visual system are disrupted, and how they are disrupted. When a given part of the eye is affected, the practitioner can make basic predictions about visual consequences by knowing the contribution of that part of the eye to vision. For example, it is well known that damage caused by macular degeneration affects the part of the retina that supports central vision, and, therefore, does not cause loss of peripheral vision.

Knowing which vision disorder is present, however, is usually insufficient to predict an individual's visual functioning. Even among individuals with the same condition, there can be critical differences in severity of disruption of a particular visual function. As a result of differences in detail vision, one person with macular degeneration might still be able to read small print in the newspaper while another might not even be able to read headlines. There can also be critical differences in the pattern of disruption of visual functions. Two individuals with macular degeneration might have the same amount of loss of detail vision, but one of them might be further disabled by things looking "washed out." As a result, performances might differ greatly between these individuals on tasks such as reading, handwriting, and detecting steps and curbs.

CLINICAL TESTING

Information derived from clinical tests of vision functions contribute to our knowledge about an individual's visual functioning, but the strengths and limitations of such testing must be understood. These tests were developed primarily to diagnose and monitor diseases and disorders of the eye and its neurological connections to the brain (i.e., the visual pathways). Good performance on the most common vision tests requires that the eyes and the visual pathways be in good condition. The optics must be in good focus, there cannot be any significant cloudiness of the optical elements, the retinas must be able to receive images well, the nerves must transmit the images well, and the brain must process them well. Finding that a person performs accurately on a range of vision tests greatly reduces (but does not eliminate) the possibility that significant vision-threatening disorders are present or imminent. Indeed, a person can do well on a wide range of vision tests and still have a dangerous defect of the peripheral retina or have elevated eye pressure that may threaten his or her vision.

Clinical vision tests are also used to explain visual functioning on everyday tasks performed outside the examination room. There might be difficulties in accurately predicting performance because clinical vision tests are performed in highly controlled environments that may not come close to simulating the actual environments in which people spend their lives. For example, color vision tests are specifically designed to eliminate contextual clues. Thus, a person may perform poorly on a clinical color vision test but have no difficulty in naming the colors on the American flag or knowing that the illuminated top light on a traffic signal is red.

Clinical tests also differ from natural environments in that only a very narrow range of light levels are used. In contrast, people naturally encounter light levels that can vary by more than a factor of 100,000 as a function of the time of day, environment, and surface characteristics of the objects viewed. For example, clinic lighting levels are much less bright than outdoor daylight settings and much more bright than most home settings. Therefore, selection of appropriately dark sunglasses requires actual outdoor testing, because outdoor lighting conditions cannot easily be replicated in a clinic. Patients who read well in the clinic under optimal lighting conditions may therefore perform poorly at home if lighting conditions in the home are less than optimal.

Despite these shortcomings of using clinical test results to predict performance in natural settings, it is tempting to make maximum use of clinical test results since they are often readily available from medical records and clearly standardized. Improved versions of eye charts and other vision tests have been created in recent decades that make it possible to measure better the vision of people who are visually impaired (Bailey, 1976, Pelli & Levi, 1988). This has created more reliable and valid data. Moreover, recent research on how vision function tests relate to real-world performance has been instructive and encouraging (West et al., 2002).

Thus, although clinical vision data are never sufficient, they are often necessary and valuable in explaining how a visual impairment may affect an individual's ability to perform tasks in daily life and in suggesting appropriate strategies for enhancing his or her performance. The four sample profiles at the end of this chapter are provided to reflect the range of possible clinical findings and to indicate the kinds of interpretations that might follow. Understanding and using such profiles require separate discussion of each of their seven key components, which is provided in the following sections.

VISUAL ACUITY

Visual acuity is the ability to resolve fine detail. Measuring visual acuity often involves the familiar task of reading successively smaller letters on an eye chart. Eye charts can be positioned either many feet away for measurement of what is termed "distance visual acuity" or can be positioned quite close for measurement of "near visual acuity."

Snellen Fraction

The most common way to write a visual acuity score is using a Snellen fraction, in which the top number indicates how far away the eye chart was and the bottom number indicates the distance at which a person with normal vision could see the smallest letter that the test subject was able to see. In the United States, Snellen fractions are usually presented in the form "20/x" indicating a 20-foot test distance. Thus, 20/20 means a person's performance matches that expected of a person with unimpaired vision, while 20/40 means that a person with unimpaired vision could see the same size letter from 40 feet away. Thus, a 20/40 acuity is reduced by a factor of two compared to normal vision. (See Chap. 3 for more details.)

Closer test distances are routinely used with persons with visual impairments, and metric distances are routinely used in the United Kingdom and other countries. To compare an acuity measured at one distance to another acuity measured at another distance, it is often convenient to convert them both to the "20/x" format. To do this, each Snellen fraction is simply set as equal to another one with 20 as the numerator (e.g., 10/20 = 20/x). The denominator is then recalculated:

$$10/20 = 20/x = 20/40.$$

For a given eye, visual acuities measured at different distances should be equivalent if the eye is in focus for each test distance and if similar testing conditions are used for each distance. Indeed, under these conditions, distance and near acuities should be equal. When acuities are not equal at distance and near, an uncorrected eyeglass prescription or insufficient close focusing ability (accommodation) may be the cause. A confounding factor is when differences in test chart design and brightness might make it harder or easier to read a specific distance eye chart compared to a specific near eye chart. Some eye con ditions, such as macular degeneration, can be particularly sensitive to such differences.

To describe a person's true potential for seeing detail, the most useful visual acuity measurement is obtained with the person wearing his or her most effective eyeglass prescription. Therefore, careful refractive testing performed by an optometrist or ophthalmologist, as well as appropriate refractive correction, are needed prior to the determination of what is termed a best-corrected visual acuity (see Sidebar 2.1). (In this chapter, all acuities mentioned are assumed to be with best refractive correction.)

If one eye has a worse visual acuity than the other, the measurement of the better eye or both eyes together is most useful in understanding how the person functions in daily activities. In general, the acuity of the better eye determines the person's visual functioning. The visual acuity of two eyes together will not be the average of the two, but, rather, will usually be the same (or nearly the same) as the acuity of the better eye.

Inconsistent acuity data are sometimes gathered when a person with a visual impairment is examined in different settings and by different examiners. For a given individual, one eye specialist might report a moderately better acuity than another, even for a person with a stable eye condition who has been tested in the two different offices on the same day. The main reason for this is that there are more sources of variability in acuity data for individuals with visual impairments than for individuals without visual impairments.

Variations in eye chart design and test administration procedures are important sources of errors (usually underestimates of ability) in measuring the visual acuity of people with visual impairments. The widely used Snellen-type eye charts do not allow for precise measurement of poor visual acuities when they are used at the recommended distances. This is because Snellen charts have few letters at the largest sizes and often jump from 20/400 to 20/200 to 20/100. Thus, a person who cannot quite read the 20/100 line is reported to have an acuity of 20/200. If tested on a chart with more lines in this range (such as 20/100, 20/125, 20/160, and 20/200), the same person might be reported as having a visual acuity of 20/125. The projected versions of these charts are often dim and have low-contrast letters, which can degrade the performance of many individuals who are visually impaired.

Acuity can also be underestimated if the person being tested does not persist in trying to read chart letters once it becomes difficult to do so. This is particularly likely when the observer has blind spots near the very center of vision that make reading laborious. Thus, the observer's level of motivation and the amount of encouragement provided by the examiner can influence the resulting visual acuity scores.

Refractive Error

The clearest possible image is formed in an eye when light from the object being viewed passes through the optical (or focusing) elements of the eye (the cornea and the crystalline lens) and is in perfect focus when it reaches the retina (which lines the inside of the eye). Such perfect focus occurs without eyeglasses in individuals with emmetropia, the condition in which the combined focal length of the cornea and crystalline lens match the length of the eye.

Refractive error refers to a condition in which light rays are not brought into focus on the retina as a result of a defect in the shape of the eye or in its optical elements. Myopia (or nearsightedness) exists when the focal length of these optical elements is shorter than the length of the eye, while hyperopia (or farsightedness) occurs when the focal length of these optical elements is longer than the length of the eye. With uncorrected myopia, distance vision is blurred, while objects held at some close distance (determined by the magnitude of the myopia) may be clear. With uncorrected hyperopia, young people with sufficient accommodation (see discussion later in this chapter) may be able to see clearly at distance and, although less likely, at near as well.

Astigmatism results when the cornea is curved not like the surface of a sphere but more like the surfaces of a football. With uncorrected astigmatism, vision tends to be blurred for objects at all distances, with some edges or lines more blurred than others.

Certain conventions are used in specifying eyeglass prescriptions. The most basic convention is use of the units of diopters to specify lens power. The dioptic power of a lens equals the reciprocal of the focal length of the lens in metric units. The sign of the dioptric power of a lens is positive if the lens causes light to converge (i.e., a convex lens) and is negative if the lens causes light to diverge (i.e., a concave lens). The first number listed in an eyeglass prescription is usually the component of the prescription that is for nearsightedness or farsightedness, often specified with the letter "D" for diopters or "DS" for diopters sphere following the number. If a second number is listed for the same eye, it is usually the power of the correction for astigmatism. It is often followed by the letters "DC" meaning diopters cylindrical. For further information on the specification of eyeglass prescriptions, see Wakefield (2000).

The importance of wearing eyeglasses (or contact lenses, in some cases) to correct one's refractive error depends, first, on the magnitude of the prescription, with stronger prescriptions being more critical. Prescription lenses range in power from 0.00 ("plano") to as high as about +25.00 DS for hyperopia, as high as about −30.00 DS for myopia, and as high as about −10.00 DC for astigmatism. The importance of wearing any given prescription, naturally, also depends on how much it improves visual functioning. However, even if performance benefits are not observed, wearing eyeglasses may be especially important for children whose visual systems are still developing. Accordingly, the actual value of eyeglasses needs to be carefully considered on an individual basis.

For more details about refractive error, lenses, and other optical principles, see Chapter 3.

Implications of Visual Acuity Impairments

Optometrists and ophthalmologists use acuity testing mostly to gauge whether a change in eyeglass prescription is needed and whether the various parts of the visual system are intact. Although most people equate 20/20 vision with perfect vision and healthy eyes, this is a misperception. Even at 20/20, eyeglasses may still be of value, and the eyes may not be healthy and fully functional. Indeed, certain eye diseases, such as glaucoma and diabetic retinopathy, can be moderately advanced without causing any reduction in visual acuity. Thus, while good visual acuity is usually reassuring and makes it less likely that there are unresolved issues related to eyeglasses or eye health, it provides no real assurances. For a patient with a known vision disorder, acuity testing can be used as a guide to monitor the condition and suggest treatment options. For instance, by monitoring visual acuity, a surgeon might decide when to recommend cataract removal or when to suspect a postsurgical complication.

Some health care services, benefits, and privileges are only available to persons who meet certain visual acuity criteria. For example, Social Security generally requires that an individual meet its definition of "legal blindness" in order to qualify for disability benefits based on vision. To meet this standard, an individual must have a best-corrected visual acuity of 20/200 or worse in the better eye (or have a visual field that is no more than 20 degrees in diameter). An alternate, more strict standard for legal blindness used by the World Health Organization (WHO, n.d.), and many countries requires best-corrected visual acuity to be worse than 20/400 in the better eye.

A revised system for evaluating permanent vision impairment has been developed by a panel of low vision experts and published by the American Medical Association (AMA) as part of their *Guides to the Evaluation of Permanent Impairment* (5th ed.) (Cochiarella, Andersson & AMA, 2001). The new system reflects improved methods for testing vision and improved understanding of the functional implications of various visual impairments. In this system, the Visual Efficiency Scale used in previous AMA guides has been replaced by a Functional Vision Score. This score is based on combining a Functional Acuity Score (by which an acuity of 20/20 gets 100 points, 20/200 gets 50 points, and no light perception gets 0 points) with a Functional Field Score (which weights central and inferior field losses more heavily). Some consideration is also allowed for other types of visual impairments (such as contrast and glare sensitivity), but formal scales have only been developed for rating visual acuities and visual fields. Although the validity of this system has yet to be proven, there are indications that its basic structure is valid and that it is an improvement over the visual efficiency scales it replaces (Massof, 2002).

Some education and rehabilitation programs categorize individuals as "visually impaired" or having low vision when their acuity is at or below the 20/60 or 20/70 level. An acuity of at least 20/40 is required by most states in the United States for driving without restrictions. In many states, individuals with acuity below than 20/40 but as good as 20/200 can be eligible for restricted licensure (e.g., daytime only or bioptic telescope use required) (Peli, 2002).

In education and rehabilitation settings, visual acuity helps to explain an individual's visual functioning and to guide exploration of appropriate adaptations and instruction for that individual. Knowing the general magnitude of the deficit in acuity allows general predictions about visual functioning. For instance, with all other things being equal, the child with only a reduction by a factor of 5 in acuity (i.e., 20/100) would be more likely to become a visual reader than a child with a reduction by a factor of 40 (i.e., 20/800). The child with 20/800 visual acuity would more likely need to learn braille as a primary reading mode and would be more likely to need other nonvisual strategies. Determining whether or not it is appropriate for a child to be primarily a visual reader requires careful consideration of many visual and nonvisual abilities by qualified education experts, the student, and family members. Visual acuity scores can provide useful general insights about the prognosis for visual reading.

Data on visual acuity can provide guidance in making the preliminary determination of how much magnification a person needs to be able to read small print. The worse the acuity, the more magnification is required. But just how much magnification is required for a person with a given acuity—say, 20/100—to see newsprint? Methods for determining this precisely require careful clinical testing. A general estimate can, however, be made by first using the distance acuity and applying Kestenbaum's rule (Kestenbaum & Sturman, 1956). This rule says that the bare minimum magnification needed to read newsprint equals the mathematical reciprocal of the visual acuity expressed in diopters (the standard units for lens power). So, for someone with an acuity of 20/100, the calculations would be 100/20 = +5.00 diopters for reading newsprint (see Chap. 3 for a more complete explanation of these calculations).

Kestenbaum's rule gives only a minimum estimate, which usually does not allow the person to read with any significant comfort, speed, or stamina. Better performance requires what is termed a substantial acuity reserve (Whittaker & Lovie-Kitchin, 1993), meaning that what is being read needs to be considerably larger than what can just barely be seen (Cole, 1993). The magnitude of the acuity reserve required by an individual is critical to selecting appropriate magnification systems. Some have proposed an acuity reserve of 2 (Cheong, Lovie-Kitchin, & Bowers, 2002), while others have shown evidence that acuity reserves need to be closer to 5 (Flom et al., 1993). These values suggest that, for maximum reading speed, a person would be predicted to need a magnifier two to five times as strong as one that is minimally adequate (based on the reciprocal of the acuity). For a person with an acuity of 20/100, a magnifier of +5.00 diopters (i.e., 100/20 = 5) would be expected to be minimally useful with newsprint, while magnifiers in the +10.00 to +25.00 diopter range would be needed to allow the best possible comfort, speed, and stamina in reading newsprint.

Despite the value of estimating required acuity reserve, simple clinical testing of actual reading performance with different levels of magnification can be used to determine the acuity reserve needed by a given individual (see Chap. 6). An important exception to this is when the individual cannot perform the reading test (e.g., a child who has not learned to read) (see Chap. 5).

Limitations of Visual Acuity Scores

Visual acuity scores can be misleading at times. In the extreme, it is possible to have 20/20 visual acuity and yet function much like someone with no vision at all. This could occur with a person who has severe tunnel vision that leaves only a tiny central island of vision that can eke out a 20/20 performance. A less extreme example would be two individuals, each with 20/200 visual acuity, but one of whom has many blind spots as well as reduced contrast sensitivity. The reading performance of these two people may differ vastly, with one able to use magnifiers quite effectively for reading and the other struggling to read with magnifiers.

Despite its limitations, acuity testing remains a fundamental measure. In nearly all cases, if only one test of vision function were to be performed in an attempt to understand a person's ability to function visually, acuity would be the best choice. Visual acuity remains the most powerful single predictor of visual functioning for most people and most tasks.

VISUAL FIELDS

An eye's visual field is the entire region of space off to all sides that is visible when the person is steadily looking and facing straight ahead. The absolute extent of the visual field can be plotted by determining how far away from straight ahead a light or other target can be seen before it disappears. Lights or other targets are typically presented in different directions to estimate the extent of vision in a full 360 degrees. These data are plotted to represent just how far from straight ahead an object can be and remain visible.

Normal Visual Fields

The outline of a normal visual field plot is an irregular oval extending from the point of fixation out to about 95 degrees toward one's temple, to about 60 degrees toward one's nose, to about 50 degrees above, and to about 65 degrees below one's point of fixation. The horizontal extent of the normal visual field for one eye is about 160 degrees (see Fig. 2.1).

The quality of vision within the visual field varies as a function of normal physiology, with better vision present centrally and poorer vision peripherally. A simple example of this is that a normal eye can read small print on an eye chart or a printed page only when the eye is aimed directly at the print. When the eye is aimed off to the side of the chart or page, the print becomes unreadable.

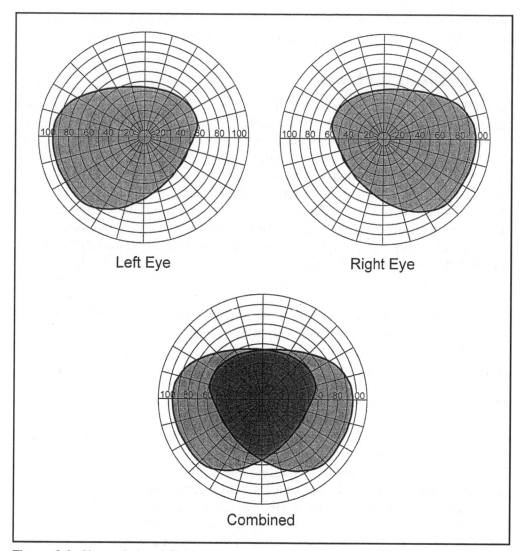

Figure 2.1. Normal visual fields.

When a person with unimpaired vision in each eye looks at the world, the visual fields of the right and left eyes tend to overlap substantially, but not completely (Fig. 2.1). Everything viewed out to about 60 degrees to the right and left of straight ahead is seen by both eyes; only the 35 or so degrees at the far horizontal limits of the visual field are seen by only one eye. The net result is that two unimpaired visual fields combine to provide about 190 degrees of continuous, uninterrupted visual field. The fact that our visual fields overlap and combine is beneficial for many people with visual field defects. If the region of visual field loss for one eye corresponds to an area of intact visual field for the other eye, the person will typically perceive no defect when both eyes are open.

Visual Field Defects

Visual field defects can be caused by many eye diseases and disorders (see the Appendix for this book). They are typically classified by their density, location, shape, and size. The most dense visual field defects, which allow no vision in the affected areas, are referred to as absolute defects. All other visual field defects allow some, albeit degraded, vision in the affected area and are referred to as relative defects. The location of a visual field defect is usually classified as either central or peripheral. This classification depends on the defect's eccentricity: how far away from straight ahead it is. Defects beyond about 30 degrees eccentricity are generally considered to be peripheral, while those at about 30 degrees eccentricity are considered to be midperipheral. Defects located within 30 degrees of straight ahead are considered to be central. These central defects are sometimes subclassified as paracentral (i.e., next to the center) or pericentral (i.e., surrounding the center). These designations indicate that the most central (and most acute) vision is not as substantially affected as adjacent areas.

Additional descriptions of field defect location would include whether the defect is to the right, left, above, or below the person's line of sight. Sometimes the defect is described as located either nasally or temporally to indicate whether it is nearer to the nose or to the side of the head. The location is often further classified as either unilateral or bilateral to describe whether visual fields are affected in one or both eyes. When a defect is bilateral, the term *homonymous* may be used to indicate that the same side of the visual field is affected for each eye. When the field defect in one eye is on the opposite side of fixation as the defect for the other eye, the defects may be described as binasal or bitemporal, depending on which parts of the field are impaired.

The shapes of visual field defects may be described in a variety of ways. A sampling of these descriptions is presented in Figure 2.2. Some midperipheral defects are described as arcuate or ring-shaped. Two common types of large peripheral field defects are hemianopias and quadrantanopias; hemianopic defects involve loss of half of the visual field (sometimes with so-called macular sparing, which allows preservation of the most central vision even on the blind side), while quadrantanopic defects involve loss of one-quarter of the visual field. Some peripheral field defects are described as altitudinal, meaning that the defect involves either the upper (i.e., superior) or lower (i.e., inferior) field. Other field losses are described as concentric, meaning that field has been lost symmetrically from all sides.

The size of a field defect may be described quantitatively in terms of degrees of field lost or degrees of field remaining. Qualitative descriptions may be used when precise testing has been impossible (such as in reporting a "tiny spared island of central vision") or when such descriptions are sufficient (such as in reporting a "complete left homonymous hemianopia").

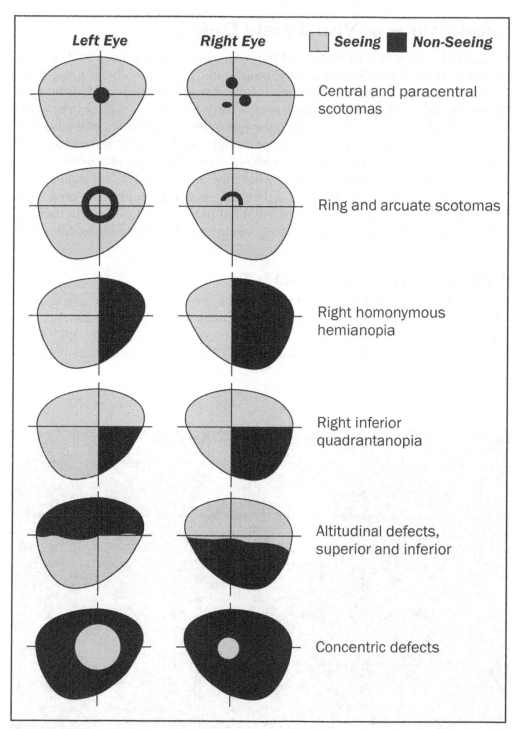

Figure 2.2. Types of visual field defects.

Implications of Visual Field Defects

Visual field testing is a fundamental part of a complete eye examination. The presence of a visual field loss and the pattern of that loss can be of great value in detecting and monitoring disorders of the visual system. Partial visual field losses are usually caused by damage to structures at the back of the eye or along the neural pathways that extend from the eye to the visual cortex at the back of the brain. The most common of these are retinal diseases, optic nerve disorders, and damage to the visual pathways or visual cortex. The specific pattern of the visual field defect can help to identify where the anatomical defect may be.

The functional implications of visual field defects vary depending on a wide range of factors, but can be grouped meaningfully in terms of the whether the defects are mainly peripheral or mainly central, as described in the following sections.

PERIPHERAL VISUAL FIELD DEFECTS

Peripheral visual field defects tend to have their greatest impact on safe, visually guided travel and driving. Orientation and mobility (O&M) performance is more closely related to visual field size than to visual acuity (Marron & Bailey, 1982; Kuyk & Elliott, 1999). When field loss is bilateral and concentric, it seems that the width

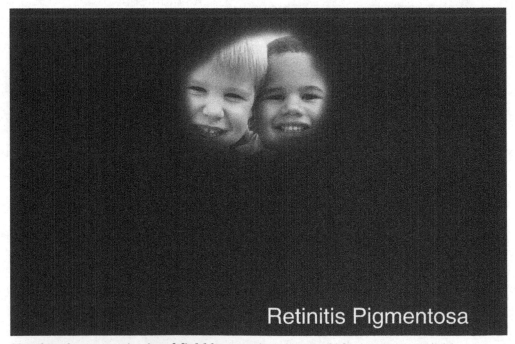

Retinitis Pigmentosa

Simulated concentric visual field loss, as in advanced glaucoma or retinitis pigmentosa. *(National Eye Institute, National Institutes of Health)*

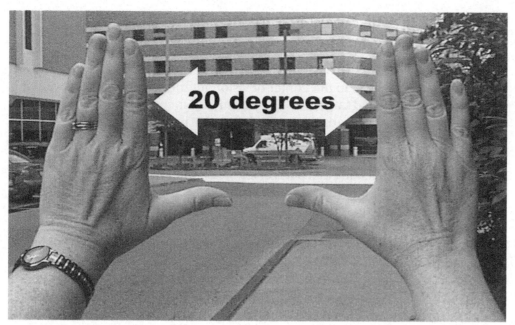

A simple way to demonstrate to oneself the approximate size of a 20-degree diameter visual field. *(Ohio State University College of Optometry Instructional Media Center)*

of the remaining visual field needs to be less than about 20 or 30 degrees before most people need to rely mainly on nonvisual travel strategies, such as long cane travel. Although determining whether or not it is appropriate for a person to be a visual traveler requires careful consideration of many visual and nonvisual abilities by qualified O&M experts, by the individual, and by family members, visual field data can provide useful general insights about the prognosis for visual travel of a particular person.

A simple way to demonstrate the approximate size of a visual field that is 20 degrees in diameter is to extend one's arms straight forward, at shoulder height with palms facing away from the face. Extend the thumbs to form a right angle with the fingers and position the thumbs so that they are separated by about one and a half inches. The distance between the fingers should represent about 20 degrees for most people.

The width of one's peripheral visual field is used to determine eligibility for some benefits, privileges, and programs. A visual field loss that leaves no more than a 20-degree-wide (in diameter) visual field meets Social Security's criteria for legal blindness. Lesser degrees of visual field loss, in combination with visual acuity loss, may be interpreted as sufficient for Social Security standards. Specific methods are available for calculating the combined effects of visual acuity and visual field losses (Cochiarella et al., 2001, p. 296). A visual field of no more than 10 degrees width meets the World Health Organization's criteria for blindness

(WHO, 1980). For driving, about half the U.S. states set some standard for minimum visual field width.

CENTRAL VISUAL FIELD DEFECTS

Visual field defects close to the center of vision interfere most with the viewing of complex and detailed targets, such as print and faces. When the visual field defect is dense and localized, it creates a blind spot in the vision known as a scotoma. People with central scotomas seldom can clearly describe the borders of their blind spot, reporting only a vague awareness of what has happened to their central vision and indicating that parts of letters or objects seem to disappear and then reappear.

Central scotomas can make reading slow and tedious even when the person is viewing print that has been made optimally large. One reason for such reading difficulties is that eye movement control is also disrupted in the presence of scotomas. People with scotomas have been found to make lots of small, inaccurate, and inefficient eye movements as they proceed through text (Bullimore & Bailey, 1995). A second reason is that the remaining, more peripheral, retinal areas have perceptual characteristics that prevent rapid reading. The ability to resolve detail (i.e., acuity) drops off rapidly for points on the retina even slightly away from the center of the macula. Even when print is enlarged enough to compensate for this reduction in acuity, peripheral retinal areas are not able to

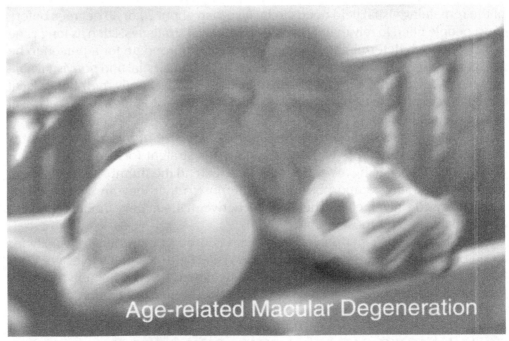

Simulated central vision loss, as in advanced macular degeneration. *(National Eye Institute, National Institutes of Health)*

support rapid reading. Studies of readers with low vision show that those with conditions that cause central visual field defects are not able to read as quickly as those with other types of eye conditions, even when high levels of magnification are provided (Legge et al., 1992). Another study (Rubin & Turano, 1992) measured how well people without vision loss could read when images of words were flashed in the center of the visual field compared to when appropriately enlarged images were flashed about 10 degrees away from center. The striking finding was that people could read about 50 times faster using their central vision than with their vision 10 degrees away from center.

It is a common misconception that the levels of magnification usually provided to assist people with central scotomas cause the scotomas to be viewed as small specks within the magnified views. This is not true. Even the higher levels of magnification achieved with optical devices and video magnification systems are insufficient to do this. This is because the magnified images remain small compared to the size of the scotomas. For instance, magnifiers in the +20.00 to +40.00 diopter range (i.e., designated as 5× to 10× by many manufacturers) only make newsprint subtend an angle of about 1.5 to 3.5 degrees on the retina in size. In comparison, the size of central scotomas can vary up to about 20 degrees. (See Chap. 3 for a discussion of optics and terms related to magnification, such as diopters.) Magnification does allow a person with a scotoma to read with an area of retina slightly more peripheral than the damaged central retina (see Fig. 2.3). Magnification makes this possible since more peripheral retinal areas naturally have worse acuity (and hence greater need for magnification) than normal central retina.

When a central scotoma occurs, a person no longer achieves best vision by aiming his or her eyes directly at a target, but must shift the gaze slightly to one side or the other, or slightly above or below the target. Shifting the gaze to use an adjoining part of the retina in this manner is called eccentric viewing. The particular part of the retina that a person chooses to use is called the preferred retinal locus (PRL). There is evidence that people with central scotomas can naturally and spontaneously adopt a consistent PRL without training, and that the retinal area they choose is fairly idiosyncratic and not always as close as possible to the area of predicted best vision (White & Bedell, 1990; Timberlake et al., 1986, 1987). Thus, the role of eccentric viewing training has not been clearly established, although it may be of significant value to some individuals. Additional interesting clinical and laboratory work with PRLs is described elsewhere by Schuchard and Fletcher (1994).

CONTRAST SENSITIVITY

The term contrast refers to small differences in brightness between an object and its background. A common way to describe the contrast of an object is to calculate the difference in brightness between the object and its background, and then divide that by the brightness of the background. This method of calculation

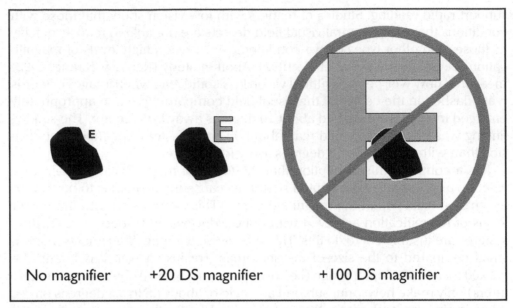

No magnifier   +20 DS magnifier   +100 DS magnifier

Figure 2.3. Using magnification with a central scotoma. When a person with a central scotoma views newsprint without a magnifier, the image subtends about 0.2 degrees. With a +20 DS magnifier, the image subtends about 1.6 degrees on the retina, usually making it readable by the slightly peripheral retina that must be used. It is impractical to provide magnification equivalent to the more than +100 DS, which would be required to make the scotoma appear very small compared to the size of the magnified image of the newsprint.

results in what is known as the Weber contrast. In everyday environments, Weber contrast levels vary as a result of surface characteristics and lighting levels, and range from a high of 100 percent to a low of 0 percent.

Contrast sensitivity refers to an individual's ability to detect various levels of contrast. The higher a person's contrast sensitivity, the lower the levels of contrast he or she can detect. Indeed, this sensitivity is usually expressed as either the reciprocal of the most subtle contrast that can be detected (i.e., contrast sensitivity = 1/contrast threshold) or as the logarithm of that reciprocal (i.e., log contrast sensitivity = log [1/contrast threshold]).

Contrast sensitivity depends on the size and detail of objects being viewed. The unimpaired eye is most sensitive to intermediate levels of detail (such as in a 20/100 acuity target) and least sensitive to high levels of detail (such as in a 20/20 acuity target). This means that more contrast is needed to see fine detail than to see gross detail. This phenomenon occurs due to limits on how perfect the optics of the eye can be for seeing fine detail. It also seems to involve the ways in which certain cells in the visual system appear to be tuned to respond more to some levels of detail (or spatial frequencies) than to others. A profile called a contrast sensitivity function can be created to describe a person's abilities across a range of spatial frequencies.

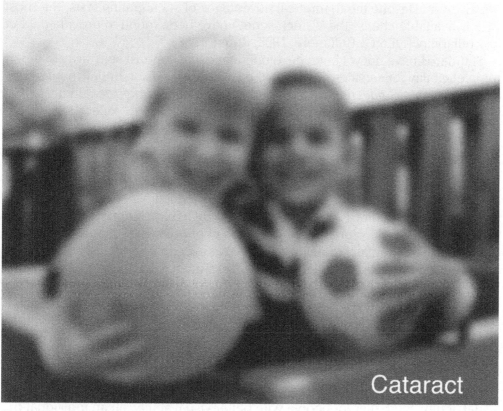

Simulation of reduced contrast sensitivity combined with blur caused by cataract.
(National Eye Institute, National Institutes of Health)

Moderate degrees of contrast sensitivity loss may result in difficulties with a wide range of tasks, but may only prompt vague complaints. More profound losses of contrast sensitivity can be severely debilitating, and may cause a person to describe vision as looking "washed out" or "misty."

Contrast sensitivity testing has not yet become a standard part of most eye examinations, but is used by some eye surgeons, many low vision care providers, and many vision researchers. Testing of contrast sensitivity need not be complicated, and, indeed, can be as simple as using an eye chart in which all the letters are the same size, but vary in contrast from black to very faint grey (Pelli, Robson, & Wilkins, 1988; Legge & Rubin, 1986; Elliott & Whitaker, 1992). (See Chaps. 5 and 6 for more information on specific eye charts.) Well-designed letter charts with a range of contrast levels, such as the Pelli-Robson chart, are quite appropriate in measuring sensitivity to middle and low spatial frequencies (Pelli et al., 1988). This testing is then complemented by standard visual acuity testing, which estimates the high spatial frequency part of the contrast sensitivity function (since visual acuity measures the smallest detail a person can see).

An alternative approach uses contrast charts with gratings (i.e., stripes) of various sizes in an effort to characterize fully the nature of any contrast sensitivity impairment. Despite the theoretical advantages of such grating tests, the most widely available charts (the Vistech series) have been found to provide data of low reliability (Elliott & Bullimore, 1993; Rubin, 1988).

Standards have not yet been developed for using contrast sensitivity to determine eligibility for services or specify the severity of a vision impairment or disability. The *AMA Guides to the Evaluation of Permanent Impairment* indicate that vision impairment ratings should be adjusted modestly to reflect any severe problems with contrast sensitivity that are not reflected by ratings solely based on visual acuity and visual field loss (Cocchiarella et al., 2001).

Contrast sensitivity is a critical component of a low vision examination. It can provide relevant information about visual abilities that is not reflected in visual acuity scores or visual field plots. Orientation and mobility performance is more highly related to contrast sensitivity than to visual acuity (Marron & Bailey, 1982; Kuyk & Elliott, 1999). More recent work has confirmed that contrast sensitivity deficits particularly affect mobility tasks such as ascending and descending stairs (West et al., 2002). Researchers (Brown, 1981; Rubin & Legge, 1989; West et al., 2002) have also shown that contrast sensitivity deficits contribute to difficulties with reading. It is easy to understand how poor print quality or use of colored paper could seriously hinder the reading ability of a person with reduced contrast sensitivity. Indeed, the evidence is that performance of a wide range of everyday visual activities can be confounded by impairments in contrast sensitivity (West et al., 2002).

Although, in general, contrast sensitivity is worse for people with more limited visual acuity and better for people with better visual acuity, on an individual-by-individual basis, visual acuity does not predict contrast sensitivity very accurately (Haegerstrom-Portnoy et al., 2000). Indeed, contrast sensitivity can be poor even when visual acuity is good (such as in people with cataract) and contrast sensitivity can be good even when visual acuity is poor (such as in people with albinism). Therefore, a strong case can be made for including contrast sensitivity as a key component of the profile of visual functioning.

LIGHT SENSITIVITY

Persons who are visually impaired are often very sensitive to light levels, although sensitivity varies by eye condition (see the Appendix to this book) and among persons with the same eye condition. This means that they must receive just the right amount of light—not too much or too little—to function optimally. The same person who may prefer very bright lighting for reading may be dazzled by bright sunlight. Thus, it is useful to differentiate between a person's preferred task lighting and preferred ambient lighting.

Preferred lighting levels for task lighting—that is, light focused directly on a near task—tend to be unusually high for persons with certain eye conditions and unusually low for others. Age-related macular degeneration often creates the need for bright task lighting (Eldred, 1992; Brown & Kitchin, 1983; Sloan, 1977).

Therefore, it is especially important to test the effect of well-directed, bright light on visual functioning (especially reading) in persons diagnosed as having macular degeneration.

Some eye conditions cause people to prefer low to intermediate levels of task lighting. Examples of these would include iris defects such as aniridia, a condition in which the iris is mostly or entirely absent; and oculocutaneous albinism, in which the iris lacks sufficient pigment to block most light. An example of a retinal condition that leads to extreme light sensitivity is achromatopsia (also known as rod monochromacy). In this condition, extreme light sensitivity results from the abnormal predominance of rods, the photoreceptor type that functions best in dim lighting.

Preferences for ambient lighting both indoors and outdoors also vary based on a person's eye condition. In general, retinal and optic nerve disorders interfere with normal processes that allow the eye to adapt to a wide range of light levels. As a consequence, changes in light level may be especially troublesome for people with conditions such as retinitis pigmentosa or diabetic retinopathy. Veiling glare is a common problem with ambient lighting and occurs when light from one side (or above or below) is scattered, thus interfering with the clarity of the object being viewed straight ahead. The particles causing the light to scatter can be external to the eye (such as the dirt on a windshield that impedes vision when one is driving toward the sun) or internal to the eye (such as with cataract or normal, age-related clouding of the crystalline lens). Scattered light from veiling glare reduces the apparent contrast of objects, which can be especially troublesome if the person already has reduced contrast sensitivity.

A person's report of light sensitivity can help eye doctors in making the correct diagnosis, since extreme light sensitivity is characteristic of certain chronic eye conditions (such as achromatopsia or retinitis pigmentosa) and some acute eye conditions (such as inflammations). Actual testing of a person's degree of light sensitivity has not been well standardized and is not included in most eye examinations. One reason for this is that special equipment is required to produce bright enough light levels indoors to simulate accurately outdoor lighting conditions (which can be more than 1,000 times brighter than indoor light levels).

Standards have not been developed for using light sensitivity to determine eligibility for services or specify the severity of a visual impairment. The *AMA Guides to the Evaluation of Permanent Impairment* indicate that vision impairment ratings should be adjusted modestly to reflect any severe problems with light sensitivity that are not reflected by ratings solely based on visual acuity and visual field loss (Cocchiarella et al., 2001).

There are many reasons that bright task lighting is underutilized by people who benefit greatly from its use. Many simply do not realize just how important bright light is for optimal visual functioning. Once individuals and their families are aware of this, significant changes are often required in the home environment that can be difficult to accept. Most homes are furnished in ways that provide far less light for reading than is recommended, even for people with no visual impairments. Many people do not understand that they need lamps with reflectors to concentrate the light and are accustomed to the common drum shade–type living room lamp, which creates very diffuse lighting and cannot be easily positioned close to printed materials. Many people misunderstand how the brightness of a page increases as a lamp is brought closer, thinking, for instance, that if a lamp is moved twice as close to an object (e.g., 1 foot away rather than 2 feet away), it will create twice as much brightness. In fact, a basic property of lighting known as the inverse square law dictates that bringing the lamp twice as close makes an object four times as bright (i.e., 2^2). An additional problem arises when one needs to achieve adequate brightness on a page held quite close to the eyes without getting stray light directly into the eyes. Accordingly, magnifiers with built-in lighting can be attractive alternatives to lamps.

COLOR DISCRIMINATION

Most impairments in color vision occur in people with otherwise normal vision and result from hereditary disorders of the retinal photoreceptors. Color vision impairments can also be caused by more serious eye conditions that also cause reduced visual acuity and other visual difficulties. Color vision impairments are most likely to occur when the underlying eye condition affects the retina or optic nerve. Only in rare cases are they caused by a brain disorder.

Tests of color discrimination are well-established tools eye care specialists use in diagnosing hereditary color vision impairments and many other eye conditions. The most common tests are called plate tests and involve recognizing a letter, number, or shape formed by colored dots on a series of pages called test plates. The dots making up a particular figure are surrounded by a field of dots that have colors commonly confused with those forming the figure. The small size of the dots on these plates can reduce the accuracy of these tests when the viewer's acuity is worse than about 20/200. In such cases, alternative tests that involve arranging medium- or large-sized samples of different colors (such as the Farnsworth dichotomous D-15 test or the Jumbo D-15 test [Sloane, 1989]) should be substituted. (See Chaps. 5 and 6 for more information about specific tests and the Resources to this book for sources of products.)

Color vision is not a significant part of most standards for determining severity of vision impairment or disability. The *AMA Guides to the Evaluation of Permanent Impairment* indicate that vision impairment ratings should be adjusted modestly to reflect any severe problems with color vision not reflected by ratings based only on visual acuity and visual field loss (Cocchiarella et al., 2001). Strict color vision requirements are, however, in place for the military and certain forms of civil service, as well as certain vocations, such as commercial truck driving.

Knowing a person's ability to discriminate colors is of particular value in working with school age children due to the heavy use of color coding in most classrooms. Color vision is also relevant in career counseling and many aspects of functioning for adolescents, teenagers, and adults, including managing clothing, cooking, and shopping. While there are no means for restoring color perception, some tasks can be modified or alternative strategies learned to cope with color vision impairment. Occasionally, colored filters can be used to help a person discriminate between specific colors, but such applications are very specific (Peli & Peli, 2002). Even when color vision is profoundly disrupted, brightness cues can be successfully used in some practical color discrimination tasks, such as telling navy blue pants from tan ones (but not from black ones).

OCULOMOTOR CONTROL

Oculomotor control (the control of eye movement and position) is often disrupted when vision is impaired. Examples of conditions involving such disruption include nystagmus, strabismus, and gaze palsies. Some types of these disruptions pose important practical problems. Others pose mainly cosmetic or social problems, or no problems at all.

Nystagmus

Nystagmus is an eye movement disorder that often accompanies visual impairments present at birth or that develop during the first several months of life. With nystagmus, the eyes appear to be in constant motion, usually jiggling from side to side. This eye movement is involuntary and continual, although the frequency or amplitude of the nystagmus may increase under certain stressful situations. For example, most people with congenital nystagmus can describe job interviews in which they have been able to feel the eyes moving more and notice their vision to be a bit worse. For many people with congenital nystagmus, the frequency or amplitude of the nystagmus decreases If they look In a certain direction or focus on an object close to them. This is described as a null point.

If nystagmus decreases greatly at the null point, a person may benefit from surgery or special prism glasses to aid them in the use of that null point. A number of treatments for nystagmus have been considered. In one study, researchers found about one line of improvement in visual acuity for people with nystagmus who were trained to reduce eye movement via auditory biofeedback (Ciuffreda, Goldrich, & Neary, 1982). Other treatment options that have been considered include ways to cancel out image motion, methods of suppressing nystagmus (including rigid contact lens wear), and drugs (Stahl, Plant, & Lehigh, 2002). At present, however, nystagmus that begins in early childhood is seldom treated due to the absence of well-tested and effective treatment strategies.

In trying to understand why nystagmus is common among people with congenital visual impairment, people often confuse cause and effect. Although many people assume that the nystagmus causes the visual impairment, most eye care specialists would agree that the nystagmus is an effect of visual impairment occurring early in life. In infancy, development of good eye movement control and the ability to fixate steadily on an object require good vision. The misconception that the nystagmus is the main visual impairment, rather than simply a result of an underlying one, is reinforced by the fact that nystagmus is readily apparent while the underlying cause of the visual impairment is often hidden deep within the eye or visual system.

Whether or not nystagmus causes the visual world to appear as if it is jiggling depends on the perons's age at onset of the nystagmus. It is rare for nystagmus occurring in infancy to cause oscillopsia, or jiggling vision. It seems that the brain selectively samples the visual information collected so that the image is essentially stabilized. An intriguing example of this phenomenon is the common report from people with nystagmus that, when they look at their own faces in the mirror, they do not see their eyes as moving. An explanation for this is that their brains are only capturing images of their eyes when the eyes are pointed straight ahead, looking directly at themselves. When the eyes are looking a bit to one side, the views available are ignored. As a result, every time the eyes are seen, they are pointing straight ahead. This sort of successful adaptation does not occur with nystagmus that develops in adulthood, such as with multiple sclerosis. The resulting oscillopsia can be extremely debilitating and difficult to treat (Stahl et al., 2002).

Strabismus

Strabismus is a condition in which one eye points directly at the object of regard, while the other eye points in another direction. An individual's strabismus is usually classified according to the direction to which the deviating eye turns, with esotropia indicating an inward turn toward the nose, exotropia indicating an outward turn toward the ear, hypertropia indicating an upward turn, and hypotropia indicating a downward turn.

Strabismus is much more common among people with visual impairment, especially those affected since birth or early childhood. When present from an early age in children with visual impairments, strabismus does not tend to cause double vision or other major visual disabilities. It is generally thought that development of well-aligned eyes requires good visual functioning in each eye. Accordingly, for children with bilaterally reduced vision, the lack of alignment is usually a reflection of underlying visual impairment rather than a cause of it. Further vision loss, known as amblyopia, may develop in the turned eye. Unfortunately, in the presence of bilateral visual impairment, surgical efforts to align the eyes are seldom sufficient to allow recovery of the lost vision. Surgery often serves mainly to improve the individual's appearance.

People who lose vision in one or both eyes after early childhood may also develop strabismus. When an adult loses substantial vision in one eye, it is common for that eye to drift out (or sometimes in toward the nose). If the vision loss in the more severely affected eye is profound, there is unlikely to be any double vision or other vision disruption caused by the eye turn. In other cases, a prism lens may be needed in his or her eyeglasses to help avoid double vision (see Chap. 3).

Gaze restrictions occur occasionally and prevent a person from moving one or both eyes into a certain direction of gaze. They can result from eye muscle weaknesses, neurological problems, or other factors. The implication of such restrictions is that placement of objects or persons to be viewed needs to be optimized. Some optical or surgical treatment options are sometimes successful.

Observations of eye movement and position control are a standard part of eye examinations and can help doctors to identify neurological impairments or certain eye conditions. With very young children, such testing can suggest how much vision is present.

The *AMA Guides to the Evaluation of Permanent Impairment of the Visual System* indicates that visual impairment ratings should be adjusted modestly to reflect any severe problems with double vision not reflected by ratings solely based on visual acuity and visual field loss (Cochiarella & Anderson, 2001, pp. 280, 297).

Nystagmus provides evidence of a visual impairment beginning in very early childhood or a neurological condition of later origin. Nystagmus originating in early childhood seldom causes visual problems, and is usually not a contraindication for contact lens wear or use of low vision devices. Strabismus in combination with visual impairment seldom causes additional visual difficulties. Gaze restrictions may have practical implications for positioning targets of vision and are occasionally treatable.

ACCOMMODATION

To see clearly within arm's reach, people need more ocular focusing power than is required to see clearly at longer range. When a person looks at an object at close range, the brain automatically signals the eye to adjust appropriately the shape of the crystalline lens within the eye to provide the needed additional focusing power. This process is called accommodation and involves increased thickness and surface curvatures of the crystalline lens. Due to the relative flexibility of this lens in childhood, most children are readily able to accommodate and can clearly see objects held very close. Accommodative ability, however, tends to decline slowly and consistently starting at or before the age of 10 years. Most people without visual impairment need their first reading prescription by about age 43 years and have no significant accommodative ability remaining by age 55 to 60 years of age.

The first reading glasses are often needed at much younger ages for people with visual impairment. The main reason for this is not that they have abnormal accommodative abilities, but that they have abnormally high accommodative demands. Such demands are created by the close viewing distances necessitated by their visual impairments. For example, a child who has a best-corrected visual acuity of 20/100 would be expected to need to hold printed materials about five times closer than a child with 20/20 acuity. The required amount of accommodation for this extra close viewing distance would be expected to be about five times greater than that needed by the child without visual impairment who does not need to hold print as close.

Very young children may not have difficulty maintaining such levels of accommodation and may not need to see very small print or read for long periods. However, recent data on accommodation in children with and without visual impairment suggest that, past the age of 9 or 10 years, children without visual impairment cannot maintain accommodation for viewing distances as close as 4 inches from the face (Lueck et al., 2000). An encouraging finding was that children with visual impairments may not notice the blur very much when they are unable to accommodate enough for a close viewing distance. Confounding the situation for these children is the fact that, during the same grade school and secondary school years when accommodative ability is declining, reading demands are usually increasing.

Overall, it is very common for children with visual impairments who are of school age and older to experience symptoms and signs of accommodative insufficiency, such as headaches, eyestrain, and reading avoidance. Appropriately strong reading glasses or bifocals may be required to alleviate these problems. An alternative for some children is simply to remove eyeglasses or contact lenses that correct for nearsightedness (myopia) when viewing close objects. For them, their eyes are naturally in focus at some close distance determined by the degree of the nearsightedness. (See Chapter 3 for more details).

Eye examinations usually include an evaluation of accommodative abilities for children without visual impairment. It is unfortunate that accommodative abilities are seldom measured in children with visual impairments because they cannot see the usual viewing targets. In low vision examinations, these abilities and the potential role of reading lenses would usually be evaluated.

Most reading lenses provided for children and young adults with visual impairments are prescribed because these patients' abnormally high accommodative demands cannot be met by their normal accommodative abilities. Sometimes, however, the eye condition itself causes reduced accommodative abilities. For instance, there is good reason to expect hardening of the crystalline lens with resultant reduced accommodative abilities in people who are developing cataracts. Thus, children and young adults with eye conditions that tend to include cataract formation, such as diabetes and retinopathy of prematurity, are likely to have reduced accommodative abilities and may require earlier and stronger prescriptions for reading glasses.

Loss of accommodative ability is usually a normal age-related process that can be addressed simply with reading glasses. Even when it occurs earlier in life, such as in persons with the eye conditions described here, it has not been considered a significant component of permanent visual impairment in formal classification systems.

VISUAL IMPAIRMENT CAUSED BY BRAIN DAMAGE

Higher visual centers in the brain involved in perception are often disrupted in people with brain injuries or disorders (Girkin & Miller, 2001). Examples of such disorders occurring very early in life include cortical visual impairment (cerebral visual impairment) (Jan, Groenveld, Kykanda, & Hoyt, 1989; Groenveld, Jan, & Leader, 1990, Dutton & Jacobson, 2001), developmental delays, some learning disabilities, mental retardation, and autism. Later-occurring examples include cerebrovascular accidents or traumatic brain injuries (Rizzo & Tranel, 1996; Suchoff et al., 2000).

Adults who sustain a brain injury can usually only expect limited resolution of their perceptual impairments over time, while children who sustain brain damage very early in life have greater neural plasticity that may allow more substantial improvements in perception as they grow older.

It can be difficult to gather information about various aspects of visual impairment necessary in order to best modify the environment and make appropriate plans for a given individual. As a result of the brain damage, it is often difficult to measure relevant visual abilities reliably. The reliability of results from standard subjective vision testing procedures can be diminished by an individual's difficulty in concentrating on and responding to vision tasks. Furthermore, visual functioning of persons with brain damage may be especially sensitive to fatigue, minor illnesses, anxiety, medications, and suboptimal viewing conditions, such as poor lighting, low contrast, or crowding. Special testing techniques are usually required to analyze vision properly using objective methods that do not require the subject to report what he or she has seen. An example of such a test is the visually evoked potential (VEP), which uses electrodes placed on the scalp to detect brain activity in vision centers of the brain. Even such objective testing requires careful and judicious interpretation by experienced examiners.

Objective testing, combined with careful and targeted questioning, can permit skilled clinicians to identify children and adults who are likely to have special visual-perceptual problems due to brain damage and to characterize the nature of their impairment. Neuroimaging techniques, such as magnetic resonance imaging (MRI) scans, can be of particular value in learning the cause of the problems and helping to focus clinical testing, especially in predicting the location of visual field defects (Dutton & Jacobson, 2001).

Although children with early brain damage do require individual assessment, an understanding of the specific patterns of visual impairments that may result from early brain damage can facilitate the design and implementation of an appropriate developmental plan. Dutton and Jacobson (2001) provide an excellent review of the differential diagnosis and management of children with cortical (or cerebral) visual impairment.

An especially common form of perceptual difficulty among people with brain disorders is the tendency for visual functioning to be impeded by even small deviations from optimal viewing conditions. Many brain disorders create a heightened level of background neurological activity, or what is termed intrinsic noise. In order to perceive an object, its signal must be successfully filtered through this noise. For instance, children with brain damage may have more difficulty paying attention to an object or person due to high levels of background intrinsic noise in the brain. Perceptual difficulties would be made worse if additional environmental distractions or extrinsic noise were present (e.g., from moving objects or persons in the peripheral visual field). Perceptual problems would also be made worse if the intended target or signal were too weak, such as if the object were too low in contrast or contained elements too closely crowded together.

Useful strategies to overcome these challenges may involve a combined effort to increase the conspicuousness of the intended object (signal) and to reduce distractions (extrinsic noise). For instance, for reading, viewing conditions might need to be optimized by creating a perfectly focused image with the appropriate eyeglass prescription and by providing appropriate magnification, contrast, and lighting. It might be equally important to minimize the interference of visual distractions by blocking veiling glare from overhead lights, eliminating clutter on the desk, and closing a door that would otherwise allow a view of passersby.

Head trauma involving the right parietal lobe of the brain can result in left hemifield neglect. This is manifested as an impairment in attention: affected people do not notice things off to the left side unless they are deliberately paying attention to that area of vision. In typical cases, the resulting visual impairments are modest and might include misjudging the width of a narrow doorway. In rare cases, the neglect is severe, causing people to be unaware of objects, persons, or even their own body parts on the affected side.

SAMPLE PROFILES

There is great variation in the nature and severity of vision impairment among people who are classified as being visually impaired or blind. Certain patterns emerge based on diagnosis (see the Appendix to this book). However, there is considerable variation even among people with the same diagnosis and visual acuity. It is, therefore, useful to develop a profile of how the various visual abilities have been affected in any given individual.

Tables 2.1 to 2.4 provide samples of assessment findings for individuals of various ages and with different eye conditions. Key implications of those findings are described for each individual. For example, in Table 2.1, the most important issues for this child with oculocutaneous albinism are the need to ensure adequate print size (or magnification), the need to consider reading glasses for accommodative relief, and the need to review methods for lighting control.

The assessment findings for the middle-aged adult with proliferative diabetic retinopathy presented in Table 2.2 indicate that adequate print size (or magnification), contrast, lighting, and the prescription of reading glasses warrant special attention.

The specific findings for the older patient with macular degeneration profiled in Table 2.3 suggest special emphasis on alternatives to visual reading for any prolonged reading tasks and adequate print size (or magnification) for brief reading tasks. These reading requirements emerge based on specific test results showing a slow peak reading speed even with magnification, despite only a moderate acuity deficit, and are not characteristic of all individuals with macu-

TABLE 2.1

Sample Profile of Visual Functions:
12-Year-Old with Oculocutaneous Albinism

VISUAL ABILITY	FINDING	IMPLICATIONS
Visual acuity	20/200 for better eye	Likely to need detail 10–20 times larger or closer than normal
Visual fields	Normal peripherally; only slight central depression	Unlikely to have much difficulty with O&M or efficient reading (with large print or close viewing)
Contrast sensitivity	Normal	Unlikely to have much difficulty with O&M
Light sensitivity	Increased: ambient lighting Normal: task lighting	Likely to benefit from filters, visors, or environmental modifications
Color vision	Normal	Unlikely to have difficulty with color discrimination
Oculomotor control	Strabismus and nystagmus	Unlikely to have double vision or see the world as jiggling
Accommodation	Normal for age	Likely to require a reading prescription to supplement accommodation due to close reading distance needed

lar degeneration. Special attention to contrast and lighting issues are also warranted by this profile.

With the profound peripheral vision and contrast sensitivity losses described in Table 2.4 for an elderly individual with glaucoma, the focus of intervention needs to be less on adequate print size (or magnification) and more on considerations related to O&M training and environmental modifications.

As the examples in these tables illustrate, a more complete understanding of key components of vision abilities enables professionals to interpret information about the nature of a particular individual's visual impairment and to use this information to improve that person's quality of life. The assessment of the individual's visual functioning that includes a consideration of these variables lays the critical groundwork for intervention and services that support the performance of key tasks and independent living.

TABLE 2.2

Sample Profile of Visual Functions: 45-Year-Old with Proliferative Diabetic Retinopathy

VISUAL ABILITY	FINDING	IMPLICATIONS
Visual acuity	20/200 for better eye	Likely to need detail 10–20 times larger or closer than normal
Visual fields	General depression of central and peripheral fields	Unlikely to have slowed reading, but likely to have navigation problems when traveling in dim lighting
Contrast sensitivity	Moderately reduced	Likely to have difficulties seeing steps and curbs, and to benefit from environmental modifications; travel training; and, possibly, yellow or orange filters
Light sensitivity	Increased: ambient lighting Slightly reduced: task lighting	Likely to benefit from filters or visors outdoors, and moderately bright lighting for reading
Color vision	Slightly reduced	May have difficulty with some color discrimination and benefit from brighter task lighting
Oculomotor control	Strabismus (exotropia) due to very poor vision in one eye	Unlikely to have double vision
Accommodation	Reduced for age	Likely to require a stronger bifocal or near vision prescription than other 45-year-olds

TABLE 2.3

Sample Profile of Visual Functions:
75-Year-Old with Age-Related Macular Degeneration

VISUAL ABILITY	FINDING	IMPLICATIONS
Visual acuity	20/100 for better eye	Likely to need detail 5–10 times larger or closer than normal
Visual fields	General depression of central field loss, plus dense paracentral scotomas	Likely to have slowed reading even with optimized magnification and lighting
Contrast sensitivity	Moderately reduced	Likely to have difficulties seeing steps and curbs, and to benefit from environmental modifications; travel training; and, possibly, yellow or orange filters
Light sensitivity	Increased: ambient lighting Reduced: task lighting	Likely to benefit from filters or visors outdoors, and strong direct lighting for reading
Color vision	Slightly reduced	May have difficulty with some color discrimination and benefit from brighter task lighting
Oculomotor control	Normal	Unlikely to have double vision
Accommodation	Normal for age (which is zero)	Likely to require bifocals or a near vision prescription for all near tasks

TABLE 2.4

Sample Profile of Visual Functions: 65-Year-Old with Advanced Glaucoma

VISUAL ABILITY	FINDING	IMPLICATIONS
Visual acuity	20/50 for better eye	Likely to need detail at least 2.5–5 times larger or closer than normal
Visual fields	Small preserved island of vision with radius of 8 degrees	Likely to affect O&M and benefit from increased scanning with long cane as adjunct
Contrast sensitivity	Severely reduced	Very likely to have difficulties with O&M and benefit from environmental modifications; travel training; and, possibly, yellow or orange filters
Light sensitivity	Increased: ambient lighting Reduced: task lighting	Likely to benefit from filters or visors outdoors, and strong direct lighting for reading
Color vision	Slightly reduced	Likely to have difficulty with some color discriminations and benefit from brighter task lighting
Oculomotor control	Normal	Unlikely to have double vision
Accommodation	Normal for age (which is zero)	Likely to require bifocals or a near vision prescription for all near tasks

REFERENCES

Bailey, I. L., & Lovie, J. E. (1976). New design principles for visual acuity letter charts. *American Journal of Optometry & Physiological Optics, 53,* 740–745.

Brown, B. (1981). Reading performance in low vision patients: relation to contrast and contrast sensitivity. *American Journal of Optometry & Physiological Optics, 58 (3),* 218–226.

Brown, B., & Kitchin, J. L. (1983). Dark adaptation and the acuity/luminance response in senile macular degeneration (SMD). *American Journal of Optometry & Physiological Optics, 60 (8),* 645–650.

Bullimore, M. A., & Bailey, I. L. (1995). Reading and eye movements in age-related maculopathy. *Optometry & Visual Science, 72 (2),* 125–138.

Cheong, A. C., Lovie-Kitchin, J. E., & Bowers, A. R. (2002). Determining magnification for reading with low vision. *Clinical & Experimental Optometry, 85 (4),* 229–237.

Ciuffreda, K. J., Goldrich, S. G., & Neary, C. (1982). Use of eye movement auditory biofeedback in the control of nystagmus. *American Journal of Optometry & Physiological Optics, 59 (5),* 396–409.

Cocchiarella, L., Andersson, G., & American Medical Association. (2001). *Guides to the evaluation of permanent impairment* (5th ed.). Chicago: American Medical Association.

Cole, R. G. (1993). Predicting the low vision reading add. *Journal of the American Optometry Association, 64 (1),* 19–27.

Dutton, G. N., & Jacobson, L. K. (2001). Cerebral visual impairment in children. *Seminars in Neonatology, 6 (6),* 477–485.

Eldred, K. B. (1992). Optimal illumination for reading in patients with age-related maculopathy. *Optometry & Visual Science, 69 (1),* 46–50.

Elliott, D. B., & Bullimore, M. A. (1993). Assessing the reliability, discriminative ability, and validity of disability glare tests. *Investigative Ophthalmology and Visual Science, 34 (1),* 108–119.

Elliott, D. B., & Whitaker, D. (1992). Clinical contrast sensitivity chart evaluation. *Ophthalmic and Physiological Optics, 12 (3),* 275–280.

Flom, R. E., Raasch, T. W., Braudway, S. M., Rubin, G. S., & Massof, R. W. (1993). A test of Kestenbaum's rule for prescribing low vision reading devices. *Optometry & Visual Science, 70 (12s),* 128.

Girkin, C. A., & Miller, N. R. (2001). Central disorders of vision in humans. *Survey of Ophthalmology, 45 (5),* 379–405.

Groenveld, M., Jan, J. E., & Leader, P. (1990). Observations on the habilitation of children with cortical visual impairment. *Journal of Visual Impairment & Blindness, 84,* 11–15.

Haegerstrom-Portnoy, G., Schneck, M. E., Lott, L. A., & Brabyn, J. A. (2000). The relation between visual acuity and other spatial vision measures. *Optometry & Visual Science, 77 (12),* 653–662.

Jan, J. E., Groenveld, M., Sykanda, A. M., & Hoyt, C. S. (1987). Behavioural characteristics of children with permanent cortical visual impairment. *Developmental Medicine and Child Neurology, 29 (5),* 571–576.

Kestenbaum, A., & Sturman, R.M. (1956). Reading glasses for patients with very poor vision. *AMA Archives of Ophthalmology. 56 (3),* 451–470.

Kuyk, T., & Elliott, J. L. (1999). Visual factors and mobility in persons with age-related macular degeneration. *Journal of Rehabilitation Research and Development, 36 (4),* 303–312.

Legge, G. E., Ross, J. A., Isenberg, L. M., & LaMay, J. M. (1992). Psychophysics of reading. Clinical predictors of low-vision reading speed. *Investigative Ophthalmology and Visual Science, 33 (3),* 677–687.

Legge, G. E., & Rubin, G. S. (1986). Contrast sensitivity function as a screening test: A critique. *American Journal of Optometry & Physiological Optics, 63 (4)*, 265–270.

Lueck, A. H., Bailey, I. L., Greer, R., & Tuan, A. (2000). *Accommodation requirements of students with low vision. Final report.* Louisville, KY: American Printing House for the Blind.

Marron, J. A., & Bailey, I. L. (1982). Visual factors and orientation-mobility performance. *American Journal of Optometry & Physiological Optics, 59 (5)*, 413–426.

Massof, R. W. (2002). The measurement of vision disability. *Optometry & Visual Science, 79 (8)*, 516–552.

Peli, E. (2002). Treating with spectacle lenses: a novel idea!? *Optometry & Visual Science, 79 (9)*, 569–580.

Peli, E., & Peli, D. (2002). *Driving with confidence.* River Edge, NJ: World Scientific Publishing.

Pelli, D. G., & Levi, D. M. (1988). On writing grant proposals: Confessions of two grant reviewers. *American Journal of Optometry & Physiological Optics, 65 (7)*, 598.

Pelli, D. G., Robson, J. G., & Wilkins, A. J. (1988). The design of a new letter chart for measuring contrast sensitivity. *Clinical and Visual Science, 2*, 135–137.

Rizzo, M., & Tranel, D. D. (1996). *Head injury and postconcussive syndrome.* New York: Churchill Livingstone.

Rubin, G.S. (1988). Reliability and sensitivity of clinical contrast sensitivity tests. *Clinical Vision Science, 2*, 169–177.

Rubin, G. S., & Legge, G. E. (1989). Psychophysics of reading. VI—The role of contrast in low vision. *Vision Research, 29(1)*, 79–91.

Rubin, G. S., & Turano, K. (1992). Reading without saccadic eye movements. *Vision Research 32(5)*, 895–902.

Schuchard, R. A., & Fletcher, D. (1994). Preferred retinal locus: a review with applications in low vision rehabilitation. *Ophthalmology Clinics of North America, 76*, 745–757.

Sloan, L. L. (1977). *Reading aids for the partially sighted.* Baltimore, MD: Williams & Wilkins.

Sloane, M., Kuyk, T., Owsley, D., Ernst, S., & Nowakowski, R. (1989). The effect of relative size magnification of Farnsworth D15 color chips on color assessment in low vision patients. *Noninvasive assessment of the visual system.* (Technical Digest 7, pp. 140–143). Washington D. C.: Optical Society of America.

Stahl, J. S., Plant, G. T., & Leigh, R. J. (2002). Medical treatment of nystagmus and its visual consequences. *Journal of the Royal Society of Medicine, 95 (5)*, 235–237.

Suchoff, I. B., Gianutsos, R., Ciuffreda, K. J., & Groffman, S. (2000). Vision impairment related to acquired brain injury. In B. Silverstone, M. A. Lang, B. P. Rosenthal & E. E. Faye (Eds.), *The Lighthouse handbook on vision impairment and vision rehabilitation* (Vol. 1, pp. 517–539). New York: Oxford University Press.

Timberlake, G. T., Mainster, M. A., Peli, E., Augliere, R. A., Essock, E. A., & Arend, L. E. (1986). Reading with a macular scotoma. I. Retinal location of scotoma and fixation area. *Investigative Ophthalmology Visual Science, 27 (7),* 1137–1147.

Timberlake, G. T., Peli, E., Essock, E. A., & Augliere, R. A. (1987). Reading with a macular scotoma. II. Retinal locus for scanning text. *Investigative Ophthalmology and Visual Science, 28 (8),* 1268–1274.

Wakefield, K. G. (2000). *Bennett's ophthalmic prescription work* (fourth edition). Oxford, U.K.: Butterworth-Heinemann.

West, S. K., Rubin, G. S., Broman, A. T., Munoz, B., Bandeen-Roche, K., & Turano, K. (2002). How does visual impairment affect performance on tasks of everyday life? The SEE Project (Salisbury Eye Evaluation). *Archives of Ophthalmology, 120 (6),* 774–780.

White, J. M., & Bedell, H. E. (1990). The oculomotor reference in humans with bilateral macular disease. *Investigative Ophthalmology Visual Science, 31 (6),* 1149–1161.

Whittaker, S. G., & Lovie-Kitchin, J. (1993). Visual requirements for reading. *Optometry & Visual Science, 70 (1),* 54–65.

World Health Organization. (1980). *International classification of impairments, disabilities, and handicaps: a manual classification relating to the consequences of disease.* Geneva, Switzerland.

3

Basic Optics and Low Vision Devices

ROBERT DISTER AND ROBERT GREER

L ow vision optical devices can play a dramatic role in the lives of many persons with visual impairments. When based on a careful evaluation of the individual's needs and visual abilities, their prescribed use can make possible tasks and activities of vital importance in everyday life, education, and work. Because of the pivotal part they can play in the delivery of effective low vision services, these devices are the focus of this chapter. To understand the effect of any given device on an individual's vision, the practitioner also needs a basic understanding of the principles of optics and lenses.

An optical device is one that creates, manipulates, or controls light. Optical devices for people with low vision include a range of options for near magnification and distance magnification (Jose, 1983; Wilkinson, 2000). It is important to understand the optical characteristics of these devices in order to determine the reasons that a particular device does or does not function well for a particular person. This chapter begins with a discussion of basic optical principles and then applies these principles to commonly used optical devices. These devices include spectacle-mounted lenses (reading spectacles or bifocal reading segments), handheld magnifiers, stand magnifiers, and monocular telescopes. Less frequently encountered optical devices such as mirror magnifiers, prisms, and minifiers for treating visual field loss are beyond the scope of this chapter.

BASIC OPTICAL PRINCIPLES AND DEFINITIONS

The following sections review basic optical principles and define terms used in describing low vision and its causes, as well as the characteristics of selected low vision optical devices.

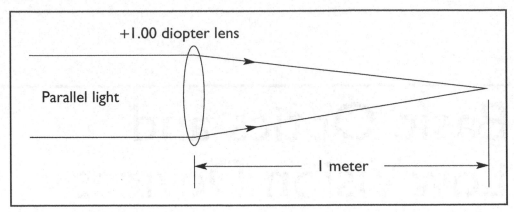

Figure 3.1. A 1-diopter lens has a focal length of 1 m.

Light

Light generated by or reflected off the surface of an object travels out in waves in a manner similar to the ripples created when water's surface is disturbed by an object thrown into it. Individual light rays normally travel in a straight line from their source. If the source of the light is very distant, the light rays from that source will be traveling essentially parallel to one another. The light rays will continue on a straight and parallel path unless that path is somehow changed.

A change in path most commonly occurs when light rays contact a transparent material such as glass or plastic at some angle other than the perpendicular (see Zimmerman, 1996, for a general introduction to light and optics). An example of this is when light rays pass through the curved surfaces of a lens. All low vision optical devices achieve their effects by using lenses with curved surfaces to refract (change the path of) light.

Diopter

The focusing power of lenses is described by a unit called the diopter (Keating, 1988). A 1-diopter lens will cause parallel light rays entering the lens from a distant object—one located at optical infinity (see the section on Handheld Magnifiers)—to converge to a point of focus 1 m away (see fig. 3.1).

Focal Length, Focal Point, and Focal Plane

If parallel light rays from a distant object enter a lens and come to a sharp focus as a result of being refracted, then the distance from the lens to that point of sharp focus is termed the focal length of that lens. Figure 3.1 illustrates the focal length of a 1-diopter lens. Principles related to focal length include the following:

➤ The focal length of a lens, in meters, is equal to the inverse or reciprocal of its power in diopters.

➤ A 4-diopter (sometimes abbreviated as *4D*) lens has a focal length of 1/4 or 0.25 m, or 25 cm.

➤ The inverse or the reciprocal of the focal length in meters is the power of the lens in diopters.

- A lens with a focal length of 1 m is a 1-diopter lens.

- A lens with a focal length of 0.20 m (or 20 cm) is a 5-diopter lens (1/0.20 = 5).

The point or plane located a focal length away from the lens is referred to as its focal point or focal plane.

Power

The power of a lens is simply its dioptric value or its focusing power. For example, a magnifier with a 6-diopter lens is said to have a power of 6 diopters.

LENSES WITH PLUS POWER

Lenses with plus power have convex surfaces and are thicker in the middle than at the edges; this causes the path of the light rays passing through the lens to converge (Fig. 3.2). The greater the plus power, the more convex the surface must be. The amount of power in a plus lens is expressed as a positive number in diopters, or the inverse of its focal length in meters.

LENSES WITH MINUS POWER

Lenses with minus power have concave surfaces and are thicker at the edges than the middle; this causes the path of the light rays passing through the lens to diverge (Fig. 3.2). The greater the minus power, the more concave the surface must be. The amount of power in a minus lens is expressed as a negative number in diopters, or the inverse of its focal length in meters.

ADD POWER

Bifocals and reading glasses are commonly specified in terms of their add (or add power). The add refers to the amount by which the extra plus power for reading exceeds the power required by the person for distance viewing tasks such as driving. For example, a person who wears 2-diopter lenses for driving and 3-diopter lenses for reading is said to be using a 1-diopter add.

Accommodation and Presbyopia

Accommodation is synonymous with focusing the eye. Accommodation is achieved through the bending of the crystalline lens within the eye. The act of accommodation adds plus power to the optics of the eye, enabling the person

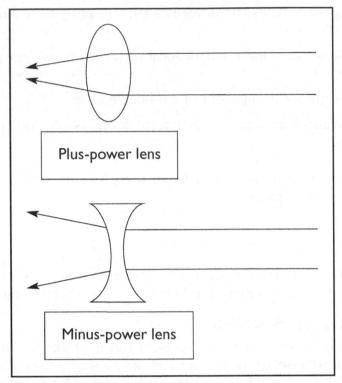

Figure 3.2. Refraction of light rays by plus- and minus-power lenses.

to focus to a closer distance than would be possible without accommodation (Grosvenor, 2002; see Fig. 3.3). (Note that accommodation can only add plus power and not minus power to the optics of the eye.) There is a limit to the amount of additional plus power that can be achieved through accommodation, and the ability to accommodate decreases with age (see Chap. 2). The loss of ability with aging to focus on near objects is referred to as *presbyopia*. Thus most people in their 40s and older need to supplement their accommodation with reading glasses or bifocals in order to see clearly at close distances.

Relationship among Focal Length, Power, and Diopters

As mentioned in the discussion of focal length, a stronger-powered lens has a shorter focal length, and a weaker-powered lens has a longer focal length. Centimeters are the most convenient unit of measurement, rather than meters, when performing magnifier calculations. The relationship between the focal length of a lens in centimeters and its power is simply that the two numbers multiplied by each other must equal 100. Thus, if D is the power of the lens in diopters and f is its focal length in centimeters, the formulas relating D to f are

$$D \times f = 100$$

$$D = 100/f$$

$$f = 100/D$$

For example, the dioptric power D of a lens with a focal length f of 25 cm is $100/25 = 4$ diopters. (Note that $4 \times 25 = 100$.) The focal length f of a lens with a dioptric power D of 2 is $100/2 = 50$ cm. (Note that $50 \times 2 = 100$.)

The Snellen Fraction

Visual acuity is normally specified by a number such as 20/40, which is termed the Snellen fraction. The Snellen fraction is determined by having the individual view a standardized letter, or optotype, from a certain distance, and it is defined as test distance/letter size (Davidson, 1991). Thus 20/40 acuity indicates that the individual is able to read at a distance of 20 ft what is somewhat confusingly termed a "40-ft letter." A 40-ft letter is not one that is 40 ft in height. For the

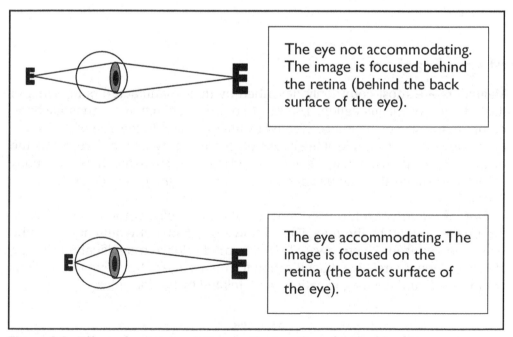

Figure 3.3. Effect of accommodation on the location of retinal image.

purposes of the Snellen fraction, letter size is defined in terms of the distance at which a letter would occupy or subtend 5 minutes of arc on the retina of the eye. (A minute is 1/60 of a degree.) Therefore, a 40-ft letter is one that would subtend 5 minutes of arc on the retina when viewed at a distance of 40 ft. A more useful indication of letter size is that a 20-ft letter is 8.87 mm in height, while a 40-ft letter is twice as large, or 19.84 mm in height.

At a given test distance, a person with 20/20 acuity can see a letter that is twice as small (8.87 mm in height from a 20-ft test distance) as one that can be seen by a person with 20/40 acuity (19.94 mm in height from a 20-ft test distance). Another way to think about this example is that a person with 20/40 acuity must move up to 20 ft to see what a person with 20/20 acuity can see from 40 ft away.

Although 20 ft is a standard test distance, measurements may be taken at other distances. For example, if a 15-ft letter were the smallest one that a person could read from 10 ft away, his or her acuity would be recorded as 10/15; this acuity is equivalent to 20/30 (by multiplying the top and bottom numbers of the 10/15 Snellen fraction by 2), and indeed, we would predict that from a distance of 20 ft (twice as far away) the smallest letter that this person could read would be a 30-ft letter (twice as large).

It is common for near acuity measurements to be taken using metric Snellen notation, which can be identified by the presence of the letter M in the denominator of the Snellen fraction. For example, an acuity measurement of 0.4/1M indicates that at a distance of 0.4 m or 40 cm, the smallest letter readable by the person was a 1M letter (approximately 8 point, or newspaper-sized print, 1.45 mm in height.)

Magnification

Magnifiers are most commonly described by their manufacturers in terms of their degree of magnification. The most common definitions of magnification compare the size of the image created by the magnifier to the size of the object being viewed. For example, if the image of an object is two times larger than the original object, then the magnification is said to be 2×. There are, however, many different formulas that can be used to determine magnification (Woo & Leung, 2001).

One of the most widely used magnification formulas compares the size of the image created by the magnifier to how big the object would appear to be when viewed from 25 cm away. This is termed relative magnification (Bailey, 1980a). When the relative magnification formula is used, the power of the lens in diopters D and the magnification M are related by the formulas

$$M = D/4$$

$$D = 4M$$

Thus, a lens labeled as having 5× magnification would have a power of 20 diopters, and a 24-diopter lens would be labeled as having 6× magnification. This formula is most commonly used for specifying the magnification of high-add spectacles.

Another widely used formula is similar but assumes that the person will hold the magnifier close to the eye and will utilize 4 diopters of accommodation to provide additional plus power. This is termed the manufacturer's magnification rating. In this case, dioptric power and magnification are related by the formulas

$$M = (D/4) + 1$$

$$D = 4(M-1)$$

Thus, a lens labeled as having 5× magnification would have a power of 16 diopters, and a 24-diopter lens would be labeled as having 7× magnification. This formula is most commonly used for specifying the power of handheld magnifiers.

It is impossible to tell which specification is being used by a particular manufacturer without measuring the power of the lens in diopters. For example, a 5× magnifier from one manufacturer may not be the same power as a 5× lens from another. Within a particular manufacturer's product line, magnifiers of the same listed magnification may have different dioptric powers. The authors are aware of one instance in which a manufacturer's 3× magnifier was actually more powerful than its 3.5× magnifier. Thus, it is much more useful for the practitioner to know the power of a magnifier in diopters; most manufacturers also provide this information.

If a practitioner encounters a magnifier with a certain labeled magnification, its power is likely to be specified by one of the two formulas described above. For example, a 5× magnifier will normally have a power of either $5 \times 4 = 20$ diopters (relative magnification) or $(5-1) \times 4 = 16$ diopters (manufacturer's magnification rating). Manufacturers occasionally will not follow either of these formulas exactly, with the result that the power may fall between those predicted (in this example, somewhere between 16 and 20 diopters).

Because both methods of describing magnification are commonly used, one cannot, with confidence, know that two different magnifiers with the same labeled magnification ratings are indeed the same power. Since there is only one definition of diopter, most practitioners use diopters rather than magnification for calculating and predicting the performance of a magnifier.

REFRACTIVE ERROR

As explained in Chapter 2, refractive error refers to a condition in which light rays are not brought into focus on the retina. The refractive status of a person—whether his or her eyes have a refractive error, and if so, what kind—is described by the terms *emmetropia, hyperopia, myopia,* and *astigmatism.* Refractive status depends on the shape and curvatures of the optical components of the eye including the crystalline lens and cornea, as well as the length of the eyeball (Grosvenor, 2002).

Emmetropia

Emmetropia is the condition in which the eye has just the correct amount of plus power to make parallel light rays from a distant object come to a focus on the retina when the eye is relaxing its accommodation. A person with emmetropia will be able to see distant objects clearly without glasses and without needing to focus his or her eyes.

Hyperopia

Also known as farsightedness, hyperopia is the condition in which an eye has too little plus power. Parallel light from a distant object entering a relaxed hyperopic eye will not have enough convergence to focus on the retina. Instead, the light rays will focus beyond the retina. Since accommodation adds plus power to an eye, an individual with a low amount of hyperopia may use his or her accommodation to make viewed objects clear at a distance. This accommodation is in addition to the accommodation required when viewing near objects. In order to see distant objects clearly without accommodating, a hyperopic individual must wear plus-powered glasses.

Myopia

Myopia, or nearsightedness, is the condition in which an eye has too much plus power, so that parallel light entering the eye from a distant object will come to a point of focus in front of the retina. This results in poor distance vision. Minus-powered spectacles that offset this extra plus power must be worn in order for the myopic individual to see distant objects clearly. Accommodation can only add plus power and therefore cannot provide focusing assistance for myopic eyes. Because the myopic eye has too much plus power, it can naturally focus at near; thus a person with myopia sees near objects in clear focus with less accommodation than a person with emmetropia or hyperopia. The greater the myopia, the closer the natural focusing distance.

Astigmatism

Astigmatism is a condition in which the focus of the eye is not at a single point because it is not the same in all directions (e.g., the power in the vertical direction may differ from that in the horizontal). This usually occurs because the surface of the cornea is not perfectly round. The differing curvatures on the surface of a football or spoon are good analogies to the curvature of the cornea that creates astigmatism. A person with astigmatism can focus on the horizontal part or the vertical part of a letter *T*, but not on both parts at the same time. The usual result is that both parts will look somewhat blurry. Astigmatism affects the clarity of objects regardless of how far away they are.

Effects of Refractive Error on Near Vision

The most common concern for individuals with low vision is the need to see detail for near tasks. Most low vision devices are prescribed to meet this need. An understanding of low vision optics needs to begin with an explanation of the effects of refractive error on a person's ability to see things up close when he or she is not wearing eyeglasses.

For an individual without refractive error (i.e., a person with emmetropia), the ability to see up close involves using accommodation to add plus power to the eye. As an emmetropic individual (or any person) ages, the ability to accommodate grows weaker (a condition known as presbyopia) and is eventually lost. A 10-year-old emmetropic person will be able to bring reading material to a closer focus than a 20-year-old, who will be able to bring it closer than a 30-year-old, and so on. As things are brought in closer to the eye, the image on the retina is enlarged (a phenomenon referred to as relative distance magnification). Thus, a young person with low vision has an advantage over an older one in that he or she can bring an object closer in order to see more fine detail.

Because the nearsighted eye naturally has too much plus power, nearsighted persons may be thought of as having built-in readers or magnifiers. The more plus power naturally present, the closer the myopic person needs to hold things for them to be in focus when he or she is not wearing eyeglasses. In comparison to an emmetropic person, an individual with myopia who removes his or her eyeglasses will be able to see more detail in an object because he or she can hold it closer and still see it in focus without needing to accommodate as much.

It is the opposite for farsighted persons, whose eyes do not have enough plus power naturally. Hyperopia may be corrected with plus-powered spectacles, or a hyperopic person can add plus power to his or her eyes by accommodating. Persons with uncorrected hyperopia must exert some accommodation at all times in order to see clearly. Because they must exert even more accommodation to see clearly at near than at distance, they will often find it fatiguing to read without their eyeglasses. Since some of their available accommodation is used up in overcoming their hyperopia, hyperopic persons whose vision is not corrected cannot move objects as close as emmetropic persons and still see them in clear focus.

NEAR VISION OPTICAL DEVICES

One way to see the small details in an object is to hold it closer, since the image on the retina increases in size as the eye-to-object distance decreases. As long as the object remains in good focus, it is easier to see details as it is moved closer to the eyes. In comparison to a person with unimpaired vision, an individual with low vision must move even closer to an object to render its details large enough to see.

As mentioned earlier, a nearsighted person can resolve detail at a very close distance by taking his or her eyeglasses off, bringing the object very close, and letting the natural plus power of the eye do the focusing. A younger person who can supply a sufficient quantity of plus power through accommodation might be able to bring an object close enough to see its fine details.

If an individual with low vision is not sufficiently nearsighted or does not possess enough accommodation, then low vision devices may be used to augment his or her available plus power to bring an object held close to the eye into clear focus. Optical devices that accomplish this may include high plus-power reading glasses, handheld magnifiers, stand magnifiers, and monocular telescopes for near viewing tasks. (Non-optical electronic magnifiers such as closed-circuit televisions may also be used by low vision individuals for reading and viewing detailed objects.)

Different types of magnifiers have different advantages and disadvantages. A person may need more than one magnifier to achieve his or her goals. The advantages and disadvantages of different types of near magnifiers are summarized in Sidebar 3.1 and are discussed in more detail throughout the rest of this chapter.

FUNCTIONAL PROPERTIES OF LOW VISION DEVICES

The following sections describe the basic optical principles and functional properties of low vision optical devices, including working distance, depth of field, and field of view.

Working Distance

The term *working distance* refers to the distance from the person's eyes to the object that is being viewed through the optical device. In the case of optical devices positioned close to the eye (e.g., spectacles and telescopes), the working distance may also be measured as the distance from the optical device to the object being viewed. Working distance depends on the type of magnifier and its power, with stronger magnifiers having a shorter working distance than weaker ones. One of the main advantages of handheld magnifiers over high-add bifocals or reading glasses is that the former provide a longer working distance which normally allows more comfortable ergonomics for the user. This is because handheld magnifiers can be positioned farther from the person's eyes than glasses. (Handheld magnifiers and reading glasses are both designed to be used with the object held at a distance from the magnifier equal to its focal length; see

Advantages and Disadvantages of Different Types of Near Magnifiers

Spectacles

Advantages

➤ Wider field of view than handheld magnifiers

➤ Binocular viewing (in powers up to about 12 diopters)

➤ Can provide relatively normal appearance to the wearer

Disadvantages

➤ Shorter working distance than handheld magnifiers

➤ No built-in illumination

Handheld Magnifiers

Advantages

➤ Longer working distance than spectacles

➤ Can have built-in illumination

Disadvantages

➤ Smaller field of view than spectacles

➤ Require one hand to be used to position magnifier

➤ Require steady grip

➤ Indicate to others that person has reduced vision (this may also be considered by some people as an advantage)

Stand Magnifiers

Advantages

➤ Do not require steady grip

➤ Can have strong built-in illumination

(continued on next page)

Disadvantages

➤ Limited range of possible working distances for presbyopic persons

➤ Indicates to others that person has reduced vision (this may also be considered by some people as an advantage)

Near Telescopes

Advantages

➤ Long working distance

➤ Leaves hands free if mounted in spectacles

Disadvantages

➤ Nonadjustable and binocular spectacle-mounted telescopes have fixed working distances

➤ Relatively heavy

➤ Relatively expensive

➤ Use indicates to others that person has reduced vision (This may also be considered by some as an advantage.)

➤ Large number of optical elements may reduce contrast and illumination reaching the eye

---

the discussion of the optical characteristics of these devices.) The main advantage of monocular telescopes used for near viewing (i.e., near telescopes) is that they provide the longest working distance of all the near optical magnifiers.

Depth of Field

Depth of field refers to the range of distances that an object can be from the magnifier lens and still appear to the observer to be in focus (Grosvenor, 2002). This depends on the optical characteristics of the magnifier as well as the sensitivity of the observer. In general, the stronger the magnifier, the shorter or more limited the depth of field. This means that for stronger magnifiers, the observer must keep the lens-to-object distance more steady and consistent, or the image will become blurry and out of focus. Limited depth of field is one factor that makes a stronger magnifier more difficult to use. An observer who is less demanding about the clarity of the image, or who has reduced visual acuity due to low vision will usually experience a greater depth of field than someone who is more demanding about image clarity or who has unimpaired visual acuity.

Field of View

The field of view of a magnifier refers to the size of the area that can be viewed through the magnifier at any one time: how big an area the magnifier takes in. Field of view depends on three factors: the diameter or width of the magnifier, the focal length or power of the magnifier, and the distance of the observer from the magnifier.

A larger magnifier will have a larger field of view than a smaller one. Due to their steeper surface curvatures, stronger magnifiers must be made with a smaller diameter, resulting in a smaller field of view. A less-powerful magnifier (i.e., one with a longer focal length) will have a larger field of view than a more powerful magnifier. The field of view will become larger as the observer moves closer to the magnifier lens, and smaller as the observer moves away from it. Individuals with low vision due to profound vision loss will often complain of the limited field of view inherent in the small-diameter, high-powered optical magnifiers appropriate for their level of acuity. It is the authors' experience that magnifiers stronger than 24 diopters are significantly more difficult to use than those with less strong lenses.

The field of view of telescopes for distance viewing is less easily predicted, and depends on a number of factors such as the basic optical design and how close the individual holds it to his or her eye. In general, stronger telescopes have a smaller field of view than weaker ones, and the field of view will decrease as the telescope is held farther from the eye.

Monocular telescopes are composed of at least two lenses mounted in a tubular housing. The lens closest to the eye is called the eyepiece, and the front lens is referred to as the objective (Fannin & Grosvenor, 1996). There are two basic telescope designs, based on the type of lens used in the eyepiece. Telescopes of Keplerian design have plus-powered eyepieces and are commonly used for telescopes of 4× magnification and higher, although 2× and 3× Keplerian telescopes are also manufactured. Galilean telescopes have minus-powered eyepieces and are most commonly used for 2×, 3×, and occasionally 4× telescopes (see Fannin & Grosvenor, 1996, for a discussion of the optics of different types of telescopes). Galilean telescopes have a smaller field of view than Keplerian telescopes, which restricts their use to low magnification devices.

The field of view in degrees of a Keplerian telescope for distance viewing can be approximated by dividing 50 by the magnification of the telescope (I. L. Bailey, personal communication August 2002). For example, a 4× Keplerian telescope would be expected to have a field of view of approximately 50/4 = 12.5 degrees. A Galilean telescope would be expected to have a field of view approximately one-half to one-third that of a Keplerian telescope of the same magnification. The field of view of telescopes for near viewing is discussed in Telescopes for Near Viewing, later in this chapter.

OPTICAL CHARACTERISTICS OF LOW VISION DEVICES

Plus-Powered Spectacles

As noted earlier, plus lenses mounted in spectacles are designated in terms of their add. Plus-add reading glasses and bifocals are designed to be used so that the wearer holds the material to be viewed at a distance equal to the focal length of the add. Thus a person wearing 4-diopter add spectacles would hold an object 25 cm from her glasses (using the formula $f = 100/D$, $f = 100/4 = 25$ cm) in order to see it clearly. (For a general discussion of the optics of near magnifiers for low vision, see Fannin & Grosvenor, 1996.) The stronger the add, the closer an object must be held for it to be in focus. For example, an individual wearing 8-diopter add spectacles would have a working distance of 12.5 cm ($f = 100/8 = 12.5$ cm). Individuals who develop low vision later in their life (e.g., due to age-related macular degeneration) often have difficulty adapting to the short working distance of high-plus spectacles.

Regardless of a person's refractive error, accommodation will add plus to the spectacles being worn and allow him or her to hold things even closer and maintain good focus. Thus, a young person who requires a larger image could bring material in closer than the focal length of his or her reading glasses by exerting accommodation. A young individual wearing 3-diopter add eyeglasses who also accommodates 2 diopters is viewing through 5 diopters of total plus power, and can hold an object 20 cm away and see it in clear focus. If this person were older and unable to accommodate, he or she would require 5-diopter add eyeglasses in order to view the object at a 20-cm distance while maintaining clear focus. When determining the appropriate working distance for reading material, practitioners must, therefore, take into account not only the focal length of the lens but also the accommodative capabilities of the reader (see Effects of Accommodation, later in this chapter).

The main advantage of spectacle magnifiers over handheld magnifiers is that the former have a comparatively large field of view because the lenses are located close to the wearer's eyes. This also creates their main disadvantage: a closer working distance. Some individuals prefer spectacles to handheld magnifiers because they do not have always to use one hand to hold the magnifier.

Prism reading glasses are available in powers up to 12 diopters. These glasses incorporate prism lenses that are thicker on the sides closer to the nose. This has the effect of enabling a person to see the object with both eyes at a close distance without having to turn the eyes inward as much as if the prism were not used.

Reading glasses stronger than 12 diopters are designed to be viewed through only one eye at a time. These eyeglasses are commonly referred to as microscopics or hyperoculars, and are usually specified in terms of relative magnification: for example, 5× microscopics have 20-diopter lenses, while 6× microscopics have 24-diopter lenses. These devices are available in magnifications up to 20×, or 80 diopters. As mentioned earlier in this chapter, the relative magnification formula is commonly applied to spectacle lenses, so that their magnification is nearly always the power of the spectacle lens divided by 4 ($M = D/4$).

Handheld Magnifiers

As with spectacle magnifiers, handheld magnifiers are designed to be used so that the object to be viewed is held in the focal plane of the magnifier. For example, a person viewing with a 3-diopter magnifier would normally hold the object to be viewed 33 cm from the lens ($f = 100/D$; $f = 100/3 = 33$ cm).

When an object is held at the focal point of a plus-powered lens, such as when one is using a handheld magnifier or spectacles, the light rays exiting the lens will be parallel. The image created is said to be at optical infinity: it is located at a point very distant from the eye. A person viewing an image at optical infinity who is emmetropic or wearing an appropriate distance spectacle correction will be able to see the image clearly without accommodating. The image will be clear and constant in size regardless of how far away the lens is from the person's eye, because light is parallel coming out of the lens and remains so regardless of viewing distance. (In most situations, a bifocal wearer using a handheld magnifier will obtain more magnification when viewing through the upper or distance portion of the glasses rather than the bifocal reading segment. See Effects of Spectacle Correction later in this chapter.)

As the lens is moved farther away from the eye, however, the field of view decreases, just as it does when looking through a knothole in a fence from several feet away (see Fig. 3.4). Because the lens of a handheld magnifier is normally positioned farther from the eye than a spectacle lens, a person using a handheld magnifier will have a smaller field of view than when using eyeglasses of the same power. However, this same person would have the advantage of a longer working distance when using the handheld magnifier. Some people prefer handheld magnifiers to plus-powered spectacles due to their longer working distance; also, handheld magnifiers can be provided with built-in illumination.

Stand Magnifiers

The optics of stand magnifiers is more complex than that of spectacles or handheld magnifiers (see Fannin & Grosvenor, 1996.) Unlike spectacles and handheld magnifiers, stand magnifiers are designed so that the object of regard is not located at the focal point of the lens when the magnifier is resting on it; rather, the

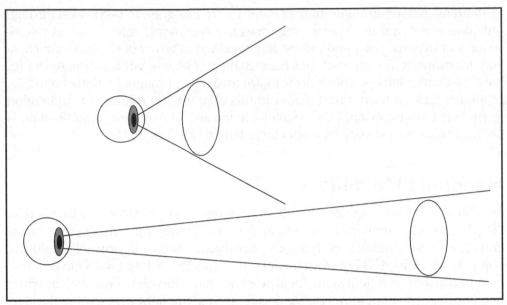

Figure 3.4. Field of view when the eye is close to a magnifier is greater than when the eye is farther away, much as it is when a person is closer or farther away from any opening, such as a knothole in a fence.

object is located closer than the magnifier's focal length. This creates a magnified image located at some finite distance beyond the lens and the object, rather than at optical infinity as with spectacles and handheld magnifiers (Bailey, 1981a) (see Fig. 3.5).

The size and location of the image depend on both the dioptric power of the lens and the length of the stand magnifier's housing. Information about image size and location is sometimes provided by the manufacturer of the stand magnifier; if not, it can be determined by means of measurements and calculations beyond the scope of this chapter (Bailey, 1983; Bullimore & Bailey, 1989).

Because the image is located at some finite distance beyond the magnifier, a younger person must accommodate in order to focus on this image. A presbyopic individual must use a bifocal add or reading glasses to focus on it. Thus a presbyopic person will normally want to view through the bifocal add when using a stand magnifier rather than through the distance portion of the glasses, as is best when using a handheld magnifier.

In order to select the best stand magnifier to meet the needs of an individual with low vision, the practitioner needs to know more than just the dioptric power of the lens; both the location of the image and how much larger it is than the original object must be taken into account. The distance from the magnifier lens to the image it creates is usually referred to as l prime (l'). The size of the image relative to the size of the object is usually termed the enlargement ratio ER. As noted earlier, manufacturers do not always provide this information.

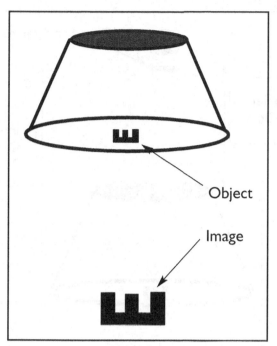

Object

Image

Figure 3.5. The image created by a stand magnifier is located on the same side of the lens as the original object and is enlarged.

A thorough discussion of the optics of stand magnifiers is complex and beyond the scope of this chapter (for more information, see Bailey, 1981a). However, a relatively simple example involves a person with presbyopia viewing an object through a stand magnifier using his or her bifocal add. In this case, the practitioner must determine the eye-to-magnifier distance that allows the viewer to see the image created by it in perfect focus. If the person is viewing from a distance such that the image created by the stand magnifier is in perfect focus, then the power of the stand magnifier is given by the following formula:

Power of the stand magnifier = Power of the bifocal add
× Enlargement ratio of the stand magnifier

Suppose a person with low vision is using 4-diopter add bifocal glasses and is viewing print through a stand magnifier with an enlargement ratio $ER = 3$ and a lens-to-image distance $l' = 15$ cm. To find the eye-to-magnifier distance for that person with the stand magnifier, one must subtract the lens-to-image distance l' of the stand magnifier from the focal length f of the person's bifocal add. Since a 4-diopter bifocal add has a focal length of 25 cm ($100/D = f$; $100/4 = 25$ cm), the person must view at a distance of 10 cm from the magnifier for the image to be in focus ($f - l'$ = eye-to-magnifier distance; $25-15 = 10$ cm; see Fig. 3.6.) When the person uses the stand magnifier from this 10 cm distance, the total power

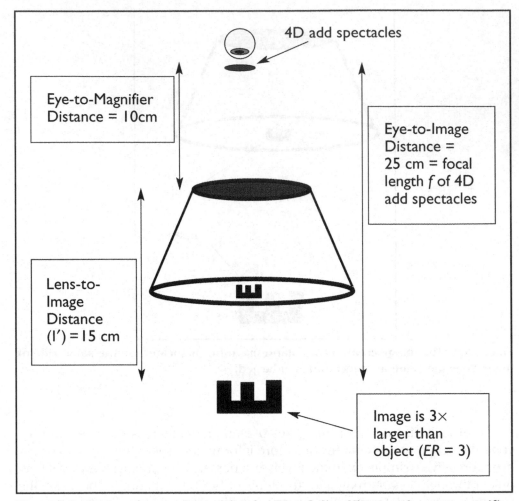

Figure 3.6. Optics of a stand magnifier for ER = 3, l′ = 15 cm, and eye-to-magnifier distance = 10 cm when used by a person wearing 4-diopter add spectacles.

obtained will be 4D × 3 = 12D (power of the bifocal add × enlargement ratio of the stand magnifier = power of the stand magnifier, as mentioned earlier). In theory, the person will be able to read the same-sized print using this stand magnifier as he or she would with a 12-diopter handheld magnifier (viewing through the top part of his or her glasses; see Effects of Spectacle Correction later in this chapter) or through 12-diopter add spectacles.

Table 3.1 may be used to determine the power of a stand magnifier for some common values of the *ER*, the magnifier-to-image distance *l′* in centimeters, and the eye-to-magnifier distance. The values in boldface type in Table 3.1 are those used in the previous example and illustrated in Figure 3.6.

The optical characteristics of stand magnifiers are more complicated than those of handheld magnifiers and high-plus spectacles. It is recommended that the low vision team work closely with the optometrist or ophthalmologist to

TABLE 3.1

Determining the Power of a Stand Magnifier

Magnifier-to-image distance (l') (cm)	15 cm			20 cm			25 cm			30 cm		
Eye-to-magnifier distance (cm)	2.5	**10.0**	25.0	2.5	10.0	25.0	2.5	10.0	25.0	2.5	10.0	25.0
Add required for image to be in focus (diopters)	5.75	**4.0**	2.5	4.5	3.25	2.25	3.75	2.75	2.0	3.0	2.5	1.75
Enlargement Ratio of stand magnifier (ER)												
2	11.5	8.0	5.0	9.0	6.5	4.5	7.5	5.5	4.0	6.0	5.0	3.5
3	16.8	**12.0**	7.5	13.5	9.75	6.8	11.3	8.3	6.0	9.0	7.5	5.3
4	23.0	16.0	10.0	18.0	13.0	9.0	15.0	11.0	8.0	12.0	10.0	7.0
5	28.8	20.0	12.5	22.5	16.3	11.3	18.8	13.8	10.0	15.0	12.5	8.8
6	33.6	24.0	15.0	27.0	19.5	13.5	22.5	16.5	12.0	18.0	15.0	10.5
7	40.3	28.0	17.5	31.5	22.8	15.8	26.3	19.3	14.0	21.0	17.5	12.3
8	46.0	32.0	20.0	36.0	26.0	18.0	30.0	22.0	16.0	24.0	20.0	14.0
9	51.8	36.0	22.5	40.5	29.3	20.3	33.8	24.8	18.0	27.0	22.5	15.8

The power in diopters of a stand magnifier is given for common values of the enlargement ratio (*ER*), the magnifier-to-image distance (l') in centimeters, and the eye-to-magnifier working distance in centimeters. The values used in the example illustrated in Figure 3.6 are in boldface type.

understand how best to use these devices when they are prescribed for individuals with low vision.

Handheld Monocular Telescopes

Many varieties of telescopes may be used by individuals with low vision. Some telescopes are designed for viewing distant objects; others are designed for viewing near objects. Some telescopes have a fixed focus and can be used to view objects at only one distance, while others have a variable focus and can be used to view objects at a variety of distances. Some fixed-focus distance telescopes can be used to view near objects by placing an auxiliary or cap lens on the front of the telescope. The following is a discussion of the different types of telescopes and their optics.

TELESCOPES FOR DISTANCE VIEWING

The optics of handheld monocular telescopes for distance viewing are relatively straightforward compared to handheld and stand magnifiers. Telescopes (and binoculars) are described using two numbers separated by an "×." The first number is the magnification rating. The second number is the diameter of the objective, or front lens, in millimeters. A commonly used telescope is labeled 4×12. It is a 4 times telescope and the objective lens is 12 mm in diameter. The magnification rating on telescopes does not vary in its definition. The magnification of a telescope causes things to appear larger (or closer) by the amount of the magnification. In other words, a 4× telescope will cause objects to appear to be 4 times larger or 4 times closer.

A typical initial goal when prescribing a monocular telescope is to provide the person with 20/40 acuity when using the telescope. This 20/40 figure is an empirical one based on the common experience of low vision practitioners. Other acuity goals may be more appropriate, depending on the circumstances and needs of the person with low vision. For example, a goal of lesser acuity may be more realistic for a person with profound vision loss, while a goal of better than 20/40 acuity might be appropriate for an individual who needs to see very small targets at a distance.

If the goal is to provide 20/40 acuity when viewing through the telescope, then a person with 20/160 acuity will require a 4× telescope to improve his or her acuity by four times and see 20/40; likewise, a person with 20/80 acuity will require a 2× telescope to improve his or her acuity by two times and see 20/40.

TELESCOPES FOR NEAR VIEWING

The optics of telescopes for near viewing are more complex than for distance telescopes. There are two types of near vision telescopes: those with continuously variable focus and those created by placing a plus-powered lens, or cap, in front of the objective lens of a distance telescope. The optics of near telescopes with continuously variable focus is especially complex and beyond the scope of this chapter (for more information, see Reich, 1995). However, the optics of distance telescopes with plus caps are reviewed below.

For near telescopes created by adding a plus-powered cap to a distance telescope, the power of the telescope is given by the following formula (Bailey, 1981b):

Power of the near telescope = Magnification of the distance telescope
× Power of the cap

Suppose that a person with low vision is using a 2× distance telescope with a 4-diopter cap placed on the objective lens. The object to be viewed must be placed at a distance from the front of the telescope equal to the focal length of the cap; in this case, 25 cm away ($f = 100/D$; $f = 100/4 = 25$ cm). The total power of the telescope will be $2 \times 4D = 8D$ (see Fig. 3.7). The theory in such a case is that the person will be able to read the same sized print using the telescope as he or she would with an 8-diopter handheld magnifier (viewing through the top part of his eyeglasses, as described in the next section) or through 8-diopter add spectacles.

The working distance advantage gained by using a spectacle-mounted near telescope in place of a pair of ordinary reading spectacles is provided by the magnification of the telescope. For example, a person using 8-diopter add reading glasses would have to hold his or her reading material at a distance equal to the focal length of the 8-diopter lenses, or 12.5 cm ($100/D = f$; $100/8 = 12.5$ cm); a person using the above-described 2× near telescope with a 4-diopter cap system would hold the material 25 cm away, which is a two-times advantage in working distance.

The field of view of near telescopes is usually expressed in terms of the lateral extent of the area that can be viewed, rather than in degrees as with distance telescopes. The field of view in meters of a Keplerian near telescope is approximately equal to the inverse or reciprocal of the power of the telescope. For the above example of a near telescope 8 diopters in power created by adding a 4-diopter cap to the objective of a 2× distance telescope, the field of view at the

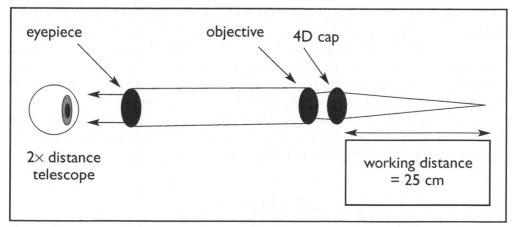

Figure 3.7. A Keplerian near monocular telescope composed of a 2× distance telescope with a 4-diopter cap. The power of this telescope is 8 diopters.

working distance of 25 cm would be approximately 1/8 m = 0.125 m = 12.5 cm. A Galilean near telescope would be expected to have a field of view approximately one-half to one-third that of a Keplerian near telescope of the same power.

PRINCIPLES FOR THE PRESCRIPTION AND USE OF LOW VISION DEVICES

Power Needed

The dioptic power of the magnifiers theoretically necessary for a person with low vision to read a particular size of print can be determined if the power of the current magnifier or spectacle add is known. The practitioner must determine the size of print that the person needs to read, as well as the size of print that the person can read with his or her current magnifier or spectacle add.

The relationship between magnifier power and the size of print that can be read is inversely proportional: if a person can read 8-point (1M, or newspaper-sized) print with a 2-diopter magnifier or 2-diopter add spectacles, then that person should be able to read 4-point print (twice as small) using a 4-diopter magnifier or 4-diopter add spectacles (twice as strong). The reader should be warned, however, that other factors such as field of view, working distance, depth of focus, and illumination might cause the person's actual performance with a magnifier to differ from that predicted. The effects of accommodation, spectacle correction, and illumination are discussed in the following sections.

When determining the power of magnifier necessary for reading a certain size of print, the practitioner should pay particular attention to how easily the person can read with his or her current glasses or magnifier. For example, suppose a person wishes to read 8-point (1M, or newspaper-sized) print. The practitioner determines that she can read 24-point (3M) print quite easily and 16-point (2M) print with difficulty using her current 2-diopter handheld magnifier. It would be more appropriate to use the 24-point figure as the size of print that the person is able to read with her magnifier when determining the power of magnifier necessary for long-term newspaper reading since this size print enables her to read with ease. In this case, the magnifier would have to be 24/8 = 3 times stronger than the current 2-diopter one (or 6 diopters) for this person to see 8-point print. On the other hand, the 16-point figure would be suitable for determining the power of a magnifier necessary for short-term reading, such as viewing price tags; in this case, the magnifier only would have to be 16/8 = 2 times stronger than the current 2-diopter one (or 4 diopters).

Effects of Accommodation

Most persons with low vision are elderly and no longer able to accommodate. For the minority of younger individuals with low vision, their ability to accommodate can have some effect on how they see through a magnifier. Since accommodation, in effect, adds plus (or magnifying) power to the eye itself, it can be used by a younger person under some circumstances to provide additional magnifying power for reading or other near viewing tasks. The result is that a younger person might be able to use a less powerful magnifier than an older person with the same visual acuity. As noted above, this is especially true when a young individual with low vision uses plus-powered spectacles when reading. A younger individual who needs a total of 7 diopters of power to read newspaper print and who can comfortably accommodate 4 diopters might be able to read effectively with 3-diopter reading glasses; if this same person were presbyopic and unable to accommodate, he or she might require 7-diopter reading glasses.

The ability to accommodate is less useful when the magnifier is further from the observer's eye, which is the usual case with handheld magnifiers. In fact, if the eye-to-magnifier distance is greater than the focal length of the handheld magnifier, the ability to accommodate is of no use at all (e.g., for a 20-diopter magnifier with a focal length of 5 cm, accommodation is of no benefit unless the magnifier is held within 5 cm of the person's eye).

Effects of Spectacle Correction

The spectacle correction worn by a person with low vision will affect his or her visual functioning with the low vision optical system being used. In most circumstances, the individual with low vision will benefit from wearing a spectacle correction. The most common exception to this general rule is that of the extremely nearsighted person, who may be able to read comfortably by removing his or her eyeglasses and taking advantage of the plus power naturally built into his or her eyes. A person who is farsighted or has a high amount of astigmatism should normally wear his or her glasses when performing demanding visual tasks.

Persons using telescopes will often find it preferable to remove the eyeglasses; this enables them to bring their eye closer to the telescope eyepiece, thus increasing the field of view. This method will work fine as long as the focus of the telescope can be adjusted to compensate for the person's refractive error. Most monocular telescopes can adjust for hyperopia and moderate amounts of myopia; however, they cannot be adjusted to compensate for astigmatism. Most telescopes of 4× power and higher are generally made in a Keplerian design (see Fannin & Grosvenor, 1996). When using such a telescope, a myopic person will gain additional power by removing his or her glasses, while a hyperopic individual will lose power by removing his or her glasses (Bailey, 1981b).

Another issue is whether a person should look through the lower, bifocal segment of his or her eyeglasses or the upper, distance portion when reading with a handheld magnifier. The answer depends on the power of the magnifier and its distance from the individual's eyes when it is being used (Bailey, 1980b). In most circumstances the person should be looking through the upper part of the glasses, unless the magnifier is being a held at a distance from the person's eyes less than the focal length of the magnifier.

A simple example can illustrate this. Suppose a person with low vision is using a 20-diopter handheld magnifier, which by definition has a focal length of 5 cm (100/20 = 5 cm). If the person is holding the magnifier more than 5 cm from his eyes, he will obtain more magnification by viewing through the upper portion of his glasses than the bifocal segment. On the other hand, if the person holds the magnifier less than 5 cm from his eyes, he should view through the lower, bifocal segment for best performance.

Since most individuals tend to hold handheld magnifiers at a relatively long distance from their eyes, they will usually benefit from viewing through the upper portion of the glasses. However, people will often tend to view through the bifocal segment because it is usually more ergonomically comfortable. Thus, the low vision practitioner should always monitor and advise the individual regarding the optimal way to view through bifocal glasses.

An individual with low vision using a handheld magnifier will normally obtain better magnification when viewing through his or her spectacles rather than removing them. The main exception to this rule is the situation in which a nearsighted person holds the handheld magnifier at a distance from his eyes less than the focal length of the magnifier. In that case, the individual will obtain more magnification by viewing through the handheld magnifier without his or her spectacles.

For example, suppose a nearsighted person with low vision is using a 20-diopter handheld magnifier with a focal length of 5 cm. If the person is holding the magnifier more than 5 cm from her eyes, she will obtain more magnification by viewing through her glasses. If the person holds the magnifier less than 5 cm from her eyes, she will obtain more magnification by viewing through the magnifier without her glasses.

Effects of Illumination

The importance of good illumination in performing tasks for persons with low vision cannot be overemphasized. A significant number of individuals may be able to read with a less powerful magnifier, or even with their current eyeglasses, if they are provided with optimal illumination. The usual goal is to provide quantities of glare-free illumination with a minimum of reflection off the material being viewed (Lewis, 1992). This is best accomplished by using a light source mounted on an adjustable arm or gooseneck. The best location for the lamp is usually close to the paper and in a position that it does not shine into the person's eyes, does not reflect off the back of his or her glasses, and does not reflect off the task directly back into his or her eyes. For an adjustable lamp using a 60- to 100-watt incandescent bulb, the optimal location is often above and to the side of the reading material and 25- to 40-cm away from it. Since this location is normally in front of the person's head, the light cannot shine directly into the person's eyes, and the location to the side minimizes reflection off the task into the person's eyes.

SUMMARY

The optics of low vision magnifiers can seem quite complex, but remembering the following 11 rules can help to make working with these devices less daunting and more effective:

1. Different types of magnifiers have different advantages and disadvantages. A person may need more than one magnifier to achieve his or her goals.

2. The power of magnifier needed by a person to read a certain size of print can be predicted by the size of print he or she can read with his or her current spectacle add or magnifier.

3. Because the term *magnification* has many definitions, it is better to describe magnifiers in terms of their dioptric power.

4. Uncorrected refractive error will affect how close a person will be able to hold an object and see it in focus. Without considering accommodative ability, a person with myopia can hold the object closer than a person with emmetropia, while a person with hyperopia must hold it farther away.

5. Younger individuals have an advantage in that they can add to the plus power of their eyes and/or a spectacle-mounted plus lens by accommodating.

6. Spectacle-mounted plus lenses and handheld magnifiers are designed to be used with the object to be viewed placed in the focal plane of the lens, creating an image at optical infinity. Because handheld magnifiers are normally held farther from the eye than glasses, they provide a longer working distance (although this is at the expense of a reduced field of view).

7. A presbyopic individual will obtain more power from a handheld magnifier by viewing through the upper or distance portion of his or her glasses than the lower, bifocal segment, unless the magnifier is held very close to the eye.

8. Stand magnifiers are designed so that the object is located closer than the focal length of the lens, creating an image at some finite distance from the lens rather than at optical infinity. Because of this, a presbyopic individual must normally look through the bifocal portion of his or her glasses to see the image clearly. The optics of stand magnifiers are much more complex than those of spectacle or handheld magnifiers, and fitting them requires knowledge of the size and location of the image created by the magnifier.

9. Stronger magnifiers have a shorter depth of field and are smaller in diameter than weaker ones, making them more difficult to use. Optical magnifiers stronger than 24 diopters are especially difficult to use.

10. The main (and only) advantage of telescopes for near use is their longer working distance.

11. The importance of good lighting cannot be overemphasized.

The understanding of the basic optical principles presented in this chapter and their application to low vision optical devices is a core element of the provision of services to individuals with low vision. Knowledge of these optical principles helps the practitioner to select the most suitable optical device and, equally importantly, ensures that the practitioner will be able to help persons with low vision use their devices in the most efficient manner.

REFERENCES

Bailey, I. L., (1980a). Magnification for near vision. *Optometric Monthly, 71 (2)*, 73–76.

Bailey, I. L. (1980b). Combining hand magnifiers with spectacle additions. *Optometric Monthly, 7 1(7)* 81–84.

Bailey, I. L. (1981a). The use of fixed-focus stand magnifiers. *Optometric Monthly, 72 (8)*, 37–39.

Bailey I. L. (1981b). Principles of near vision telescopes. *Optometric Monthly, 72 (8)*, 32–34.

Bailey I.L. (1983). Locating the image in stand magnifiers—an alternative method. *Optometric Monthly, 74 (9)*, 487–488.

Bullimore, M., & Bailey, I. L. (1989). Stand magnifiers: an evaluation of new optical aids from Coil. *Optometry and Vision Science, 66 (11)*, 766–773.

Davidson, D. W. (1991). Visual acuity. In J. B. Eskridge, J. F. Amos, & J. D. Bartlett (Eds.), *Clinical procedures in optometry*, (pp. 17–29). Philadelphia: Lippincott.

Fannin, T. E., & Grosvenor, T. (1996). *Clinical optics*, (2nd ed.). Boston: Butterworth.

Grosvenor, T. (2002). *Primary care optometry* (4th ed.). Boston: Butterworth.

Jose, R. T. (1983). *Understanding low vision.* New York: American Foundation for the Blind.

Keating M. P. (1988). *Geometric, physical, and visual optics.* New York: Butterworth.

Lewis, A. L. (1992). Lighting considerations for the low vision patient. In R. G. Cole & B. P. Rosenthal (Eds.), *Problems in optometry, patient and practice management in low vision* (Vol. 1, No. 4, pp. 20–33). Philadelphia: Lippincott.

Reich, L. N. (1995). Field of view and equivalent viewing power of near-vision telescopes. *Optometry and Vision Science 72 (6)*, 411–416.

Wilkinson, M. (2000). Low vision devices: An overview. In F. M. D'Andrea & C. Farrenkopf (Eds.), *Looking to learn: Promoting literacy for students with low vision* (pp. 117–136). New York: AFB Press.

Woo, G. C., & Leung, M. L. (2001). The term magnification. *Clinical and Experimental Optometry, 84 (3)*, 113–119.

Zimmerman, G. J. (1996). Optics and low vision devices. In A. L. Corn & A. J. Koenig (Eds.), *Foundations of low vision: Clinical and functional perspectives* (pp. 340–362). New York: AFB Press.

Part 2

EVALUATION OF FUNCTIONAL VISION

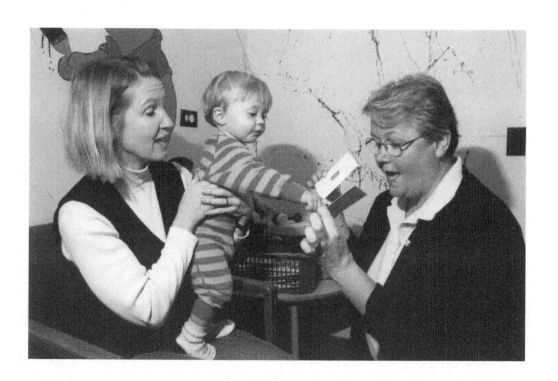

4

Overview of Functional Evaluation of Vision

AMANDA HALL LUECK

Individuals with low vision usually enter the comprehensive low vision care system when the results of their initial eye examination indicate that their vision cannot be corrected through typical surgical, medical, or optical treatments. (See Chapter 1 for more information on the comprehensive low vision care process.) At that point an ophthalmologist or optometrist conducts a low vision evaluation. The low vision evaluation refines many of the measurements made during the general eye examination and also addresses functional aspects of visual performance through evaluations of the individual's basic visual functions and through the application of these visual capacities in specific functional tasks. This functional evaluation is accomplished through the administration of standard tests that relate to functional activities such as reading and through the direct measurement of the visual parameters of tasks identified as critical activities for a specific person, such as reading a designated newspaper, textbook, recipe book, or medicine labels (Jose, 1983). Additional functional evaluations of vision performed primarily by health, education, and rehabilitation professionals, ideally in natural settings, provide information about a person's visual abilities and the ways in which he or she applies visual skills and behaviors in usual tasks of daily life. These professionals who participate in the evaluation of functional vision are designated by several interchangeable terms in this book: assessors, evaluators, or examiners. The major goal of these evaluations is to obtain detailed information about an individual's current visual performance on functional tasks carried out in the home, school, workplace, and community in order to determine the most effective compensatory methods to improve performance and, as a consequence, increase his or her independent participation in those tasks.

As discussed in more detail later in this chapter, functional vision evaluations ideally are performed after the general vision evaluations and the assessment of visual functions in low vision evaluations performed by ophthalmologists or optometrists to ensure that all refractive errors and accommodative anomalies have been addressed to optimize a person's visual performance. The functional vision evaluation includes an analysis of a person's performance with any low vision devices.

Chapters 5 and 6 of this book will focus on initial evaluation of functional vision, with the understanding that assessment of functional vision is a continuing process, since visual functions and functional tasks can change over time. Re-evaluation occurs during regularly scheduled low vision evaluations, during functional vision evaluations in educational or rehabilitation settings whenever changes in vision are noted, and when there are major changes in activities of daily life (such as making the transition from school to work, changing work assignments, or taking up a new hobby upon retirement).

USING INFORMATION FROM FUNCTIONAL EVALUATIONS

Educators and rehabilitation specialists conduct functional vision evaluations in order to design appropriate educational and rehabilitation intervention programs and cannot use functional vision assessment information to diagnose medical conditions. Visual diagnosis is a primary responsibility of ophthalmologists or optometrists. Information from the assessment of functional vision obtained from low vision evaluations and functional vision evaluations performed by health, rehabilitation, and education professionals can be used, in combination with other assessment data (in such areas as reading, writing, mathematics, home management, personal management, and mobility), to determine the extent and form of education or rehabilitation services required (Ponchilla & Ponchilla, 1996; Lewis & Allman, 2000).

Functional evaluation results provide the following:

➤ a baseline to measure changes in vision use over time in selected school, work, home, or leisure tasks,

➤ data for the determination of the range of compensatory methods to consider for a particular person,

➤ critical information for assistive device recommendations including optical device prescription and instruction,

➤ data for determining areas of visual functioning that may be amenable to direct instruction of visual skills and behaviors as well as specific methods for this instruction (most often skills related to reading performances are addressed in low vision evaluations [Freeman & Jose, 1991]),

➤ data for making recommendations regarding specific environmental adaptations.

TOOLS TO ASSESS FUNCTIONAL VISION

Standard tools that measure or record observations of the visual demands of real-world tasks for a specific individual are used to assess functional vision. These methods will be discussed in detail in Chapters 5 and 6. There may be some overlap in the tools used to assess visual functioning in clinical settings and functional vision evaluations performed by professionals in non-clinical settings (e.g., tools that measure visual discrimination at near distances using letter, word, and text reading charts). In the latter situation, these tools are used to characterize a person's performance in natural settings rather than the isolated environment of a clinic or medical office. They may yield different results from those found in a clinical setting, where environmental factors can be controlled more easily. Differences in performance on tasks administered in clinical settings compared to natural settings may be related to variety of factors, including variations in lighting, differences in the materials used for assessment of function and vision, and the presence or absence of other people who may contribute to a more or less stressful atmosphere. In addition, a person's behavioral state (e.g., level of anxiety, illness, fatigue, hunger, effect of medications), familiarity with surroundings, familiarity with the examiner, and familiarity with assessment tasks may also contribute to performance differences.

Standard tools that relate to functional tasks can be used to provide a systematic method for observing and documenting ways in which a person approaches functional tasks in addition to documenting actual response errors. For example, performance on a standard near vision task—in which a person is asked to read a series of sentences of gradually decreasing size—relates to real-life reading tasks, as the following example shows:

During a functional vision evaluation in his school, a teenager felt comfortable expressing fear when asked to complete this task, and he mentioned to his vision teacher that he had "failed" similar tests in the past. The student was not comfortable mentioning this concern during the low vision evaluation. His remark gave the low vision team insight into the student's psychosocial concerns related to visual functioning. Also during the functional vision evaluation, this teenager became excited when his performance improved after his vision teacher placed directional lighting on the near vision task; he had not realized that such lighting might help with reading tasks in school. He was shown the effect of lighting during his low vision evaluation, but he was quite nervous at that time and was not able to take in all that was happening. In the familiar school setting, his vision teacher was able to impress upon her student the importance of lighting using the example of a standard task that illustrated to the student his performance differences quite clearly. The student's performance on the near vision task also provided valuable information beyond data on his near visual acuity: reading fluency, reading speed, ability to follow words on a line and method of doing so, ability to locate the next line of print on the page and method of doing so, and use of head and eye movements while reading.

PREPARING FOR THE EVALUATION

Have Necessary Optical Prescriptions in Place

As noted earlier, before any evaluation of functional vision can be conducted, it is essential that a basic eye examination and low vision examination are performed. These will determine the best refractive correction and the most appropriate low vision optical devices for a particular individual. Any issues related to accommodation should also have been addressed. If a person has a refractive error that can be corrected with eyeglasses or contact lenses, the prescription should be in place during functional vision assessment procedures. Without this prescription, his or her ability to see details at distance or near may be less than optimal, and visual performance can be seriously affected. Low vision optical devices evaluated during the functional vision assessment should be ones that have been determined based on results of the low vision evaluation. Substitution of other devices outside the low vision evaluation is not advisable without checking with the individual's eye care specialist to be sure that the substituted device is of equivalent power to the prescribed device. This is because manufacturers may use different systems to determine the degree of magnification (e.g., a device rated as 2x magnification by one manufacturer may be the equivalent in power to a device labeled 3x magnification by another manufacturer since they may have used different formulas to arrive at these ratings). This is not the case when diopters are used to predict the performance of a magnifier. Even more caution is advised when substituting one category of optical device for another, especially handheld magnifiers for stand magnifiers (Bailey, et al., 1994). See Chapter 3 for more information on the specifics of optical devices.

Review Existing Records

A careful and critical review of the individual's records is necessary prior to conducting an assessment of functional vision. The information obtained from an individual's records needs to include the following:

➤ history of visual condition(s), other medical conditions, and treatments

➤ current medications

➤ current eyeglass or contact lens prescription

➤ history of eyeglass or contact lens use

➤ types of assessments previously performed and previous assessment results

➤ previous methods used to adapt or modify assessment protocols to facilitate the individual's participation

➤ previous education or rehabilitation services, including orientation and mobility

Records may include eye examination findings or other available documents describing visual function or factors affecting a person's overall performance. Ophthalmologists or optometrists conducting low vision evaluations usually administer assessments related to basic visual functionings and necessary optical corrections prior to conducting assessments of functional vision. Other health, education, and rehabilitation personnel conducting functional vision evaluations, however, must rely on an individual's recent records or recent communications from team members to obtain this critical information.

It is important to determine whether any spectacle correction or low vision devices have been prescribed so that their use can be evaluated. If a correction for refractive error has been prescribed, and the individual with low vision is not using it, every effort should be made to encourage its use. If the individual or family reports that the prescribed correction does not appear to be helpful, the eye care specialist should be contacted to determine if further testing is required.

Prior records can provide information about basic visual functioning and the types of assessments previously performed. These, in turn, can serve as a starting point for the assessment of functional vision. For example, descriptions of the successful administration of specific assessment instruments in the past can be particularly helpful in making decisions about which tools to administer during a current evaluation of functional vision, especially when working with people of any age with multiple disabilities. In addition, if changes in functioning over time are found in a person's records, this would raise the possibility that additional changes may have occurred since the last reports were made.

An inspection of previous records is important, but it is also critical not to make the assumption that previous findings are still accurate or that they will be the same in different testing environments. It is important to commence an evaluation by investigating areas of functional vision previously assessed, whenever possible. This is particularly important if a long time has elapsed since the last functional vision evaluation. Conducting thorough evaluations of visual functioning also provides a way to become more familiar with the visual performance of the person being assessed.

Establish Rapport

Establishing and maintaining rapport with the client or student and family members throughout the functional vision evaluation process is vital. Encouraging optimal performance is the desired outcome. An examiner must strive to create a supportive and positive assessment situation, since many assessment tasks may require great effort and may lead to feelings of frustration on the part of the person being assessed. A child or adult may have experienced previous failures with visual tasks similar to those in the functional vision evaluation. These can elicit strong emotional reactions, which may lead to decreased task performance. To provide a supportive atmosphere, service providers can

➤ Make the individual as physically comfortable as possible in the evaluation setting. In some natural settings it may be difficult to control some environmental variables such as lighting or background noise.

➤ Explain the role of each service provider in the current evaluation setting.

➤ Review the overall evaluation process so that the individual knows what to expect.

➤ Show genuine interest and listen carefully to the individual's concerns in an accepting manner.

➤ Explain each assessment procedure in clear terms, using language that the person understands.

➤ Encourage questions to clarify information throughout the evaluation, checking periodically to see if further explanations are needed.

➤ Present assessment procedures in ways that reduce frustration (e.g., present larger target items first to create initial success, and then move to smaller items).

➤ Involve family members, as appropriate, being certain that they also understand the evaluation process, the goal of each assessment procedure, and evaluation results.

Include Family Members and Key Professionals

Evaluation of functional vision is likely to be more valuable and provide more useful information when families and key professionals are included throughout the process. This includes their participation in a formal interview when evaluating a young child or school age youngster or participation in portions of the interview of an adult. These individuals can also be involved in others aspects of the evaluation process. When watching an observation session, for example, a family member or key professional may be able to indicate whether an individual's behaviors are routine or unusual. Often family members or teachers can provide appropriate language or motivators that encourage an individual's performance on visual tasks during the evaluation process. They may also indicate to an examiner when a person is "trying" or "holding back" on specific tasks, so that the testing process can be modified accordingly. With this fuller involvement, family and significant others can benefit from seeing a person's performance on the many assessment tasks. Sometimes significant people are not aware that an individual is able to do so much with their vision or, conversely, that a person's visual skills and behaviors are so limited. Watching the assessment prepares families and key professionals to receive the report of the final results, since they have observed the evaluation process.

The presence of family members and key professionals often provides a calming influence on the person being assessed, although sometimes the opposite is the case. For example, an elderly woman may be concerned that her son may reduce his daily visits if he observes that she is able to read medicine labels on her own. A child may show different behaviors in a play session at school when his or her mother is present. When family members or key professionals appear to be distracting the person with low vision from performing optimally, it can tactfully be suggested that they step farther away, to another area in natural settings, or to another room in clinical settings. For example, another team member can offer to take the family member or professional to another area to obtain more background information, or to discuss informational brochures or other materials. It is important to determine if family members or key professionals affect performance during the assessment process, either positively or negatively, since this information can be used in the design and implementation of intervention strategies.

STEPS IN THE EVALUATION PROCESS

There is a general sequence for conducting an evaluation of functional vision that applies for individuals of all ages. The five steps are

➤ observation

➤ interview

➤ assessment

➤ report writing

➤ conveying information in person

These steps are detailed in the following sections.

Step 1: Observation

Watching a person function in his or her usual activities and across different environments is a critical part of the evaluation of functional vision. It is a luxury not readily available to eye care specialists in medical settings. However, even in those settings the way a person walks into a room, reaches for objects, reacts to activities, and maintains eye contact can be very helpful in understanding his or her visual functioning. When conducting observations, the examiner looks for behavioral indicators of underlying visual functions and their application to functional tasks that will be more directly assessed later using specific assessment techniques. For example, a person may hesitate when walking across a floor where a carpet stops and a slightly lighter color of linoleum begins, reaching more carefully with his or her foot before moving from one surface to the other. The examiner will note this performance and will later check to determine if this hesitant movement was likely related to reduced visual acuity, reduced depth perception, reduced contrast sensitivity, visual field limitations, or a combination of factors. Observation can take place in natural settings in the school, home, workplace, or community to provide information about critical activities and how a person uses his or her vision to complete them. Observation of functional vision during daily routines, including play, of young children with visual impairments or students with visual and multiple disabilities can provide valuable information about how these children use their vision in usual tasks and also helps to determine appropriate materials and methods to use in more formal testing procedures (Erin, 1996). Sidebar 4.1 provides a general guide for recording observational assessment data. Examiners may find that adapting this guide helps them to meet the needs of the specific population they are serving.

SIDEBAR 4.1

Guide to Observational Assessment of Functional Vision

Observations of an individual's use of functional vision during everyday routines can include the following behaviors and characteristics:

➤ **Reading ability and efficiency:** Describe reading characteristics noted, such as preferred print size, distance from eyes to page, lighting required, reading fluency, and reading speed.

➤ **Reading or close-viewing behaviors:** Describe any head tilts, eccentric viewing, finger pointing, place keeping, or reading letter by letter.

➤ **Pictures:** Describe size of pictures viewed and seen and whether they are black and white or color, photographs or line drawings, pictures with complex backgrounds, or single objects.

➤ **Preferred viewing distances for near and far work:** Describe target, including its size and distance.

➤ **Preferred or optimal positioning for viewing:** Describe target and its position—held below, above, to one side or the other.

➤ **Use of writing equipment:** Describe use of pens, pencils, markers, and any specific writing guides.

➤ **Writing:** Describe use of print and cursive letters, their size and legibility. Does the person read his or her own writing? What size writing can he or she read?

SIDEBAR 4.1 CONTINUED

➤ **Copying, drawing, cutting or other relevant eye-hand coordinating tasks:** Describe task(s) and any information pertinent to task completion such as slow performance or errors noted. For young children, determine if they can color within lines or cut along lines.

➤ **Color identification and use:** Describe viewing of primary colors, pastels, and any color preferences.

➤ **Lighting requirements; performance in different lighting conditions:** Describe performance variations in different lighting conditions, adaptation from light to dark or dark to light, effects of glare, lighting conditions of daily environments.

➤ **Contrast needs:** Describe examples of performance with low-contrast and high-contrast materials.

➤ **Mobility and distance tasks:** Describe walking, running, and ability to locate large objects. Describe any unusual behaviors such as tripping or bumping into objects below, above, or to one side; hesitant gait; hesitation on stairs; or slowing down in bright light or dim light.

➤ **Near object location and reach:** Describe ability to locate desired small objects, and their size, search techniques, direct or indirect reach for objects, overreaching or underreaching for objects.

➤ **Use of eyeglasses:** Are eyeglasses kept clean, in good condition, and easy to locate? Describe use: wears regularly or for specific activities, takes off all the time, takes off to read or to see at distance, looks over the top regularly, pulls outward to look through when carefully examining objects.

➤ **Use of optical devices:** Are devices kept clean, in good condition, and easy to locate? Describe use: used for prescribed purposes, not used at all, used for other purposes, how they are held in relation to visual target and eyes.

➤ **Use of special equipment:** Describe specific type and use of computer, closed-circuit television magnifier, adaptive devices such as bold-lined paper, reading stand, reading lamp, adaptive sports equipment.

➤ **Requests for assistance:** Are they appropriate or unusually demanding? Is the person not able to request?

Step 2: Interview

Learning about the history of a person's visual impairment, changes in visual functioning over time, personal concerns related to visual functioning, and what a person would like to be able to do using his or her vision are among the types of information that can be obtained from an insightful interview. Interview questions should address a person's visual abilities and performance across tasks that address the full range of components of functional vision. Figures 4.1 and 4.2

FIGURE 4.1

Caregiver Interview Guide for Evaluation of Functional Vision for Young Children

QUESTIONS TO ASK	INFORMATION THAT ANSWERS PROVIDE
History	
1. Please tell us about the cause of your child's visual impairment and what you know about it.	Information about early history and caregiver's understanding of visual condition.
2. Has your child's vision changed in any ways?	Whether there has been any change in vision functioning over time.
3. Has your child had any eye surgeries?	Additional medical history.
4. What medications is your child currently taking?	Whether medications may affect the child's visual functioning.
5. When was your child's last eye exam?	Verification of date of exam and that latest reports are available in records.
6. What type of educational or other services is your child now receiving?	Information about educational and other services.
7. Do you notice any difference in your child's vision on different days or different times of day?	Whether the child's vision fluctuates.
8. What are your major concerns about your child's vision?	Identification of caregiver's priorities.
Favorite Things	
9. What are your child's favorite toys? How does your child play with them?	Whether the child shows any interests in toys that have a visual component; how the child interacts with toys.
10. What are your child's favorite activities?	Whether the child shows any interests in activities that have a visual component.
11. What are your child's favorite colors?	Whether the child sees colors.

Source: Adapted, with permission, from A. Hall, D. A. Orel-Bixler, and G. Haegerstrom-Portnoy. "Special visual assessment techniques for the multihandicapped," *Journal of Visual Impairment & Blindness*, 85, 23–29 (1991).

Figure 4.1. Sample interview guide for use with caregivers of young children, including explanations of the information that answers provide.

FIGURE 4.1 CONTINUED

Visual Activities

12. What types of objects does your child reach for? Please describe this. Are they of any particular color?

Information about color and eye-hand coordination.

13. Does your child have any favorite picture books? Please describe them.

Whether the child looks at pictures and, if so, what types.

14. Does your child recognize people when they first enter a room without making any sound? How far away are they?

Whether the child has enough vision to recognize faces at a distance.

15. When watching television, how far does your child sit from the screen?

Whether the child can see well enough to view television images and what size images can be seen from what distance.

16. Does your child use a computer at all? What types of things does your child do and how far away from the screen does your child sit?

Whether the child sees computer screen images, what size images can be seen from what distance, and whether the child prefers moving or stationary images.

17. When riding in a car, is your child interested in looking out the window, or does your child usually do other things?

Whether the child attends to distant objects.

18. Does your child seem to look more at still or moving objects?

Whether the child is more likely to look at stationary objects or objects in motion.

19. Have you noticed your child squinting when playing in bright sunlight, or does your child turn away from bright lights coming in windows or from lamps?

Any glare sensitivity.

20. Does your child like to look at room lights or at windows for a relatively long time?

Whether the child has light perception and whether the child perseverates in staring at lights.

21. Some children with visual impairments hold their hands near or against their eyes in unusual ways. For example, some children wave a hand in front of one or both eyes; others press their hands against an eye. Have you noticed your child doing anything like this?

Whether the child has any light perception and whether the child has any unusual visual behaviors that require further investigation.

22. Does your child appear to tilt his or her head in unusual ways to look at things?

A head tilt may indicate a field loss or eccentric viewing due to central scotoma or finding the null point of nystagmus.

(continued on next page)

FIGURE 4.1 CONTINUED

23. Does your child have any difficulty moving about the house? Please explain.	Travel skills can provide varied information about visual abilities.
24. Is your child more hesitant to explore or move about in unfamiliar places? Please explain.	If the child moves about more freely in familiar places, vision could be a factor.
25. How does your child use his or her vision to locate and move on stairs?	Whether there are visual acuity, depth perception, visual field, or contrast sensitivity problems.
26. Please describe your child's outdoor play activities.	Information about child's use of vision outdoors or ways that child interacts with environment: i.e., likes more active games, prefers to sit in one spot.
27. How does your child locate things that he or she drops on the floor? Please give an example.	Whether the child uses vision to locate lost objects and how.
28. Describe your child's coloring, drawing, cutting, writing. (Obtain a sample if possible.)	Whether the child uses vision on these tasks, such as seeing lines as guides.

For Children with Eyeglasses

29. Does your child wear his or her glasses all the time? If not, why not?	Whether the child will wear eyeglasses and whether his or her glasses are the correct prescription.
30. Does your child move his or her glasses forward on the nose or look over the glasses often?	Whether glasses are the correct prescription. The way the child adjusts the glasses may alert the optometrist or ophthalmologist to the correct prescription.
31. How long has your child had his or her present pair of glasses?	Whether it is time to be evaluated for a new pair of eyeglasses.

present separate sets of interview questions that can be used with caregivers of young children and with adults, with explanations about the type of information provided by each interview question. Blank copies of these interview guides can be found in Appendix 4.1 and 4.2 for readers' use. Examiners should feel free to adapt these interview guides to meet the needs of the specific population and person they are serving.

In any interview, input from family and key professionals should be encouraged. With young children or some persons with additional disabilities, this input

FIGURE 4.2

General Interview Guide for Evaluation of Functional Vision

QUESTIONS TO ASK	INFORMATION THAT ANSWERS PROVIDE
History	
1. Please tell us about the history of your visual impairment.	Information about the visual impairment, how much the person understands it, and his or her reactions to it.
2. What have you been told about your visual impairment?	Understanding of visual condition.
3. Have you noticed any change in your vision in the past month, year, or several years?	Change in visual condition.
4. What eye surgeries have you had and when?	More information on medical history.
5. When did you get your last pair of eyeglasses and are they helpful to you?	Utility and age of eyeglass prescription.
6. Have you ever used optical devices such as telescopes or magnifiers? If so, what do you use them for and do they help you at all? Do you have any at home? Could you bring them in, if possible?	Familiarity with optical devices.
7. Do you have any additional major health concerns?	Additional factors affecting functioning.
8. Are you currently taking any medications? Which ones?	Medications that might affect visual functioning.
Home/Work/School Situation (as appropriate)	
9. What is your current living situation?	Whether there is a readily available support system at home.
10. What type of work do you do?	Occupational information.
11. What visual tasks do you do on your job?	Visual demands at work.
12. What kind of help would you like with visual tasks related to your job?	Whether the person has realistic expectations and is receptive to help.
13. What kind of school program are you in?	School information.

Figure 4.2. Sample interview guide for use with adults, including explanations of information that answers provide.

(continued on next page)

FIGURE 4.2 CONTINUED

14. What kind of help would you like with your vision related to school or work?	Whether the person has realistic expectations and is receptive to help.
15. Have you ever had any special training related to your vision: special education, rehabilitation, orientation and mobility? Please describe.	Whether the person is familiar with, has used, or is receptive to specialized services.

Visual Status

16. Do you watch television? At what distance?	Whether the person can see well enough to view television images and of what size.
17. Do you use a computer? Do you happen to know the size of the screen? What size font do you use, and how far away do you sit from the screen?	Whether the person can see computer screen images, and of what size from what distance.
18. Can you recognize faces? At what distance? Can you see my face?	Information about ability to see details and detect low contrast details.
19. Is your vision different on different days or at different times of the day?	Whether the person's vision fluctuates.
20. Is your vision better on a bright day, an overcast day, at night, at twilight?	Effects of lighting on visual functioning.
21. Does a lamp help you for near work?	Effect of lighting on visual functioning.
22. Do you wear sunglasses?	Effect of glare on visual functioning.
23. Is glare a problem for you? For example, do you have more difficulty seeing when you face a bank of windows?	Effect of glare on visual functioning.
24. Can you recognize colors? Do some pose more problems for you than others?	Information about color vision.

Usual Daily Activities

25. What activities do you typically do each day at home?	Activity level and activities to target for instruction or adaptations.
26. Do you have any hobbies or other things that you like to do?	Activity level and activities to target for instruction or adaptations.
27. What do you typically read: novels, magazines, newspaper, *TV Guide,* recipes?	Reading needs to target for instruction or adaptations.
28. How do you usually get about indoors? Do you bump into any particular things?	Information on indoor mobility. Performance and activities to target for instruction or adaptations.

FIGURE 4.2 CONTINUED	
29. How do you usually get about outdoors? Do you have any particular problems we should know about?	Outdoor mobility performance and activities to target for instruction or adaptations.
30. Do you have any trouble with curbs or steps outdoors?	Outdoor mobility performance related to low-lying objects.
31. Do you have any trouble seeing traffic signs and lights?	Outdoor mobility performance.
32. Do you take public transportation? Do you have any difficulty seeing bus numbers?	Transportation capabilities and needs.
33. Do you drive? Where do you go and at what times of day?	Transportation capabilities and needs.
Summary Question	
34. We've talked a lot about your vision and the things you do each day. What do you consider the most important things for us to address related to your visual activities?	The person's priorities.

is vital. Behavior can be quite different in different environments and any differences can be elucidated in the interview process. For example, it might come out in an interview that a young child actively explores his or her classroom visually, although the same child is shy and inactive during a functional vision evaluation conducted by a stranger. This behavioral difference should be carefully noted, since functional vision evaluation results may not accurately reflect this child's true abilities.

Initial interview questions should be phrased in ways that do not immediately highlight a person's visual deficits, starting with open-ended questions about visual functioning. Often interviews bring up issues with strong emotional overtones. A careful examiner should attempt to balance these issues with ones that emphasize qualities or activities that a person and the family value. For example, rather than asking an adult if he or she is having difficulty seeing at night, the interviewer can ask if he or she sees differently at different times of day. If the person becomes agitated when mentioning that he or she has very little vision at night, the examiner can shift to a question about favorite activities that the person enjoys. The examiner can return to a review of the individual's night vision later in the interview, when the person is calmer and feels more rapport with the examiner.

Step 3: Assessments of Visual Functioning

After pertinent information from a person's records, observations, and interviews has been collected, it is time to conduct assessments of his or her visual functioning. Which methods to use will be determined from the information gathered to this point and modified as testing progresses. Detailed descriptions of assessment methods for children and adults can be found in Chapters 5 and 6. Family members and key professionals should be involved in this part of the process. They can contribute valuable assistance in determining appropriate test materials and communication methods, interpreting responses of young children or individuals with multiple disabilities, providing encouragement for individuals to complete difficult tasks, and helping to explain assessment findings clearly to the person with low vision.

In addition to administering the assessment tasks and evaluating specific test results, the examiner needs to be sensitive to the manner in which an individual with low vision completes each assessment task. This provides valuable information about such aspects of vision as coordination of vision with other sensory input, eye-hand coordination, use of head, and eye movements, among others. Sidebar 4.2 presents a list of behaviors to look for while individuals are completing an assessment task. An examiner's confidence in the assessment findings is also important to record. For example, if a person is sick on the day of testing, he or she may stop responding to items on a test prematurely, resulting in an inaccurately low measurement of visual functioning.

Step 4: Report Writing

Although there are many ways to organize a report, two methods are most often used: a checklist of items assessed, with a brief summary provided in text format and a list of recommendations; or a report written entirely in text format with recommendations listed. The first method saves time and is the most efficient way to present evaluation findings. The second method, preferred by this author, paints a more complete picture of the assessment process and a person's visual functioning. However, it takes more time and may not always be feasible. Examples of both methods of report writing are provided in the appendixes of Chapters 5 and 6.

Whether a report or checklist, or both, are used, the writer must provide a synopsis of assessment methods, findings, and recommendations, delineating areas of strength and weakness that can be incorporated into intervention programs and providing guidance in the selection of appropriate adaptations. Both types of report should include any material, verbal, or behavioral adaptations made during testing and indicate the examiner's level of confidence in the findings for each evaluation component. An introduction to any report should provide background information and a history of the individual's earlier vision evaluations. Reports must be free of jargon and, if technical terms are used, they should be explained in parentheses: ". . . diagnosed with myopia (nearsighted-

SIDEBAR 4.2

Behavioral Factors Affecting the Evaluation of Functional Vision

Consider the following questions about an individual's behavior while observing him or her complete an assessment task that may provide additional clues to the individual's visual functioning.

➤ Does the person respond slowly or rapidly during testing, and what appears to be the reason for the speed of response (e.g., inability to discriminate details visually, unfamiliarity with materials, lack of understanding of test demands)?

➤ Does the person exhibit any unusual head positions or movements when responding to all or portions of the test material?

➤ Does the person attempt to move forward to see the test material?

➤ Does the person squint when attempting to look at test material?

➤ Does the person take off his or her glasses or look over them to view test material?

➤ Does the person respond better when the test materials are moving?

➤ Does the person make consistent errors on line acuity charts? What are these consistent errors?

➤ Does the person appear to be easily frustrated and to give up on tasks before his or her visual limits are reached?

➤ Does the person understand the task requirements?

➤ Does the person tire easily and need rest time between performing tasks?

ness) . . ." Reports should present facts only and must be free of judgments about the individual assessed. They need to be organized so that a reader can find information easily, with a clearly written summary of findings. Use of "person first" language is desirable in any reports (e.g., "student with low vision," rather than "low vision student"). Sample functional vision reports are included in the appendixes to Chapters 5 and 6.

Step 5: Conveying Information in Person

It is usually necessary and valuable to report evaluation findings in face-to-face situations. Interactions among the examiner(s), the individual with low vision, the family, and other significant professionals should be encouraged at this time. The primary aim is to relay major assessment results and recommendations and to be certain that they are understood by all parties involved. Recipients should be given opportunities to ask questions if points are unclear or if areas of concern to them have not been addressed sufficiently. This verbal explanation of assessment findings should be supported by the written evaluation report.

ADDITIONAL ISSUES

Additional concerns may arise as functional vision assessments are performed. New issues related to visual functioning or other nonvisual abilities may be detected. The examiners must be prepared to make appropriate adjustments in the assessment process or make appropriate referrals as these emerge, as in the following two examples:

A 6-year-old boy was referred for a low vision evaluation by a low vision eye care practitioner and for a functional vision assessment by the teacher of students with visual impairments to gather information about the most appropriate reading medium for him. During the low vision evaluation, it was discovered that the child was not able to differentiate colors. More assessments were recommended and performed. The child's teacher was alerted to the need to collect more information regarding his use of color cues at home and when performing educational tasks during the functional vision evaluation scheduled to follow the low vision evaluation.

———

A 40-year-old lab technician had recently experienced some vision loss due to glaucoma, and was under the continuing care of her ophthalmologist. She wanted to retain her present employment, and contacted her state Department of Rehabilitation for assistance. The agency referred her to an optometrist for a low vision evaluation and for a functional vision evaluation by a rehabilitation teacher specializing in visual impairments. The latter would assess her visual skills and behaviors in relation to the visual demands of her work tasks. This information would be used to determine the most appropriate rehabilitation plan. During the functional vision evaluation, her rehabilitation teacher noticed that the woman had difficulty hearing comments from her co-workers when laboratory equipment was running in the background, although others in the room heard the remarks without difficulty. He referred her for a hearing evaluation, which determined that she had a mild bilateral hearing loss unrelated to her visual impairment.

CONCLUSION

Evaluation of functional vision can be undertaken by a variety of professionals in the low vision care process to determine and implement methods that allow individuals with low vision to participate more fully in functional and meaningful tasks of daily life. The overview in this chapter considered issues and methods that can be applied for individuals of all ages to accomplish this goal. Chapter 5 reviews methods to assess functional vision that are applicable to young children with visual impairments and individuals with visual and multiple disabilities who have cognitive challenges. These children and adults need to use assessment techniques that require limited knowledge of letters or words, place limited cognitive demands on them, and require responses at a simple verbal or nonverbal level. Chapter 6 reviews in detail functional assessment techniques applicable to schoolchildren and adults who are able to read letters and words, who can complete tasks with moderate cognitive demands, and who can respond verbally.

REFERENCES

Bailey, I. L., Bullimore, M. A., Greer, R. B., & Mattingly, W. B. (1994). Low vision magnifiers—Their optical parameters and methods for prescribing. *Optometry & Vision Science, 71,* 689–698.

Erin, J. (1996). Functional vision asssessment and instruction of children and youths with multiple disabilities. In A. L. Corn & A. J. Koenig (Eds.), *Foundations of low vision: Clinical and functional perspectives* (pp. 309–330). New York: AFB Press.

Freeman, P. B., & Jose, R. T. (1991). *The art and practice of low vision.* Boston: Butterworth-Heineman.

Hall, A., Orel-Bixler, D., & Haegerstrom-Portnoy, G. (1991). Special visual assessment techniques for multiply handicapped persons. *Journal of Visual Impairment & Blindness, 85,* 23–29.

Jose, R. T. (1983). Clinical examination of visually impaired individuals. In Jose (Ed.). *Understanding low vision* (pp. 141–185). New York: American Foundation for the Blind.

Lewis, S., & Allman, C. B. (2000). Educational programming. In M. C. Holbrook & A. J. Koenig (Eds.). *Foundations of education* (2nd ed.). *Vol. 1. History and theory of teaching children and youths with visual impairments* (pp 218–246). New York: AFB Press.

Ponchilla, P. E., & Ponchilla, S. V. (1996). *Foundations of rehabilitation teaching with persons who are blind or visually impaired.* New York: AFB Press.

Caregiver Interview Guide for Evaluation of Functional Vision for Young Children

Child's name _____   Birthdate _____

Examiner _____   Date of interview _____

Person interviewed _____   Relationship to child _____

QUESTIONS	RESPONSES

History

1. Please tell us about the cause of your child's visual impairment and what you know about it.

2. Has your child's vision changed in any ways?

3. Has your child had any eye surgeries?

4. What medications is your child currently taking?

5. When was your child's last eye exam?

6. What type of educational or other services is your child now receiving?

7. Do you notice any difference in your child's vision on different days or different times of day?

8. What are your major concerns about your child's vision?

Favorite Things

9. What are your child's favorite toys? How does your child play with them?

10. What are your child's favorite activities?

11. What are your child's favorite colors?

Visual Activities

12. What types of objects does your child reach for? Please describe this. Are they of any particular color?

13. Does your child have any favorite picture books? Please describe them.

14. Does your child recognize people when they first enter a room without making any sound? How far away are they?

15. When watching television, how far does your child sit from the screen?

16. Does your child use a computer at all? What types of things does your child do and how far away from the screen does your child sit?

17. When riding in a car, is your child interested in looking out the window, or does your child usually do other things?

18. Does your child seem to look more at still or moving objects?

19. Have you noticed your child squinting when playing in bright sunlight or does your child turn away from bright lights coming In windows or from lamps?

20. Does your child like to look at room lights or at windows for a relatively long time?

21. Some children with visual impairments hold their hands near or against their eyes in unusual ways. For example, some children wave a hand in front of one or both eyes; others press their hands against an eye. Have you noticed your child doing anything like this?

22. Does your child appear to tilt his or her head in unusual ways to look at things?

23. Does your child have any difficulty moving about the house? Please explain.

(continued on next page)

24. Is your child more hesitant to explore or move about in unfamiliar places? Please explain.

25. How does your child use his or her vision to locate and move on stairs?

26. Please describe your child's outdoor play activities.

27. How does your child locate things that he or she drops on the floor? Please give an example.

28. Describe your child's coloring, drawing, cutting, writing. (Obtain a sample if possible.)

For Children with Eyeglasses

29. Does your child wear his or her glasses all the time? If not, why not?

30. Does your child move his or her glasses forward on the nose or look over the glasses often?

31. How long has your child had his or her present pair of glasses?

General Interview Guide for Evaluation of Functional Vision

Name _____   Birthdate _____

Examiner _____   Date of interview _____

QUESTIONS	RESPONSES

History

1. Please tell us about the history of your visual impairment.

2. What have you been told about your visual impairment?

3. Have you noticed any change in your vision in the past month, year, or several years?

4. What eye surgeries have you had and when?

5. When did you get your last pair of eyeglasses and are they helpful to you?

6. Have you ever used optical devices such as telescopes or magnifiers? If so, what do you use them for and do they help you at all? Do you have any at home? Could you bring them in, if possible?

7. Do you have any additional major health concerns?

8. Are you currently taking any medications? Which ones?

Home/Work/School Situation

9. What is your current living situation?

10. What type of work do you do?

11. What visual tasks do you do on your job?

12. What kind of help would you like with visual tasks related to your job?

(continued on next page)

13. What kind of school program are you in?

14. What kind of help would you like with your vision related to school or work?

15. Have you ever had any special training related to your vision: special education, rehabilitation, orientation and mobility? Please describe.

Visual Status

16. Do you watch television? At what distance?

17. Do you use a computer? Do you happen to know the size of the screen? What size and type font do you use, and how far away do you sit from the screen?

18. Can you recognize faces? At what distance? Can you see my face?

19. Is your vision different on different days or at different times of the day?

20. Is your vision better on a bright day, an overcast day, at night, at twilight?

21. Does a lamp help you for near work?

22. Do you wear sunglasses?

23. Is glare a problem for you? For example, do you have more difficulty seeing when you face a bank of windows?

24. Can you recognize colors? Do some pose more problems for you than others?

Usual Daily Activities

25. What activities do you typically do each day at home?

26. Do you have any hobbies or other things that you like to do?

27. What do you typically read: novels, magazines, newspaper, *TV Guide*, recipes?

28. How do you usually get about indoors? Do you bump into any particular things?

29. How do you usually get about outdoors? Do you have any particular problems we should know about?

30. Do you have any trouble with curbs or steps outdoors?

31. Do you have any trouble seeing traffic signs and lights?

32. Do you take public transportation? Do you have any difficulty seeing bus numbers?

33. Do you drive? Where do you go and at what times of day?

Summary Question

34. We've talked a lot about your vision and the things you do each day. What do you consider the most important things for us to address related to your visual activities?

Evaluation Methods and Functional Implications: Young Children with Visual Impairments and Students with Visual and Multiple Disabilities

GUNILLA HAEGERSTROM-PORTNOY

Early identification and correction (if possible) of ocular and visual abnormalities are critically important for the visual and overall development of infants. Most visual development in infants occurs during the first year of life. Early correction of abnormalities minimizes the damage to the developing visual system. Early identification of abnormalities that cannot be corrected allows for appropriate intervention strategies to maximize function and overall development.

This chapter provides detailed information about the assessment of functional vision for young children with visual impairments as well as for students with both visual and multiple disabilities. Young children (under age 2 or 3 years) are nonverbal and so are many older children with multiple disabilities, so that the assessment techniques and the need for alternative communication methods are similar for both groups.

Assessment of the components of functional vision discussed in Chapter 2 is covered. In addition, background information is provided concerning the reasons for recommending specific methods, the need to consider how assessment results fit together for this complex population of children, and the variety of factors to consider when planning an assessment. A functional vision evaluation report form is included in Appendix 5.1 at the end of the chapter. This form summarizes much of the information gathered using the tests described.

PLANNING THE ASSESSMENT

Selection of Assessment Methods

Some additional considerations must be addressed early in the evaluation process by examiners when working with young children and students with visual and multiple disabilities. Evaluation of the presence or absence of light perception should be conducted early in the assessment process when it is apparent that children are not responding visually to their environment. In addition, for children who are nonverbal, an evaluation of oculomotor function (i.e., eye movement and position) early in the assessment process is necessary to determine if eye movements can be used as a way to determine an individual's responses to assessments of vision functions. Young children or students with visual and multiple disabilities may exhibit unusual behaviors that provide important clues to their vision functioning. Information about these behaviors should also be gathered early in the assessment process. Finally, it should be determined, based on findings from records, interviews, and observation, if the individual should wear prescribed eyeglasses during the evaluation.

It is also critical that assessment tasks for young children and students with visual and multiple impairments be within their communicative, cognitive, and experiential capabilities. Since many concepts and skills are learned through the visual channel, any limitation in this sensory modality can lead to limitations in conceptual and performance skills. It is also important to provide the optimal environment for assessment. When adapting or administering any tests for these youngsters, it is important to consider the following questions:

➤ *Are tasks within the child's visual capabilities?* When administering tests of vision, the tasks presented should be close to the student's abilities as determined through observation, so that the student is not discouraged and actively participates in the assessment process.

➤ *When administering a standardized test, is the perceptual basis of each task within the student's experience and of equivalent difficulty to the group used in determining the test's norms?* In any normative test of visual perception, for example, task items need to be within the student's background of experience in order for the results to be valid for comparison purposes. (See Chapter 6 for a discussion of visual perceptual skills assessment.)

➤ *Is the child familiar with objects used in the task?* The examiner cannot take for granted that a student is familiar with task objects, particularly when they are models of larger objects. For example, a toy car is not especially similar tactilely to a real car. This is particularly important for students with severely limited vision.

➤ *Are items involving imitation within the student's visual capabilities?* For a student to imitate actions, sufficient vision is required to take in the necessary information.

➤ *Is the language used in the assessment process understood by the child?* Young children with visual impairments and students with visual and multiple impairments may have unique communication needs (Rowland & Schweigert, 1998; Lueck, Chen, & Kekelis, 1997). It is important to present tasks using language that the student understands and to interpret the student's communicative attempts as accurately as possible. For example, pronouns must be used carefully with students who have difficulty with them. Often caregivers can provide valuable assistance.

➤ *Are any gestures used in testing within the student's visual capabilities?* Does the student need to be able to see the examiner point, smile, raise a hand to indicate stop, shake his or her head yes or no, and so forth?

➤ *Are substituted items testing equivalent underlying processes?* If items or objects on any standardized tests are changed, the examiner must be certain that the substituted items or objects test the same underlying cognitive and visual processes as the original.

➤ *Has the student been given enough time to respond?* Many youngsters, especially those with physical impairments, require time to integrate incoming information and to plan and execute their responses. Patience is crucial.

➤ *Has the student responded in an unusual way that has meaning for him or her?* The examiner should be alert to very subtle responses such as quieting, stiffening, small movements of one or more fingers, small foot movements, and eye or head movements.

➤ *Has the environment been prepared to optimize the student's participation in the assessment process?* Many young children with visual impairments and students with visual and multiple disabilities are easily distracted by highly visible objects, movement, noise, smells, and even rushing air in their environment. It is important to note in the assessment report stimuli that serve as distractions. It is important to eliminate or reduce these distractions in the assessment process to maximize the student's performance on assessment tasks.

➤ *Are the materials used for observational assessment optimal for the child?* When working with young children who are visually impaired or students with severe disabilities, it is often difficult to elicit visual behaviors. Determine, based on observation and interview results, the types of materials a child prefers and is familiar with so that you have an idea of what to present before you begin to work with the child. The following are examples of materials that can be used for assessment purposes:

● Flashlights with colored caps

● Penlights with colored caps

● Cheerleader's pompom

- Shiny material such as decorative Christmas tree tinsel ropes
- Soft sound toys such as a medium-sized squeezable duck toy that quacks
- Small toys of varying textures (porcupine, furry material, soft cloth bracelet)
- Light box to use as a background for some students
- Directional lamp to focus student's attention for some students
- Toy with buttons that make sound or create movement when pressed
- Picture books with pictures that vary in complexity, size, and contrast.

While certain visual behaviors may only be elicited by highly conspicuous stimuli such as colored lights or shiny material, it is important to differentiate the need to elicit responses for assessment purposes and the goal of intervention strategies. Eliciting responses to materials used in the assessment process should not become the goal of intervention strategies. Rather, intervention goals and practices must be linked to meaningful outcomes related to cognitive growth, exploration, or the performance of functional activities (see Chap. 8).

Before conducting any evaluation of vision functioning, it is necessary to determine which assessment materials will be most appropriate, given a student's developmental capabilities and physical limitations, and how selected assessment materials will best be administered. It is also critical to determine alternative ways in which a young child or a student with multiple disabilities may respond during evaluation procedures. These methods are determined from observation and interviews with family members, caregivers, and other professionals before the start of the evaluation process and can be refined as the evaluation progresses.

Communication and Test Limitations

A major concern when performing visual assessments of infants, young children, and students with multiple disabilities is communication. The type of communication (verbal, pointing, eye fixation) has to be established before the assessment is begun. This will determine how best to administer assessment procedures and elicit and interpret a child's responses to them. The following questions are particularly applicable to children with multiple impairments:

➤ Does the child have normal hearing?

➤ What expressive verbal language does the child have?

➤ What verbal directions does the child understand? Can you determine the level of understanding through interaction with the child?

➤ If the child is nonverbal, is he or she physically capable of pointing?

➤ Children with cerebral palsy frequently have limited physical capabilities. If the child cannot point, is he or she capable of responding "Yes" and "No" using head movements or other established signals?

➤ What kind of hand control does the child have?

➤ If no other communication mode is possible, will you be able to make judgments of vision function through the child's use of eye movements? Can the child use his or her eyes to look at objects when requested?

➤ Does the child have any oculomotor limitations that prevent visual fixation in some fields of gaze?

➤ Is the child known to have a significant field defect that would make it inappropriate to place a visual target in some part of his or her visual fields?

Light Perception

If the child appears to be very visually inattentive, light perception should be assessed prior to attempting formal vision testing. This assessment is usually not necessary if observation of the child has clearly established that vision is present. If no light perception is present, further vision testing is not necessary.

PUPIL RESPONSES TO LIGHT

If a bright light is shone in one eye of a person without visual impairment, the pupils of both eyes will constrict and remain constricted as long as the bright light is present because the pupil responses of the two eyes are linked. The same size of pupil response should occur in both eyes, and the responses should be maintained. In a child with no light perception in either eye due to optic nerve or retinal disorders, there will be no pupil response to light. If one eye has light perception but not the other, both pupils will respond when light is shone in the seeing eye, but no pupil responses will be seen in either eye when the light is shone in the nonseeing eye. In cases of significantly reduced vision, the pupil responses may be very sluggish and hard to see. Performing the test with a bright penlight in a dim room will make the evaluation easier. However, the presence of normal-appearing pupil responses does not guarantee that the child has light perception. If the retinas and the optic nerves are normal but there is damage at the level of the visual cortex, pupil responses may be present but the child may have no light perception.

BLINK REFLEX

The blink reflex can be used as an indication of light perception. When an object, such as a hand, is moved rapidly towards the eye as if about to hit the person, an involuntary blink reflex closes the eye. In eyes without light perception, there is no such blink reflex. To assess the blink reflex, the examiner moves his or her hand rapidly toward the child's face without touching any part of the face and observes the blink response. This can be done with both eyes and for each eye alone. The hand movement needs to be fast enough to appear menacing but not so fast that the movement causes air movement, which the child can feel and may respond to even if he or she has no light perception.

Oculomotor Function

A quick assessment of oculomotor function should be done prior to any other measurements of vision function. Since these measurements will depend on eye movements and accurate fixations in nonverbal children with physical limitations, it is essential to establish the quality of eye movements prior to any visual assessment.

Is the child able to move his or her eyes around in all directions? Children who have sustained brain damage may, in addition to their visual problems, also have oculomotor abnormalities that make it difficult for them to move their eyes voluntarily in certain fields of gaze. Some may not be able to elevate their eyes, while others may have difficulty looking to one side. Is the child capable of fixating with either eye alone? When presented with a visual target, does the child fixate centrally (look directly at it) or does he or she look to the side or above or below the target (use eccentric viewing)? Is fixation steady or can the child maintain fixation on a target for only a brief moment when only one eye is allowed to see.

Children with visual impairments frequently have eye turns (see the Eye Turns section later in this chapter). One eye may turn in or out or there may be a vertical deviation. Is there a large eye turn present that makes judgments of fixation difficult? Is the eye turn constant (the same eye turns all the time) or does the child alternate which eye is fixating? A child may prefer to fixate with one eye for distance and the other eye when viewing at near distances. The child may also rapidly switch fixation between the two eyes at any one distance. Does the child use one eye when looking to the right and the other when looking to the left? These are important distinctions to make since the observation of the "wrong" eye during vision testing might lead to incorrect conclusions about the child's visual responses.

Is there nystagmus (involuntary movements of the eyes), which can make it difficult to judge where the child is looking? Nystagmus can be horizontal, vertical, or rotary. Nystagmus varies in the amount of movement (amplitude) and rate of change of movement cycles (frequency). It can be very difficult to determine fixation in a child with a large amplitude nystagmus. The amplitude of nystagmus often varies with viewing distance and tends to be of lower amplitude for near viewing distances. In addition, at any one distance, there may be a null point where the nystagmus is minimal (and vision is optimal). Null points are frequently associated with habitual head turns to place the null point in the direction of the visual target. If such a null point exists, it is important to establish where it is and to allow the child to hold that posture during vision testing.

FIXATION

Many eye care practitioners (optometrists and ophthalmologists) limit their assessment of vision function in infants and other nonverbal patients to determining whether the child's fixation is definable as central, steady, and maintained in the two eyes. A child without visual impairment is assumed to fixate on an interesting object (move his or her eyes toward the target), look directly at the target (have central fixation), maintain fixation on the target for some time (have steady fixation), and follow that target when it is moved across the visual field. A child's vision is considered "normal" if he or she is able to do these tasks with either eye. If fixation is not central, steady, and maintained, the assumption is made that an ocular, visual, or oculomotor abnormality exists.

There are several reasons why a child may have difficulty fixating a steady target or tracking a moving target.

➤ Oculomotor limitations, either neural or muscular, may prevent the child from following the target in certain fields of gaze.

➤ The child may have a visual field defect that causes the target to disappear from view as it is moved.

➤ The target may not be of sufficient contrast or size to be seen except in certain parts of the child's visual field.

➤ The child may lose interest in the task.

The assessment of fixation should initially be done with both eyes open and then with each eye in turn. The behavior of the child when each eye is covered can alert the examiner to differences in vision function between the two eyes if the child objects to one eye being covered but not the other. Whether fixation is central can be most easily estimated with a penlight. The reflex on the cornea is normally centrally or slightly nasally located and should be symmetrical in the two eyes.

Differences in the fixation behavior in the two eyes indicate the presence of some abnormality (see the Appendix to this book for more information on specific eye conditions). Children with eye turns and amblyopia (reduced visual acuity associated with eye turns) may have noncentral or eccentric fixation in the amblyopic eye. Eccentric fixation refers to the use of a nonfoveal retinal area for fixation. The fovea is the part of the retina that has the best visual acuity. Usually the amounts of eccentric fixation associated with amblyopia are so small (a few degrees at most) that they are very difficult to detect using simple methods such as fixation on a penlight. An eccentric fixation that is quite obvious, either through nonsymmetrical locations of the light reflex in the two eyes or noncentral location of the reflex in both eyes, usually indicates the presence of significant central scotomas (i.e., blind spots).

Determining whether fixation is maintained or not can be difficult in young children due to attention difficulties. A large selection of visually interesting toys, some with associated sounds, is useful in this situation.

Steadiness of fixation is easier to assess than whether fixation is central. Provided the attention of the child is drawn to the fixation target, there should be no movements of the eye and the fixation should be maintained for several seconds at least. The presence of nystagmus (involuntary movements of the eyes) always indicates either a motor or a sensory anomaly (see Chap. 2).

In general, there are two types of nystagmus: sensory and motor. Sensory nystagmus is the result of eye and vision disorders, while motor nystagmus is caused by an abnormality of the oculomotor control systems. Motor nystagmus will usually, in turn, reduce vision functioning since the eyes are not steady. Whatever the cause, the fact that the eyes are not steady in both motor and sensory nystagmus will decrease an individual's visual acuity. In children with sensory nystagmus, in general, the larger the size (amplitude) of the eye movements and the more erratic the movements, the less the acuity. Sensory nystagmus is only present if vision is affected from an early age in both eyes. A child with a severe abnormality in one eye but with normal vision in the other eye will not have sensory nystagmus. Damage to both eyes in an adult will not result in nystagmus. If nystagmus is present, and the determination is made that it is sensory in nature (associated with ocular abnormalities), the visual abnormality was present from infancy. Children with acquired abnormalities, such as Stargardt's disease, with onset in the primary grades, generally do not have nystagmus.

Like eye turns, sensory nystagmus can be caused by many different disorders, including some that are life-threatening, such as brain tumors. For this reason, a specially trained eye care practitioner should always assess a child with nystagmus. The eye movements in children with nystagmus can include horizontal, vertical, and rotary movements, and, in rare cases, the nystagmus may only be seen in one eye.

Latent nystagmus, which is only evident when one eye is covered, is associated with early onset inward eye turns (infantile esotropia). If it is necessary to measure vision function in each eye in a child with latent nystagmus, rather than covering each eye the examiner can blur one eye with lenses to avoid precipitating the latent nystagmus, which will reduce visual acuity. Holding a cover a few inches away from the eye and allowing light into the eye sometimes also prevents the latent nystagmus.

The absence of nystagmus does not guarantee normal vision. Children with normal retinas and optic nerves will show no nystagmus even though damage may exist at the level of the visual cortex. Children with bilateral cortical visual impairment from infancy usually do not have nystagmus unless they also have optic atrophy.

EYE TURNS

The majority of children with multiple disabilities have eye turns (e.g., Orel-Bixler et al., 1989; Hall et al., 1991). Eye turns can be caused by many different conditions including visual impairment, refractive anomalies, neurological anomalies, systemic diseases, and brain tumors, among others. Because of the complexity of assessment and the multitude of causes, some of which may be life-threatening, this type of assessment should only be done by optometrists or ophthalmologists with specialized training in this area.

Unusual Visual Behaviors

Some innate behavioral adaptations to visual impairment serve to compensate for loss of function (Good & Hoyt, 1989), while other behaviors may be detrimental. It is important to identify these behaviors and to understand their behavioral significance. Such behaviors can provide important clues to the child's level of visual impairment and may guide the evaluation process if the examiner has the opportunity to observe them prior to the exam. If the examiner has not directly observed these behaviors, family members should be questioned about their occurrence.

HOLDING ITEMS CLOSE

A commonly observed behavior that frequently causes parents to bring a child to a visual assessment is that the child holds objects closer when looking at them than what would be expected for the age of the child. The child may also like to sit very close to the television. It should be noted that any child who shows any visual interest in television at all has significant residual vision functioning. Most often, holding these items close indicates reduced visual acuity but, rarely, this might indicate that the child has a high nearsighted refractive error that is uncorrected.

Children with reduced visual acuity hold items close to provide magnification. If the target of interest is too small for the child to resolve, he or she will naturally bring it closer to his or her face. An object of fixed size (most things in the physical world) that is moved closer to the eyes will subtend a larger visual angle and will therefore be easier to see (see Chap. 3). Children usually hold things of interest at such a distance that the visual task becomes possible. The more difficult the task, the closer the child will hold the object. Children with visual impairments should be allowed to hold materials as close as they need. This includes allowing a child to sit close to the television to see; nose touching, if necessary. For children with multiple disabilities who may be physically unable to move close enough to the object of interest, the object needs to be moved close enough to the child. This may require attachments to wheelchairs and other environmental adaptations. More information on viewing at near distances appears in the Accommodation section later in this chapter.

HEAD TURNS AND HEAD TILTS

Children may habitually turn or tilt their head or they may adopt unusual head postures when asked to do a visually demanding task. There may be several reasons for this behavior. The head turn or tilt may be present because it allows single binocular vision if the child can minimize or eliminate an eye turn by turning or tilting his or her head. In other fields of gaze and when the head is straight, he or she may be seeing double. The head posture may also result from efforts to slow down or eliminate nystagmus movements. Nystagmus frequently varies in different fields of gaze and often has a null point where it is reduced. The child will attempt to place this null point toward the visual target using head turns or tilts. In this case, the improved visual acuity when the nystagmus is minimized is the driving force.

Visual field limitations may also lead to unusual head postures. For example, if the inferior visual field is missing, the child may look down much of the time to place the seeing part of the visual field toward the objects of interest. Head turns and tilts can also be caused by nonvisual factors such as muscular or spinal abnormalities. If the purpose of the head posture is to allow binocular vision, the child will straighten up so that the head turn disappears when one eye is covered. If the purpose is to minimize nystagmus or to compensate for visual field loss, or if it has a nonvisual origin, covering one eye will have no effect. In most cases, head turns or head tilts represent a functional adaptation to an abnormality. The child should be allowed to maintain this adaptation if the underlying cause cannot be repaired.

Certain head shaking behaviors may also be visual in origin: the child is using his or her head to counteract movements of the eyes caused by nystagmus (Jan, Groenveld, & Connolly, 1990; Jan, 1991). In children with some disorders, and particularly cortical visual impairment, adding motion seems to improve vision function.

ECCENTRIC FIXATION AND ECCENTRIC VIEWING

Significant eccentric fixation usually indicates the presence of a central scotoma or blind spot. If the child is aware that he or she is not looking straight ahead, the term eccentric viewing is used. The child is using an area of intact retina to see an object, by moving the central scotoma out of the way. This always results in decreased visual acuity since it involves fixating with the parafoveal retina (the area next to the fovea) or the peripheral retina, which inherently has worse visual acuity.

EYE POKING AND EYE PRESSING

Children with severe visual impairment, usually only those with retinal abnormalities (such as Leber's congenital amaurosis), may press on or poke their eyes repeatedly (Jan et al., 1983). Children who experience pain in their eyes from undiagnosed glaucoma may also press on them. Children with optic nerve disorders (optic nerve atrophy, optic nerve hypoplasia) and children with cortical visual impairment do not usually poke their eyes (Jan et al., 1987). These behaviors should be discouraged since the continuous poking can damage the eyes and disfigure the area around the eyes, causing a sunken appearance. This is assumed to be a form of self-stimulation, since it does not occur in children whose optic nerves are not functioning well.

LIGHT GAZING AND FINGER FLICKING

Children with visual impairment frequently stare at bright lights, including the sun (Jan, Groenveld, & Sykanda, 1990). The reason may be that these bright light sources are the only targets with high enough contrast to attract their visual attention. Staring at the sun should be strongly discouraged since it can damage the eyes. Most artificial light sources are not bright enough to cause damage if stared at.

Children may also flick their fingers in front of their eyes. It may be related to other motion-producing activities; as already noted, a moving stimulus may be more visible to children with certain types of disorders such as cortical visual impairment. Children with congenital visual anomalies may engage in these types of behaviors at very young ages when their vision function is at its worst. As their vision improves with their overall development, these behaviors may stop. Older children who persist in these behaviors usually have severely reduced vision functioning. Body rocking, jumping, or obsessions with particular objects are also signs of severely reduced vision function and may reflect lack of stimulation by other means (Fazzi et al., 1999; Van Dijk, 1983).

Using Eyeglasses During an Evaluation

Eyeglasses can be prescribed by eye care specialists based on results of objective techniques such as retinoscopy or through the use of automated refractors. The light reflected back from the eye will travel differently depending on the focusing error of the eye. The eye care specialist uses lenses to neutralize the movement. These lenses correspond to the focusing error of the eye. No response is required from the child. It is thus possible to correct the refractive errors without any cooperation from the child.

The following questions should be answered before performing any assessment of vision:

➤ Does the child have eyeglasses?

➤ What is the primary purpose for the eyeglasses?

➤ How strong is the child's refractive error?

➤ If a child's eyeglasses are not available, will the child be able to focus at the distance where visual targets will be presented?

➤ Is the refractive error the same in the two eyes or is the prescription much stronger in one eye than the other?

➤ How old are the glasses? How old is the prescription?

➤ Were the eyeglasses prescribed primarily for distance use or for reading?

➤ Were the eyeglasses prescribed primarily to align the eyes?

In children with outward eye turns, eyeglass prescriptions often include a stronger minus correction than the refractive error in order to force the child to accommodate (change focus). This may maintain eye alignment through the connection between accommodation and convergence. Many children with cerebral palsy (and Down syndrome), however, have poor accommodative abilities, which may defeat the purpose of such prescriptions, contribute to the child not wanting to wear the glasses, and/or make vision worse with the glasses than without.

A child may object to wearing prescribed eyeglasses for visual or tactile reasons. Even children with very high refractive errors whose vision clearly benefits from wearing glasses will sometimes object because of the fit of the glasses or the feeling of something on their faces.

If the child has been given eyeglasses for full-time wear fairly recently, the assessment should be done with the eyeglasses in place. If it is known that the child has a very strong prescription, and for some reason, the eyeglasses that are normally worn are unavailable, it may be better to wait and perform the assessment when the eyeglasses can be used. As an alternative, if the prescription is known and is for nearsightedness, the visual targets can be placed at the appropriate distance to be in focus by using the following equation (see Chap. 3).

$$\frac{100}{\text{diopters}} = \text{measurement in cm}$$

(To convert to inches, 2.5 cm = 1 in.) For example, if the prescription is –10.00 diopters, an object will be in focus at a distance of 10 cm (4 in) from the individual without correction. For a –5.00-diopter correction, targets will be in focus at 20 cm (about 7.8 in). This equation is applicable only for prescriptions for nearsightedness, not for farsighted refractive errors.

TESTS OF VISUAL FUNCTIONS

The following sections describe tests of vision functions that can be used to evaluate functional vision in very young children or those with multiple disabilities, including visual acuity, visual fields, contrast sensitivity, light sensitivity, color vision, depth perception, and accommodation.

Visual Acuity

The measurement of visual acuity, or detail vision, is commonly used by eye practitioners and others for many different reasons (see Chaps. 2 and 6). Visual acuity may appear to be a simple measurement but is, in fact, very complex and is affected by numerous factors including stimulus variables, environmental variables, behavioral variables, the task chosen, as well as disorders in the individual's visual system. For a person with unimpaired vision, whether visual acuity is measured with symbol or letter charts, single lines, single symbols, gratings (striped patterns), or words, the results will be little affected by the task chosen. This is not the case with patients with low vision, however, for whom each of these target types can yield dramatically different results. In general, the more complex the task, the worse the measured visual acuity in persons with low vision. Single-symbol acuity will be better than line acuity; whole-chart acuity will be worse; use of crowded symbols, such as those found on standard reading charts, will result in the worst acuity.

Grating acuity is measured by presenting gratings or stripes using a two-alternative forced-choice method. Teller acuity cards are commercially available for measurement of grating acuity (McDonald, 1985). A grating is presented together with a blank field and the child is asked to point or look at the patterned field (the grating). When the grating is suprathreshold (above threshold), the child will usually rapidly look at the pattern rather than the blank field. The size of the stripes is decreased until threshold is reached. The size of the threshold grating is recorded as well as the test distance (e.g., 20-ft stripe at 4 ft, consistent with a grating acuity of 4/20. The Snellen equivalent is 20/100). Detecting the presence of a grating is a different and easier task than identifying symbols, and grating acuity is known to overestimate acuity for optotypes in patients with reduced acuity. In other words, many ocular disorders generate a significant discrepancy between grating acuity and optotype acuity, with grating acuity always better than the acuity measured with symbols. Some specialists do not consider it appropriate to convert grating acuity to optotype acuity. In some practice settings, a conversion is used to predict optotype acuity from grating acuity. At the University of California, Berkeley, School of Optometry, for example, this conversion is approximately a factor of 3 when grating acuity is less than 10 cycles per degree (i.e., Snellen equivalent acuity is worse than 20/60). Others report the grating acuity as measured compared to age norms for grating acuity and emphasize that the acuity measured is a grating acuity (Mayer, 1995).

TASK COMPLEXITY

Visual acuity should always be measured using as complex a task as possible for the individual being tested. It is possible to miss the presence of a visual impairment if too simple a task is used. If the child is able to read letters, use a letter chart to assess visual acuity. (Issues related to chart design are discussed in Chap. 6.) The Resources section of this book describes many different visual acuity tests, and provides information about their availability. If the individual's reading capability is of primary importance, and the child is able to read words, use a word-reading chart. Letter charts and word-reading charts are usually too difficult for young children as well as for many children with multiple disabilities. If the child is able to identify symbols, it is preferable to use a line chart with symbols, such as the Lea Symbol Tests, rather than a test using single symbols. Pointing to each letter on a chart or isolating a single line on a chart simplifies the task and may give a different acuity result than if the child is required to find the letters by himself or herself.

A child recently examined exemplifies the importance of using as complex a task as possible:

An 8-year-old child with cortical damage who was nonverbal had been tested using single symbols and was found to have a visual acuity of 20/30. On the basis of this test, he was declared to be not visually impaired; however, he could not learn to read. Measurement with single symbols confirmed the acuity of 20/30. When an isolated line on an acuity chart was used, his visual acuity was 20/60. When the whole chart was presented, his acuity decreased to 20/120; when a chart with crowded symbols was used, his visual acuity was 20/200. This child definitely had visual impairments. When letters were presented to him at the appropriate size for a visual acuity of 20/200 (discussed later in this chapter), he was able to learn to read.

TEST ADMINISTRATION

The recommended steps for administering visual acuity tests are detailed in the following paragraphs.

➤ Always make sure that the child can easily read the first row of symbols presented. If the child struggles to read them, move the chart closer to the child.

➤ Ask the child to continue reading down each row until his or her reading slows down or the child states that he or she cannot read any more. To speed up the process, you can ask the child to read only one letter on each row (preferably the middle letter) until the reading becomes difficult, then move up one whole line and ask the child to read all the letters on that line. Continue testing, asking the child to read all the letters until the child refuses or makes errors. At that point, encourage guessing to make sure that the child's threshold (smallest visible size) has been reached.

➤ Record the size of the symbols in the last line in which at least three of five symbols have been read correctly. Record the distance from the eyes to the chart in the same units as the symbols. For example, on the Lea Symbol Test, if the child reads the 30-ft line at threshold and the distance is 1.5 ft, his or her acuity is 1.5/30.

To convert to Snellen equivalent acuity, divide the denominator by the numerator ($30/1.5 = 20$). This is the minimum angle of resolution (MAR) in minutes of arc. Multiply this number by 20, to give the Snellen 20-ft denominator. In this case the equivalent Snellen acuity is $20/(20 \times 20)$ or 20/400. (See Sidebar 6.1 for more details.)

If the child is verbal, he or she can name the symbols. If the child is nonverbal, use a matching task. To do this, a template with the four symbols that are quite large can be placed in the child's lap. He or she is asked to match the symbol that the examiner is pointing to with the same one on the template. This is a slightly different (and less difficult) task than reading the chart without the adapted assistance. If use of a chart is impossible because it is too difficult or the child cannot communicate adequately, single symbols can be used at a close viewing distance. Two symbols of a size expected to be easily visible are first presented at a near distance, such as 1 ft. The child is asked to point to or look at the symbol that matches the one the examiner is displaying, or the child is asked to locate one of the symbols.

If the child's response is rapid and obvious, only one presentation of symbols this size needs to be made. As sizes are decreased and the child's responses become more hesitant, a sufficient number of presentations must be made to ensure that the effects of guessing are taken into account. Since only two symbols are presented, there is a 50/50 chance that the child will point to the correct one even if he or she cannot see it. Table 5.1 shows the total number of presentations that must be made to make sure that the effects of guessing have been taken into account in such forced-choice tests. For the examiner to be confident of the measurement, the percentage of correct choices when corrected for guessing

TABLE 5.1

Interpreting Forced-Choice Results: Correction for Guessing

NUMBER OF PRESENTATIONS IN A TWO-ALTERNATIVE PROCEDURE	NUMBER CORRECT	PERCENTAGE CORRECT, CORRECTED FOR GUESSING
4	2	0
4	3	50
5	3	20
5	4	60
6	4	33
6	5	67
8	5	25
8	6	50
8	7	75

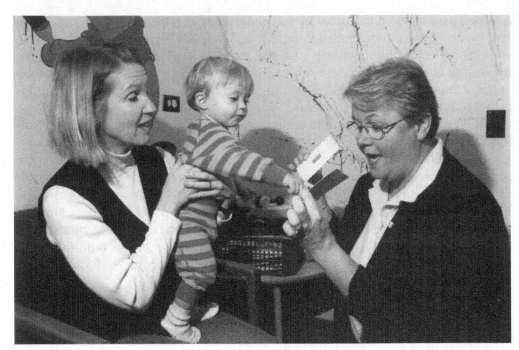

Administering the Bailey-Hall Cereal test, a test of visual acuity, to a young child. *(Peg Skorpinski)*

must be at least 50 percent, which means that three out of four, four out of five, five out of six, or six out of eight presentations must be correct. Table 5.1 shows that four correct out of five presentations corresponds to 60 percent, while three correct out of four represents 50 percent corrected for guessing. Five presentations are recommended if possible, with four correct taken as the threshold (i.e., 60 percent). This threshold corresponds to reading three out of five letters correct on a linear letter chart. Since there are theoretically 26 possible letters on a chart, guessing effects are negligible when letter charts are used.

SPECIAL CONSIDERATIONS IN ASSESSING VISUAL ACUITY

TEST ADMINISTRATION DISTANCE. For a person whose vision is appropriately corrected for distance and near and who is able to focus normally, the measured visual acuity should be the same at distance and near. Standard acuity measurements in adults are always done at a distance—usually of 20 ft or 6 m. However, measures of visual acuity in young children or children with multiple disabilities with low vision are frequently done at near viewing distance (within arm's reach) for the following reasons:

➤ Reduced acuity necessitates the use of larger symbols: The acuity may be so reduced that no symbols large enough are available for distance testing.

➤ The examiner may find it easier to attract and maintain the child's attention at a close distance. Testing should be done at near if the child will not attend to distant targets.

➤ The measured visual acuity may also differ between distance and near distances due to factors such as nystagmus, oculomotor control, accommodative ability, and uncorrected refractive error.

➤ Even though an individual's visual acuity is the same at distance and near, visual field limitations may make the measurements more difficult at a particular distance.

If possible, testing should be done at distance as well as at near. If quantitative visual acuity measurements have been done by the child's eye care specialist, and the functional assessment yields significantly different values from those found previously, it is important to contact the eye care professional to discuss the findings before discussing the results with parents and other teachers. In the case of children with multiple impairments, frequently no quantitative assessments exist.

EFFECTS OF LIGHTING AND GLARE. Lighting will have a much greater influence on results of visual acuity testing in children with low vision than in children who do not have visual impairment. The effects will also vary depending on the underlying cause of the individual's low vision. Children with retinal disorders will be more affected by lighting than children with optic nerve disorders or cortical visual impairment because the retina controls light and dark adaptation. For some children, vision function will improve as more light is provided, while for others the reverse is true. Some have a very specific optimal light level at which their vision is best.

Glare is primarily a problem for children with eye conditions that cause light to be scattered, such as corneal opacities, cataracts, colobomas or other large retinal scars, and retinal edema.

In general, lighting should be diffuse and even in the room where the test is administered. The child should be allowed to adapt to the room environment prior to testing. Even though many parents or caregivers, or the child himself or herself, are aware of the optimal light level for maximum vision, frequently they may not be conscious of fluctuations in vision that occur with changes in light level. Observation, careful questioning, and perhaps testing at two different light levels can reveal the influence of lighting.

TWO-ALTERNATIVE FORCED-CHOICE TESTING. When children, even newborn infants, are presented with two targets, one of which is blank and the other containing a visible pattern, they prefer to look at the patterned target. Most vision tests for young children and nonverbal children with multiple impairments rely on this preferential looking behavior. Two targets are presented, one of which is blank. The detail (or contrast or color) of the patterned target is made more difficult to see as the test progresses. At some point, the pattern is no longer visible, and the child shows no preference for either target. The stimulus that is just larger than the one no longer visible is the threshold—the smallest visible pattern in the case of acuity measurements or the lowest contrast in the case of contrast sensitivity measurement.

Presenting two alternative targets, such as two kinds of single symbols, and asking the child to point or look at a particular one appears to be a simple activity. It is, in fact, quite difficult. It is quite easy to be fooled into thinking that a child sees a lot more than he or she actually does due to examiner errors. The same is true for grating acuity tasks that present two alternatives: a grating and a blank field. The examiner should be conscious of the cues provided to the child. Presentations should not be alternated in a regular manner (such as right, left, right, left). Children learn to anticipate very quickly and the examiner can seriously overestimate the vision functioning of a child who makes accurate guesses based on the expected pattern of presentation.

The following suggestions are useful in optimizing the results of task presentations:

➤ Mix vertical presentation with horizontal. Vertical presentations are particularly useful if judgments are based on observation of the child's fixation and the child has strabismus (eye turn) or horizontal nystagmus: the vertical eye movement is easier to see.

➤ Some children keep looking back and forth until they are rewarded for looking at or pointing at the correct target. Feedback should be avoided until the child has made a final choice.

➤ Some examiners unconsciously place the correct target closer to the child. Be aware of where the correct target is placed.

➤ It is important for practitioners to be aware of their behavior. Even children with reduced vision pick up on subtle cues. It is sometimes helpful to have a second examiner present to make a judgment about the child's correct or incorrect choices.

➤ The child should be rewarded verbally or with food items (as appropriate) for making the effort, whether or not the child gets the correct answer. Some children are very hesitant to guess and need considerable encouragement to participate in the task, particularly close to their visual threshold.

➤ When approaching the child's visual threshold, the examiner needs to keep track of how many presentations have been made at a particular target size and how many correct responses the child has given.

➤ It is helpful to present even smaller sizes than the expected threshold to verify that the child, cannot, in fact see the smaller size.

➤ If the test distance is varied instead of the size of the target, it is helpful to adjust the distance to carefully improve the accuracy of the measurement. For example, if a child correctly identifies a 20-ft symbol at a distance of 2 ft four out of five times; identifies the same symbol two out of four times at 4 ft; and is able to point correctly to the same target three out of four times at 3.5 ft,

TABLE 5.2

Converting Raw Visual Acuity Measures to Equivalent Snellen Notation

TEST DISTANCE (FT)	NUMBER OF PRESENTATIONS	NUMBER CORRECT	PERCENTAGE CORRECT, CORRECTED FOR GUESSING	VISUAL ACUITY	MINIMUM ANGLE OF RESOLUTION	SNELLEN 20-FT NOTATION EQUIVALENT
2	5	4	60	2/20	20/2 = 10	20/200
3.5	4	3	50	3.5/20	20/3.5 = 5.7	20/114
4	4	2	0	4/20	20/4 = 5	20/100

Example uses a 20-ft letter presented at different test distances.

what does this mean? Table 5.2 shows that the measures at 2 and 4 ft indicate that the child's acuity is at least 20/200 but not as good as 20/100. The measure at 3.5 ft shows that the actual acuity is closer to 20/100, and the child's acuity in Snellen equivalent notation is 20/114.

OPTIMAL SYMBOL SIZE. Visual acuity is usually represented by a threshold measure of the smallest detail that a person can resolve. To read text comfortably or repeatedly and easily identify symbols such as those on a communication board, the text and the symbols cannot be at threshold size but must be suprathreshold (well above threshold and thus clearly visible). There is no agreed upon multiple of threshold size for comfortable viewing. Multiples of three times and five times the size at threshold have been suggested—three times threshold size for adults and five times threshold for children—and are used in the Low Vision Clinic and the Special Visual Assessment Clinic, University of California, School of Optometry at Berkeley.

OBJECT SIZE AT A FIXED VIEWING DISTANCE. Table 5.3 shows how to convert from a visual acuity measure to an object size at a fixed viewing distance for a series of visual acuity values. Table 5.3 presents recommended object sizes for both three times and five times threshold size. These values were determined as follows for five times threshold size:

➤ The first step is to determine the MAR from the acuity. For example, if a child's acuity is 20/200, the MAR is 10 minutes of arc. This is calculated, as noted earlier, by dividing the Snellen denominator 200 by the Snellen numerator 20 (200/20 = 10).

TABLE 5.3

Estimate of Object or Symbol Sizes from Visual Acuity Measurements

VISUAL ACUITY SNELLEN NOTATION	THRESHOLD SIZE AT 1 FT (IN)	3× THRESHOLD SIZE AT 1 FT (IN)	5× THRESHOLD SIZE AT 1 FT (IN)
20/50	0.04	0.13	0.22
20/60	0.05	0.16	0.26
20/70	0.06	0.18	0.31
20/80	0.07	0.21	0.35
20/100	0.09	0.26	0.44
20/150	0.13	0.39	0.66
20/200	0.17	0.52	0.87
20/300	0.26	0.79	1.31
20/400	0.35	1.05	1.76
20/600	0.53	1.58	2.67
20/800	0.69	2.11	3.59
20/1000	0.87	2.66	4.57
20/1200	1.04	3.22	5.60
20/1600	1.40	4.37	7.89
20/2000	2.14	5.60	10.68

Rule of thumb at 12 in (assumes three times smallest visible or threshold size):
20/100 = 1/4-in object
20/200 = 1/2-in object
20/300 = 3/4-in object
20/400 = 1-in object

➤ The MAR refers to the detail of the smallest resolvable symbol. The symbol itself is five times that size, so the symbol has an angular size of 50 minutes of arc ($5 \times 10 = 50$).

➤ The recommended symbol size for educational use should be five times larger than the threshold size, which means that symbol size will be 250 minutes of arc in this example ($50 \times 5 = 250$).

➤ This corresponds to an angular size of 4.17 degrees ($250/60 = 4.17$ degrees), since there are 60 minutes of arc in a degree.

➤ To determine what size this symbol should be in inches for a particular viewing distance, take the tangent of the angle and multiply by the distance. In this example, to determine the size of the recommended symbol for a viewing distance of 12 in, take the tangent of 4.17 degrees and multiply by 12, which gives 0.87 in ($\tan 4.17 = 0.07291$; $12 \times 0.07291 = 0.87$).

➤ How large would the symbol need to be at a distance of 3 ft? In order to maintain the same angular size, the symbol has to be three times larger, or 2.6 in ($0.87 \times 3 = 2.62$).

Visual Fields

Visual field loss can be caused by abnormalities of the eye itself, damage to the optic nerve or the pathways leading to the brain, or damage to areas of the brain that process visual information. Some disorders produce specific and predictable visual field loss. For example, a child with large bilateral colobomas will have a superior visual field loss since the colobomas affect the inferior retina. A person with damage to the right visual cortex will have a left hemianopia; loss of the left visual field in both eyes. If there is visual field loss in one eye only, and the testing is done binocularly, the field loss will not be detected since most of the visual field overlaps between the two eyes. There is a small temporal crescent for each eye, which is only seen by that eye.

TWO GENERAL MEASUREMENT TECHNIQUES

Two distinctly different techniques are used clinically to assess the quality of the visual field. One estimates the extent of the peripheral visual field using different sized moving targets. It is called kinetic perimetry and is performed using a Goldman perimeter. The other method measures the sensitivity of the central and midperipheral visual field by finding the threshold for detection of a light of a fixed size presented on a fixed intensity background in various fixed locations within the central 30 to 60 degrees. It is called static perimetry and is used by most automated perimeters.

It is almost impossible to perform static perimetry in young children or children with multiple disabilities since it requires accurate and maintained central fixation and the ability to respond to the lights by pushing a button. This task is too difficult even for some adults.

CONFRONTATION FIELD TECHNIQUE

It is possible to assess the extent of the peripheral visual field crudely in young children or children with multiple impairments using confrontation visual field techniques similar to kinetic perimetry. The general method is as follows:

➤ The child's attention is directed by the examiner to a central target while another person presents the test target by moving it with uniform speed from a location behind the child.

➤ A small light in a dim room is a high-contrast target. If presented to a child with a normal visual field, this target will elicit an almost involuntary eye movement to pick up fixation on the light.

➤ The examiner then must judge the angle between the child's eyes and the test light when the child noticed the light. See the section on Peripheral Visual Fields in Appendix 5.1, Functional Vision Evaluation Report, at the end of this chapter for more information on estimating the angle.

➤ The light is presented to various locations in the child's peripheral visual field from above, below, the right and left sides, and, sometimes, from positions in between these orientations. It should be moved from behind all the way in front of the face until the child responds.

➤ It is important for the examiner and others in the room not to give auditory cues to the location of the test target, such as the clicking made when turning the test light on and off.

➤ Because of the inexactness of the method, multiple presentations must be made for each orientation. This provides the examiner with a reasonable estimate of the extent of visual field and the reliability of the results.

➤ Measurements of visual field in adults are normally monocularly (with each eye alone); for the purpose of functional visual assessment, binocular testing is used.

Since children with multiple impairments frequently have irregular fixation, nystagmus, variable eye turns, and take a long time to respond to a stimulus (have long latencies), this method is at best a crude measure of their peripheral visual field. However, it is possible to detect serious field losses due to pathological conditions of the eyes or visual pathways. The extent of the field will depend primarily on the light level in the room, as well as the size and the contrast of the test target. The author uses a flashing small light (a diode) mounted on a fairly long black stick, which is moved slowly starting behind the child until the child makes an eye movement to fixate the target.

LIGHT LEVEL

In persons with retinal disorders, the extent of visual field loss and its dependence on light level are closely related to the type of receptor affected. An example of extreme light level dependence of the visual fields can be found in patients with retinitis pigmentosa and in children with Usher's syndrome, a disorder involving congenital deafness and retinitis pigmentosa. The field measurements tested under conditions of very dim lighting will show the earliest abnormalities, since this disorder affects rods initially. Measures at higher light levels can be completely normal, while very dim conditions document severely reduced fields. As the disease progresses, the light level at which the field is affected increases until field abnormalities are seen at light levels equivalent to outside daylight.

Figure 5.1 shows the extent of the peripheral visual field for children with Usher's syndrome tested at several different light levels (Haegerstrom-Portnoy, 1998). A 1 cm black target was presented on rear-illuminated backgrounds of different light levels. Testing was done binocularly. An observer free from ocular disease would have the same size of visual field at all these light levels (indicated

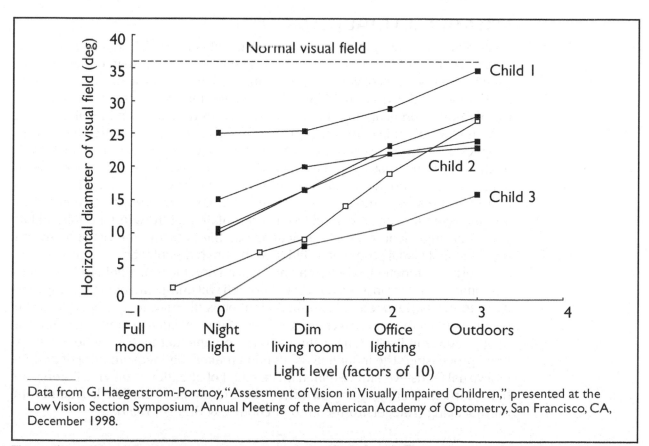

Data from G. Haegerstrom-Portnoy, "Assessment of Vision in Visually Impaired Children," presented at the Low Vision Section Symposium, Annual Meeting of the American Academy of Optometry, San Francisco, CA, December 1998.

Figure 5.1. Effect of background light level on peripheral visual field in children with Usher's syndrome. The size of the horizontal diameter (in degrees) is shown as a function of background light level for several children with Usher's syndrome. The dashed line indicates normal visual fields for these testing conditions. The normal visual field is shown to be unchanged for these light levels. The small value of the maximum size of the visual field for the normal observers was determined by the testing conditions.

by the dashed line). The test conditions used in Figure 5.1 only allowed measurements of the field indicated by the dashed line, even though the normal visual field, of course, is much larger than indicated.

The results indicated by Child 1 in Figure 5.1 show a fairly large horizontal diameter at the highest light level corresponding to outdoor conditions. The field decreases only slightly with decreasing light levels. The child represented by line 2 (open symbols) has a horizontal diameter of about 27 degrees when tested at outdoor light levels, but the visual field constricts dramatically with decreasing light level. At night light levels, the field has essentially collapsed. These results indicate the difficulty of categorizing patients as legally blind on the basis of the extent of the visual field (see Chap. 2), since the size of the visual field depends dramatically on the light level used for testing.

Children with other retinal disorders such as albinism and achromatopsia will prefer lower light levels and their vision functioning will be worse in outdoor environments.

ATTENTIONAL VISUAL FIELDS

Visual field loss normally refers to loss of the field caused by organic pathology. There are parts of the visual field where a target cannot be seen or can only be seen if it is very bright or very large, or both. Even though some diseases produce fluctuations in the visual field loss, these fluctuations are modest compared to the phenomenon of attentional visual field loss frequently seen in children with various types of brain damage. In many of these children, if they are attending to a central task directly before them, they frequently do not respond at all to very bright, very large, moving or flashing targets presented in their peripheral visual field. They have no functional peripheral visual fields when a central task is required at the same time that the peripheral targets are presented. When they are not asked to fixate a central target, presentation of the same peripheral target results in a clear response, indicating that the eyes and the visual pathways up to the first visual processing station in the brain are intact.

In terms of function, whether a child has an organic visual field loss or an attentional visual field loss is irrelevant. The child will bump into objects or trip over them to the same extent if his or her attention is diverted to another task as he or she would if the loss was caused by brain damage. Such an unusual influence of attention is in itself an indication of other organic damage at higher levels of brain processing. The influence of attention makes the measurement of peripheral visual fields even more difficult. The effect of attention seen in children with brain damage is an exaggerated form of the attentional visual field loss seen with normal aging (Haegerstrom-Portnoy, Schneck, & Brabyn, 1999).

Contrast Sensitivity

Contrast sensitivity is the ability to detect and discriminate subtle differences in brightness between an object and its background. In clinical use, it relates to detecting subtle shades in large objects compared to their backgrounds. It is another aspect of spatial vision (see Chap. 2) that is different from visual acuity. Visual acuity describes the smallest detail that a person can discriminate; contrast sensitivity describes the smallest amount of contrast needed for a person to see large objects. Examples of tasks in daily life that depend on good contrast sensitivity include edge detection of stairs and curbs, general aspects of mobility, and face discrimination.

IMPORTANCE

In the normal eye, there is a strong correlation between contrast sensitivity, as it is measured clinically, and visual acuity. This has caused many to state that measurements of contrast sensitivity are unnecessary and redundant when measurement of visual acuity is provided. In people with abnormal vision function, however, the correlation, even though still present, is much weaker. In one study involving measurements of several hundred children with optic nerve disorders, there was a statistically significant correlation between contrast sensitivity and visual acuity, but the range of values was enormous (Orel-Bixler, Haegerstrom-Portnoy, & Dornbusch, 1993). For any value of visual acuity, the range of contrast sensitivity values varied by a factor of 50. In addition, for any value of contrast sensitivity, visual acuity varied by a factor of 50. For example, children whose visual acuity varied from 20/40 to 20/2000 all had the same contrast sensitivity. These results emphasize that, for an individual, it is impossible to predict contrast sensitivity accurately on the basis of measurements of visual acuity. In addition, in the author's experience of over 15 years of assessment of children with multiple disabilities at the University of California, evaluating acuity, contrast sensitivity, and general visual attentiveness, contrast sensitivity has proven to be a better predictor of visual attentiveness than visual acuity (Orel-Bixler et al., 1993).

Children with the same visual acuity, for example 20/200, can function quite different visually. One child, even though legally blind, can appear very visually alert, interact visually with the environment, and have no problems maneuvering in his or her environment. Another child can appear to have more visual limitations, hesitate when moving around, and not explore his or her world visually. The measurable visual factor that differs between these two children is usually contrast sensitivity.

It is possible to have normal contrast sensitivity even though visual acuity is severely impaired, depending on the cause of the visual impairment. For example, a child with a large central scotoma who is legally blind can have normal parafoveal and peripheral retinal function, and therefore have normal contrast sensitivity for large objects.

In addition to assessing contrast sensitivity for the purpose of a quantitative relationship to visual attentiveness, as well as predicting mobility, contrast sensitivity measurements can also provide information on whether magnification would be helpful for a child. If contrast sensitivity is poor, magnification may not be particularly helpful. However, if an adaptive magnification system also changes the contrast sensitivity function (through, for example, increased illumination), magnification may still be helpful.

Figure 5.2 shows the inverse of the smallest amount of contrast (contrast sensitivity) needed to detect a target (on the *y*-axis) as a function of the size of the target (on the *x*-axis). Larger size targets are represented on the left side of the *x*-axis. The solid line without symbols represents the human contrast sensitivity function for stationary objects of a person with unimpaired vision. This curve shows that much less contrast is needed to see large objects than small ones. The point where the curve crosses the x-axis is a measure of high-contrast visual acuity or detail vision. The peak of the curve shows the smallest contrast that can be detected and represents contrast sensitivity for large targets as measured clinically. It is also possible to measure other points on this function. When measuring low-contrast visual acuity using, for example, the Bailey-Lovie Low Contrast

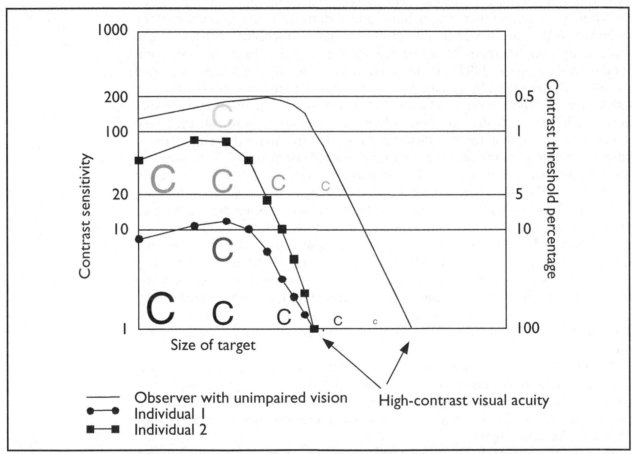

Figure 5.2. Contrast sensitivity and visual acuity. Contrast sensitivity functions are shown in stylized form for an observer with unimpaired vision (line without symbols) and two individuals with reduced contrast sensitivity (circles, squares). The inverse of the smallest visible contrast (left vertical axis) and the contrast threshold in percentage contrast (right vertical axis) is plotted on a logarithmic scale as a function of size of the target. The intersection of the curves with the *x*-axis (at 100 percent contrast) represents the smallest detail that can be resolved (visual acuity). Both observers with reduced contrast sensitivity have the same visual acuity, while their contrast sensitivity for large objects differs significantly.

Chart (see the Resources section), the contrast is set at some level and the size of the targets (letters in this case) is decreased until the location of the curve is identified. This size is then specified as the low-contrast acuity value.

Two additional curves in Figure 5.2 indicated by solid circles and squares, are theoretical examples of abnormal contrast sensitivity functions from two different individuals. The two curves converge to the same point on the x-axis, which indicates that these two people have the same visual acuity for high-contrast targets. The height of the curve is distinctly different in each. If magnification is given to Individual 1, his contrast sensitivity is so poor (he requires such high contrast even for large targets) that magnification may not help him particularly. Individual 2 has near-normal contrast sensitivity for large objects, and would significantly benefit from magnification of objects. Magnification in this context should be viewed as moving to the left on the x-axis (increasing size of target).

MEASUREMENT

In most contrast sensitivity tests used clinically, the size of the test target is constant (and large) and the contrast is varied in small steps from very high (black on white) to very low (light gray on white). Different types of targets have been used. Large letters are used in the Pelli-Robson chart (see Chap. 6 and the Resources section for information on specific tests), gratings (stripes) are used in the Cambridge Low Contrast Gratings test, and faces are used in the Mr. Happy test and the Hiding Heidi test, described below. Unfortunately, these different measurement tools use different units to describe the test results. The Pelli-Robson chart (Pelli, Robson, & Wilkins, 1988) results are expressed in log (Weber) contrast sensitivity units. Weber contrast is defined as the difference in luminance (brightness) between the target (the letter) and the background divided by the luminance of the background. The contrast sensitivity is the inverse of the smallest visible contrast and the log contrast sensitivity is taken as the logarithmic value of the contrast sensitivity.

The Cambridge Low Contrast Gratings (Wilkins & Robson, 1988) and the Mr. Happy test express the results in Michelson contrast units (not contrast sensitivity, which is the inverse of the smallest visible contrast). The Hiding Heidi test uses Michelson contrast units (expressed as a percentage) as well. Michelson contrast is defined as the difference in luminance (brightness) between the target (the letter) and the background divided by the average of the luminances of the target and the background. Table 5.4 shows the relationship among all these units. It is important to be aware of these different units in order to evaluate whether contrast sensitivity has deteriorated over time if different tests have been used for measurement at different times.

NORMAL CONTRAST SENSITIVITY. For young adults, on the Pelli-Robson chart the value of 1.8 log contrast sensitivity was found to be the average, with a standard deviation of 0.15. (Elliott, Sanderson, & Conkey, 1990) This indicates that values below 1.5 are considered abnormal (average value minus 2 times standard deviation). Testing was done at a 1 m distance. For the Cambridge Low Contrast

TABLE 5.4

Relationship Among Units of Contrast Sensitivity

MICHELSON CONTRAST PERCENTAGE	WEBER CONTRAST PERCENTAGE	MICHELSON CONTRAST SENSITIVITY	WEBER CONTRAST SENSITIVITY	MICHELSON LOG CONTRAST SENSITIVITY	WEBER LOG CONTRAST SENSITIVITY
99.9	99.9	1.0	1.0	0.0	0.0
80.0	88.9	1.3	1.1	0.1	0.05
50.0	66.7	2.0	1.5	0.3	0.2
20.0	33.3	5.0	3.0	0.7	0.5
15.0	26.1	6.7	3.8	0.8	0.6
10.0	18.2	10.0	5.5	1.0	0.7
5.0	9.5	20.0	10.5	1.3	1.0
4.0	7.7	25.0	13.0	1.4	1.1
3.0	5.8	33.3	17.1	1.5	1.2
2.0	3.9	50.0	25.5	1.7	1.4
1.0	2.0	100.3	50.7	2.0	1.7
0.5	1.0	199.0	100.0	2.3	2.0
0.3	0.7	299.0	150.0	2.5	2.2
0.1	0.2	999.0	500.0	3.0	2.7

Gratings test (and Mr. Happy test), a value of 0.5 percent Michelson contrast is considered as a normal level (corresponding to Weber log contrast sensitivity of 2.0). Under specialized laboratory conditions, contrast thresholds for large gratings can be considerably better than 0.5 percent but for clinical use this value is reasonable. The threshold for the grating test is lower (better) than the average results on the Pelli-Robson chart due to the sizes of the targets and the easier task on the grating (and on the Mr. Happy test).

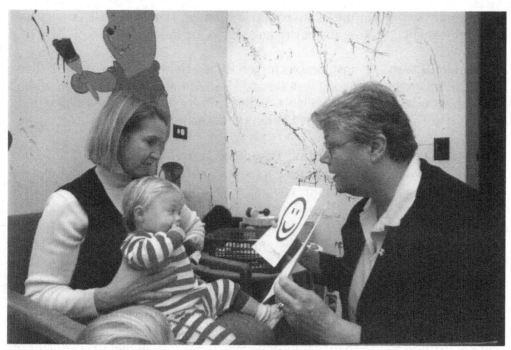

Administering the Mr. Happy Test to a young child. *(Peg Skorpinski)*

The same factors that affect visual acuity will also affect measurement of contrast sensitivity; for example, light level, complexity of the task, and the size of the target. Because the targets used in clinical contrast sensitivity tasks are fairly large, blur from uncorrected refractive error has much less of an effect on this measure than it does on visual acuity. If the child has a very high refractive error, he or she should wear any prescribed eyeglasses for tests of contrast sensitivity. If the refractive error is modest, no eyeglasses are required. Issues relating to the number of presentations, effects of guessing, and strategies related to two-alternative presentation discussed in the section on visual acuity also apply to the tests of contrast sensitivity described in the following sections.

TEST ADMINISTRATION. Mr. Happy Test. The target is used at near. The child is asked to point to or look at the picture of the face, which is presented together with a blank page in a forced-choice presentation. The contrast of the face is then decreased until the child shows no preferential looking.

The distance at which the test is done—whether 1, 2, or 3 ft—makes no significant difference to the result as long as the angular size of the targets is fairly large. The test should not be done at 10 ft, however, because at this distance, the angular dimension of the target is no longer "large."

The same caveats and concerns discussed in the section on Visual Acuity regarding two-alternative forced-choice testing apply to tests of contrast sensitivity that use this format of presentation. Contrast sensitivity testing of this type is frequently the first in the examination sequence, since the task is easy and children with all cognitive abilities relate well to the face targets.

Hiding Heidi Test. The instructions for the Hiding Heidi test are similar to those just provided for the Mr. Happy Test. Detailed instructions for the use of the Hiding Heidi Low Contrast test are available on the website that describes all the pediatric tests designed by Dr. Lea Hyvarinen (www.lea-test.fi).

Cambridge Low Contrast Grating Test. The Cambridge Low Contrast Grating Test is also a two-alternative forced-choice test, which presents gratings of fixed size but varying contrast in combination with a blank page. The test distance needs to be short (2 to 5 ft) to allow pointing or judgment of eye movements. However, the test is invalid if the child's visual acuity is good enough to resolve the individual dots that make up the gratings (stripes). Presentations are made until threshold is reached. Most young children or children with significantly delayed development do not relate well to stripes, but may be able to respond to the faces in the Mr. Happy or Hiding Heidi tests.

Table 5.5 classifies the severity of contrast threshold levels. In general, a contrast threshold of around 5 percent or less is considered severely reduced. This value is 10 times worse than the normal expected value, similar to 20/200 representing acuity, which is 10 times worse than the normal 20/20.

Light Sensitivity

With young children, each measure of vision function is dependent on the level of lighting used during testing as noted previously. Unusual behaviors related to

---

TABLE 5.5

Classification of Contrast Threshold Severity

CATEGORY	REQUIRED MICHELSON CONTRAST PERCENTAGE
Normal	≤0.5
Near-normal	≤1.0
Slightly reduced	1.0–2.0
Moderately reduced	3.0–4.0
Severely reduced	≥5.0

light often seen in young children and children with visual and multiple disabilities have also been discussed earlier in this chapter (see the section on Light Gazing and Finger Flicking). The examiner needs to use observation and interview methods to determine if a child has special sensitivity to light manifested through any of the following behaviors:

➤ excessive squinting in bright light

➤ consistent turning away from bright light sources such as lamps or windows

➤ an unusually long adjustment time when moving from dimly lit to bright environments or vice versa (e.g., moving indoors to outdoors on a sunny day)

➤ changes in performance levels for usual tasks in different lighting environments.

Color Vision

Color vision abnormalities are of two types: congenital and acquired due to diseases of the eye or visual pathway.

CONGENITAL COLOR VISION DEFECTS

Congenital color vision defects vary in severity from mild (most cases) to severe. Since these red-green color vision defects are due to a sex-linked recessive trait, they are more common in boys than girls. Blue-yellow color vision defects are extremely rare in the inherited form. The red-green defects occur with a frequency of 8 percent in white males and 0.5 percent in white females. The inherited blue-yellow defects have a prevalence of less than 0.007 percent (Adams & Haegerstrom-Portnoy, 1987). Most standard clinical tests of color vision, such as the Ishihara test, only test for red-green defects, (Adams & Haegerstrom-Portnoy, 1987). In such tests the person is asked to identify numbers against a different colored background. The book tests commonly used are all screening tests and are very sensitive; they will detect the mildest as well as the most severe defect but will not differentiate between them. Failure on a book test, even failing every plate, does not provide any information about the severity of the person's color defect.

The vast majority of boys with a congenital color vision defect have a mild to moderate defect (about 6 percent of the male population). Severe defects occur in only 2 percent of the male population. Only boys with moderate to severe defects will have difficulties with color vision in daily life, such as differentiating between colors and naming colors correctly.

A very small proportion of the population (less than 0.003 percent) has a congenital condition called achromatopsia or rod monochromacy caused by a loss of cone photoreceptors. This condition is associated with reduced visual acuity, photophobia (aversion to light), nystagmus beginning in infancy, and severely reduced or absent ability to discriminate colors.

ACQUIRED COLOR VISION DEFECTS

Acquired color vision defects are commonly of the blue-yellow variety but can also be red-green and may be caused by retinal, optic nerve or cortical disorders. In the more advanced forms of ocular or visual conditions, loss of color discrimination can affect all color combinations. When all color vision has disappeared, the child is diagnosed as having acquired achromatopsia.

TEST ADMINISTRATION

For children with congenital and with acquired color vision defects, their color discrimination will be more difficult with lower light levels and smaller test targets. A child with an acquired defect may be unable to discriminate between crayon marks made with different colors, but may have no problem correctly naming and discriminating those same colors when the area of color is larger.

No commercially available tests of color discrimination can be used for assessing very young children or children with multiple disabilities. Tests such as sorting colored blocks into groups of the same color are so insensitive that they may not even identify children with complete achromatopsia. The blocks have different levels of brightness, which can be used as a cue for sorting. The author has therefore developed a series of color vision tests that can be used to assess color discrimination in young children and children with multiple disabilities if they are able to point.

MODIFIED F2 PLATE. The first test is a screening test, which is a modification of a test designed by Farnsworth called the F2 plate. The modification consists of two test plates each containing a square (either solid or outlined) in a color different from the background and a blank plate containing only the background color. One of the test plates contains a blue square presented on a purple background; this is a screening plate for red-green color vision anomalies. The other test plate contains a green square presented on the same purple background; this is a screening plate for blue-yellow color vision anomalies. The plates are made by hand using Munsell papers. Detailed descriptions of how to create this test can be found elsewhere (Adams, Bailey, & Hardwood, 1984; Haegerstrom-Portnoy, 1990).

RED-GREEN SCREENING PLATE. The red-green screening plate is considerably more sensitive to color defects than the blue-yellow plate. One test plate and the blank plate are presented together at near in a forced choice method and the child is asked to point to the square. A minimum of four presentations should be made; three correct responses represent 50 percent correct answers, when corrected for guessing. The test distance is not important as long as it is close enough for the child to point to the plates. If a child fails either of the screening plates, further test plates are used to determine the severity and type of color vision anomaly.

PORTNOY PLATES. The Portnoy plates consist of six plates each with four colored disks. On each plate, three of the disks are the same color (green) and one is different. The child is asked to point to the one that is different. The colors are chosen along color confusion lines for deutan, protan, and tritan color defects from the Farnsworth D-15 color test (Farnsworth, 1943, 1947). Three plates contain desaturated colors while the other three contain saturated colors, which allows determination of the severity of the defect. If a child fails the F2 screening plate but passes the desaturated and saturated Portnoy plates, the child has a fairly mild defect. If a child also fails the desaturated plates but passes the saturated ones, the child's defect is moderate to severe, and the child is likely to experience difficulty with color discrimination in daily life. If the child fails the saturated plates as well, the child has a very severe defect. The Munsell papers used for the Portnoy plates are described elsewhere (Haegerstrom-Portnoy, 1990).

MODIFIED BERSON TEST. The final set of plates used if the child fails the Portnoy plates is the modified version of the Berson test (Berson & Sandberg, 1983). This test consists of four disks and is designed to identify achromatopsia. The disks are chosen to have the same brightness to someone who is lacking all cone function. People with rod monochromacy (congenital achromatopsia) as well as those with acquired achromatopsia cannot discriminate the purple disk from the three green disks since they have no color vision and all brightness cues have been eliminated. The Berson test will clearly discriminate between persons with rod monochromacy and those with blue cone monochromacy (Haegerstrom-Portnoy et al., 1996). The Portnoy plates and the Berson test all use four alternative forced-choice procedures for which 25 percent of the presentations could be correct with guessing. At least four presentations should be made. Three correct out of four presentations represents 67 percent correct, when corrected for guessing.

Depth Perception

Caregivers and teachers of children with visual impairments often observe hesitation on a child's part when walking downstairs, at a curb, or at a border between two materials such as concrete and grass. The caregiver or teacher often reports that "The child has a problem with depth perception." Most often, this hesitation is related to reduced contrast sensitivity rather than faulty depth perception (although the two are correlated, since good depth perception requires good contrast sensitivity). Visual field limitations may also contribute to difficulties in accurately identifying curbs and borders. There are many cues to depth including perspective, texture gradient, interposition, haze, relative size, shadows, and motion parallax (determining the relative location of objects by moving back and forth or sideways). All of the cues require only one eye; however, a particular form of depth perception is possible when using both eyes. This cue is called stereopsis and depends on the fact that one eye's image is slightly different from the other. The brain translates this disparity into a perception of depth.

STEREOPSIS

Stereopsis is a kind of depth perception that requires the use of both eyes, with equal and good vision function in both and normal ocular alignment (straight eyes). A child who has constant strabismus will have no stereopsis. Any child with a significant abnormality in one eye only will have reduced or absent stereopsis. A child with equal but poor vision in both eyes will also have poor stereopsis, even if his or her eyes are aligned. Stereopsis as a cue to depth is only useful within a few feet from the person (Schor & Flom, 1969). Beyond that distance, the other monocular cues to depth take over. Examples of tasks for which good stereopsis is helpful include fine near point tasks such as threading needles, pouring liquids, or reaching for objects within arm's reach. For activities such as walking, climbing stairs, and stepping down from curbs, the major cause of reported difficulties is poor contrast sensitivity rather than poor stereopsis.

People who are born with constant eye turns learn to rely on other cues to depth, even for near tasks, since they have no stereopsis. The majority of children with multiple disabilities also have eye turns, so measurement of stereopsis is low on the list of priorities in their visual assessment (Orel-Bixler et al., 1989). Many of these children are also visually impaired and have reduced acuity and reduced contrast sensitivity.

BINOCULAR FUNCTION

Stereopsis is usually measured as an indicator of binocular function and is commonly tested in children who have disorders of eye alignment (such as strabismus or eye turns). Standard clinical tests for stereopsis usually involve methods for presenting slightly different images to the two eyes through the use of either red-green or polarized eyeglasses.

STEREO-SMILE TEST

The Stereo-Smile test (Ciner, Schanel-Klitsch, & Herzberg, 1996) presents faces that are seen in depth through the use of polarized glasses. This is the only currently available test of stereopsis for young children or children with multiple disabilities. The contrast of the test face is fairly low and some children may fail the test because their contrast sensitivity is too poor to detect the face. The target consists of two slightly different images: one is polarized in one direction and the other in the orthogonal direction. By wearing the polarized glasses, each eye sees only one of the two images; the slight difference in the images in the two eyes is translated into a perception of depth. The face is presented on one side of a card in a two-alternative forced-choice method in which the examiner asks the child to point to or look at the face. The Stereo-Smile test includes a demonstration card as well as cards with two different disparities. The exact disparity (depth angle) will depend on the test distance (for a 55 cm test distance, the disparities are 120 and 480 seconds of arc, which means that they are 60 seconds and 240 seconds at a distance of 110 cm). A normal value for clinically measured stereopsis is 40 seconds of arc.

FRISBY TEST

Other tests of stereopsis do not require special red-green or polarized eyeglasses to generate the disparity but instead use a physical disparity. The Frisby test (Frisby, Davis, & McMorrow, 1996), is a four-alternative forced-choice test. The child is asked to identify in which of four squares a circle is seen. This test can only be used by children who are asked to point to the circle.

Accommodation

In order to see at near, everyone has to change the focus of the lens inside their eyes: they must accommodate. Accommodation allows near objects to be seen clearly. Accommodation is also linked to convergence: the two eyes move together so that they now point at the near target. The closer the object, the more accommodation is required to see it clearly and the more convergence is required. Young children usually have very large amounts of accommodative ability. Even though a young child who is visually impaired holds materials close, he or she normally has sufficient accommodation to maintain this close focus without experiencing problems or symptoms. Holding things close is frequently the only low vision "aid" needed by young children with visual impairment until the visual demands increase and accommodative ability decreases (usually around fourth grade or age 9).

The ability to accommodate decreases with age from infancy, even though most people are only conscious of older adults needing reading glasses. Teenagers and preteenagers with visual impairment may not have sufficient accommodation to maintain clear viewing of very close objects comfortably. Reading glasses or bifocals can help them. In addition, young children with cerebral palsy and Down syndrome may have severely reduced accommodative abilities (Leat, 1997; Ross et al., 2000; Cregg et al., 2001). A young child with cerebral palsy who is also visually impaired may need to bring objects close to magnify them but may not have sufficient accommodation to keep the objects in clear focus at these close distances. This child may benefit from reading glasses.

In adults and cooperative children, accommodative or focusing ability is normally tested by moving text closer to the person and having him or her indicate verbally when it becomes blurry. The inverse of the distance (in meters) at which text blurs is the accommodative amplitude (in diopters). For example, if text blurs at 0.25 m (25 cm), the accommodative amplitude is 1/0.25 or 4 diopters. This test is usually done with each eye in turn. In nonverbal children and children with multiple disabilities, this kind of subjective test is often not possible. Instead, if the examiner suspects that the child has poor accommodative abilities, vision function can be remeasured with extra reading prescriptions (additional plus lenses that make close near objects clearer without the need for accommodation) to determine whether the child's vision measures improve. The examiner may suspect poor accommodation due either to the child's clinical condition (e.g. Down syndrome or cerebral palsy) or to the child's behavior (e.g., rubs eyes after close work, avoids looking at near, dislikes reading, etc.). Such testing is best completed by an optometrist or ophthalmologist, since it involves the use of additional plus lenses, which should be placed in front of the current eyeglasses (if any). The additional plus power should be inversely related to the distance at which the child is holding the near material. For example, if the child is holding near material at 20 cm (0.2 m), the additional plus power should be 1/0.2 or 5 diopters.

SUMMARIZING INFORMATION

When a functional visual assessment has been completed, a tremendous amount of information has been gathered. Considerable experience is required to consolidate and translate this information for parents and teachers and other interested parties. Of course, the most important information to convey will depend on the individual child being assessed. In general, the following five points are commonly discussed in the context of making optimal use of the child's vision for communication and learning:

➤ How large a symbol size is required for the child to discriminate it reliably and easily from others?

➤ How high must the contrast be in order for the child to see learning material easily?

➤ What is the appropriate placement of materials within the child's visual field?

➤ Can the child discriminate color? Are there any limitations?

➤ Does lighting need to be modified to maximize the child's functional vision?

The optimal size for symbols or text should be calculated from the measured visual acuity, using the conversions discussed earlier in this chapter. If a particular distance is of importance—such as the distance to the tray on a wheelchair—the optimal size should be calculated for that distance. The optimal size for two different distances should be presented (i.e., if the optimal size for a distance of 1 ft is 2 in, the optimal size for a distance of 2 ft is 4 in). Understanding this angular relationship explains why the child does not pay attention to materials in the far distance if they are not large enough. Frequently, people who work with a child who is visually impaired with other disabilities are not sure whether the child's lack of response to a visual stimulus is due to the object not being seen clearly or the result of some other behavioral reason. Specifying the child's abilities in a conservative manner should clarify this situation. If in doubt of which size to recommend, err on the side of the larger size.

The more limited a child's contrast sensitivity is, the higher the contrast needed for materials used for education and communication. If a person's contrast sensitivity is moderately or significantly reduced, for example, photographs should not be used for communication; they tend to have much lower contrast than drawings done with bold markers. Contrast sensitivity and visual acuity can be poorly correlated, and it is not possible to predict one from the other on an individual basis. A child with normal contrast sensitivity but reduced visual acuity may appear so visually attentive and visually alert that parents and teachers find it difficult to believe that his or her detail vision is affected in any way. This applies particularly to young children who are not yet reading. A careful explanation of the difference between tasks that require good contrast sensitivity and those that require good detail vision is usually necessary. A common objection when parents are told that their child has significantly reduced visual acuity is: "But he can find the smallest things on the floor!" Detecting an object of any size against its background is a contrast sensitivity task; discriminating the shape of the object (e.g., whether it is a circle or a square) is a visual acuity task. Contrast sensitivity addresses the question, "Is anything there?" whereas acuity addresses the question, "What is it?"

A child may have only moderately reduced visual acuity and contrast sensitivity but may still show erratic visual behavior, responding to visual targets at some times but not at others. This variability in behavior may be explained by the presence of a visual field defect. If a visual field defect has been found, it is important to explain to parents and teachers where materials should be placed in order to be most easily seen by the child. Vision problems due to placement may also be caused by oculomotor limitations. If a child has difficulty moving his or her eyes in downgaze, materials should obviously not be placed in that portion of the visual field, but should be placed instead on typing stands or on a computer at eye level. The child's physical limitations and use of visual adaptations, such as head turns and tilts, also need to be considered when deciding where to place educational materials.

If the child's color vision is found to be poor, it is important to communicate that to his or her teachers, to minimize the frustration experienced by both the child and the teachers if the child is asked to make choices on the basis of color.

If questioning or testing has revealed unusual lighting requirements (whether more light than normal or less) for optimal vision functioning, clearly these requirements should be included in the discussion with parents, caregivers, and teachers. Sunglasses, colored filters, and environmental modifications to increase or decrease available light can optimize vision for someone with light aversion. Extra lights and sometimes lighting in all rooms can be helpful for those who need high light levels. Concerns about glare should also be addressed.

Providing a written summary of what is explained to the caregivers or teachers is essential, since many questions usually arise after the evaluation when everyone has had a chance to digest the verbal information. The summary form for providing a functional vision reports that appears in Appendix 5.1 can serve as an aid for organizing and summarizing evaluation data. The form is comprehensive, covering a wide range of assessment areas. Not all items need to be completed for every child. The information included in the form can also be used as the basis for the more extensive and complete written version of the assessment findings. See Chapter 4 for information about writing a final report. Appendix 5.2 provides a sample report documenting an 8-year-old girl with multiple disabilities.

CONCLUSION

Vision functioning of children who are visually impaired changes, and usually improves, with age unless the cause of the impairment is a progressive disease. The vision functioning of children with congenital visual impairment frequently shows improvement up until the age of about 8 or 10 years. In view of their changing vision function, infants and young children should be examined frequently—every six months or annually—while children over the age of 8 or 10 years usually need assessments every two years. Individual needs and different causes of the visual impairment (stationary or progressive) will determine the appropriate frequency for examinations.

Students with multiple handicaps involving one or more sensory anomalies, physical limitations, or cognitive abnormalities require the cooperation of many different professionals with different skills for optimal care. Communicating the extent and details of a student's visual abilities can help others involved in the student's care to match material used for assessment and education to the student's abilities.

REFERENCES

Adams, A. J., & Haegerstrom-Portnoy, G. (1986). Color deficiencies. In J. F. Amos (Ed.), *Diagnosis and management in vision care* (pp. 671–714). Boston: Butterworth.

Adams, A. J., Bailey, J. E., & Harwood, L. (1984). Color vision screening: A comparison of the AOH-R-R and the Farnsworth F-2 tests. *American Journal of Optometry & Physiology Optics 61,* 1.

Berson, E. L., Sandberg, M. A., Rosner, B., Sullivan, P. L. (1983). Color plates to help identify patients with blue cone monochromatism. *Journal of Optical Society of America [A] 95,* 741.

Ciner, E. B., Schanel-Klitsch, E., & Herzberg, C. (1996). Stereoacuity development: 6 months to 5 years. A new tool for testing and screening. *Optometry and Vision Science, 73*(1), 43–48.

Cregg M., Woodhouse, J. M., Pakeman, V. H., Saunders, K. J., Gunter, H. L., Parker, M., Fraser, W. I., & Sastry, P. (2001). Accommodation and refractive error in children with Down syndrome: Cross-sectional and longitudinal studies. *Investigative Ophthalmology and Visual Science, 42*(1), 55–63.

Elliott, D. B., Sanderson, K., & Conkey, A. (1990). The reliability of the Pelli-Robson contrast sensitivity chart. *Ophthalmic and Physiological Optics 10*(1), 21–24.

Farnsworth, D. (1943). The Farnsworth-Munsell 100 hue and dichotomous tests for color vision. *Journal of Optical Society of America, 33,* 568–578.

Farnsworth, D. (1947). *The Farnsworth dichotomous test of color blindness—Panel D-15.* New York: Psychological Corporation.

Fazzi, E., Lanners, J., Danova, S., Ferrarri-Ginevra, O., Gheza, C., Luparia, A., Balottin, U., & Lanzi, G. (1999). Stereotyped behaviours in blind children. *Brain Development, 21*(8), 522–528.

Frisby, J. P., Davis, H., McMorrow. K. (1996). An improved training procedure as a precursor to testing young children with the Frisby Stereotest. *Eye. 10* (Pt 2), 286–290.

Good, W. V., & Hoyt, C. S. (1989). Behavioral correlates of poor vision in children. *International Ophthalmology Clinics, 29* (1), 57–60.

Haegerstrom-Portnoy, G. (1990). Color vision. In A. Rosenbloom & M. Morgan (Eds.), *Pediatric optometry* (pp. 449–466). Philadelphia: J. B. Lippincott.

Haegerstrom-Portnoy, G . (1998, December). Assessment of vision in visually impaired children. Low vision section symposium conducted at the annual meeting of the American Academy of Optometry, San Francisco.

Haegerstrom-Portnoy, G., Schneck, M., Hewlett, S., Verdon, W., & Fisher, S. (1996). Clinical vision characteristics of the congenital achromatopsias. II. Color vision. *Optometry and Vision Science, 73*(7), 457–465.

Haegerstrom-Portnoy, G., Schneck, M., & Brabyn, J. (1999). Seeing into old age: Vision function beyond acuity. *Optometry and Vision Science, 76*(3), 141–158.

Hall, A., Orel-Bixler, D., & Haegerstrom-Portnoy, G. (1991). Special visual assessment techniques for multiply handicapped persons. *Journal of Visual Impairment & Blindness, 85:* 23–29.

Jan, J. E. (1991). Head movements of visually impaired children. *Developmental Medicine and Child Neurology, 33*(7),645–647.

Jan, J. E., Freeman, R. D., McCormick, A. Q., Scott, E. P., Robertson, W. D., & Newman, D. E. (1983). Eye-pressing by visually impaired children. *Developmental Medicine and Child Neurology, 25*(6), 755–762.

Jan, J. E., Groenveld, M., & Connolly, M. B. (1990). Head shaking by visually impaired children: A voluntary neurovisual adaptation which can be confused with spasmus nutans. *Developmental Medicine and Child Neurology, 32*(12), 1061–1066.

Jan, J. E., Groenveld, M., & Sykanda, A. M. (1990). Light-gazing by visually impaired children. *Developmental Medicine and Child Neurology, 32*(9), 755–759.

Jan, J. E., Groenveld, M., Sykanda, A. M., & Hoyt, C. S. (1987). Behavioural characteristics of children with permanent cortical visual impairment. *Developmental Medicine and Child Neurology, 29*(5), 571–576.

Leat, S. J. (1996). Reduced accommodation in children with cerebral palsy. *Ophthalmic and Physiological Optics, 16*(5), 385–390.

Leat, S. J., & Woo, G. C. (1997). The validity of current clinical tests of contrast sensitivity and their ability to predict reading speed in low vision. *Eye 11*(Pt 6), 893–899.

Lueck, A. H., Chen, D., & Kekelis, L. (1997). *Developmental guidelines for infants with visual impairment: A manual for early intervention.* Louisville, KY: American Printing House for the Blind.

Mayer, D. L., Beiser, A. S., Warner, A. F., Pratt, E. M., Raye, K. N., & Lang, J. M. (1995). Monocular acuity norms for the Teller Acuity Cards between ages one month and four years. *Investigative Ophthalmology & Vision Science, 36*(3), 671–685.

McDonald, M. A., Dobson, V., Sebris, S. L., Baitch, L., Varner, D., & Teller, D. Y. (1985). The acuity card procedure: a rapid test of infant acuity. *Investigative Ophthalmolgoy & Vision Science, 26*(8), 1158–1162.

Orel-Bixler, D., Haegerstrom-Portnoy, G., & Dornbusch, H. (1993). Relationship between attentiveness and vision function in multihandicapped patients with optic nerve disorders. *Investigative Ophthalmology & Visual Science, 34*(4), 790.

Orel-Bixler, D., Haegerstrom-Portnoy, G., & Hall, A. (1989). Visual assessment of the multiply handicapped patient. *American Journal of Optometry & Physiological Optics, 66*(8), 530–536.

Pelli, D.G., Robson, J.G., & Wilkins, A.J. (1988). The design of a new letter chart for measuring contrast sensitivity. *Clinical Vision Science, 2,* 187–199.

Ross, L. M., Heron, G., Mackie, R., McWilliam, R., & Dutton G. N. (2000). Reduced accommodative function in dyskinetic cerebral palsy: A novel management strategy. *Developmental Medicine and Child Neurology, 42*(10), 701–703.

Rowland, C., & Schweigert, P. (1998). Enhancing the acquisition of functional language and communication (pp. 431–439). In S. Z. Sacks and R. K. Silberman (Eds.), *Educating students who have visual impairments with other disabilities.* Baltimore, MD: Paul H. Brookes.

Schor, C. M., Flom, M. C. (1969). The relative value of stereopsis as a function of viewing distance. *American Journal of Optometry and Archives of the American Academy of Optometry, 46*(11), 805–809.

van Dijk, J. (1983). Effect of vision on development of multiply handicapped children. *Acta Ophthalmologica Supplement, 157,* 91–97.

Wilkins, A. J., & Robson, J.G. (1988). *Cambridge low contrast gratings. Instructions for use.* London, UK: Clement Clarke International, Ltd.

Functional Vision Evaluation Report:
Young Children and Students with Additional Disabilities

Assessor _____   Assessment date _____

Student's name _____   Birth date _____

School or program _____   Grade _____

Visual diagnosis: _____

Visual prognosis: ☐ Stable   ☐ Deteriorating   ☐ Capable of improvement   ☐ Unknown

Eye Care Specialist: Name _____   Phone _____

                          Address _____

                          Date of most recent evaluation _____

Visual acuity without correction from specialist's report: Right eye ____ Left eye ____ Both eyes ____

Visual acuity with correction from specialist's report: Right eye ____ Left eye ____ Both eyes ____

Visual field from specialist's report _____

Eye care specialist's recommended activity limitations _____

Summary and Recommendations (based on information gathered for this evaluation)

_____

_____

_____

_____

_____

_____

_____

_____

_____

_____

_____

_____

Source: Adapted with permission by Amanda Lueck, from Functional Vision Assessment Report, prepared by Stephen Sanders, Judith Norton, and Programs for Students with Visual Impairments staff, San Diego Unified School District, San Diego, CA.

1

(continued on next page)

Conclusion (for educational services only)

☐ Student has a visual impairment that adversely affects educational performance.

☐ Student does not have a visual impairment that adversely affects educational performance.

Other Evalulations Recommended

☐ Low vision evaluation   Reason _____

☐ Ophthalmological evaluation   Reason _____

☐ Orientation & mobility evaluation   Reason _____

☐ Other _____

Suggested Viewing Distances

☐ Chalkboard: _____   Prefers: ☐ Blackboard   ☐ White dry-erase board

☐ Television (screen size _____) _____

☐ Computer (screen size _____) _____

☐ CCTV (screen size _____) _____

☐ Class activities _____

☐ Wall clock _____

☐ Faces _____

☐ Sign language _____

☐ Movies _____

☐ Other (specify) _____

2

Contents

(continued on next page)

Checklist of Evaluation Findings

1. Optical Correction Information

Wears: ☐ Distance glasses   When prescribed? _____   Improves performance: ☐ Yes   ☐ No
                                         Wears regularly ☐ Yes   ☐ No

      ☐ Contact lenses   When prescribed? _____   Improves performance: ☐ Yes   ☐ No
                                           Wears regularly ☐ Yes   ☐ No

      ☐ Reading glasses   When prescribed? _____   Improves performance: ☐ Yes   ☐ No
                                           Wears regularly ☐ Yes   ☐ No

      ☐ Bifocals   When prescribed? _____   Improves performance: ☐ Yes   ☐ No
                                           Wears regularly ☐ Yes   ☐ No

      Condition of eyeglasses? _____   Adequate? ☐ Yes   ☐ No

2. Other Relevant Health/Medical/Educational Information

_____

_____

_____

_____

3. Additional Information Gathered from Student and Family about Areas of Difficulty and Preferences

_____

_____

_____

4. Social Behaviors Dependent on Visual Cues

☐ Identifies people from distance (specify distance) _____

☐ Identifies facial expressions (specify distance) _____

☐ Maintains appropriate social distance when talking (specify distance) _____

☐ Uses appropriate gestures (for school age students)

☐ Recognizes gestures of others

☐ Uses eye contact

5. Behavioral Impressions

☐ Responds to simple verbal requests

☐ Communicates verbally ☐ Communicates nonverbally only

☐ Responds more readily to familiar people

☐ Responds more readily in familiar places

☐ Has limited hand use (specify) _____

☐ Has limited mobility (specify) _____

☐ Requires minimal environmental distractions to stay on task

Comments: _____

_____

_____

6. Appearance of Eyes

List any unusual appearance of the eyes that should be evaluated by an eye care specialist.

_____

_____

7. Oculomotor Control

List any unusual muscle imbalance (eye turn). This can include esotropia (eye turn inward), or exotropia (eye turn outward). Muscle imbalances must be evaluated by the eye care specialist.

Right eye _____ Left eye _____

8. Sensory Nystagmus

☐ Present ☐ Not present Increases under stress: ☐ Yes ☐ No

Student naturally uses null point: ☐ Yes ☐ No

Describe head position for null point. _____

_____

9. Blink Reflex

Move your hand toward student's face with fingers spread apart, being careful not to move hands too quickly. (Fast hand movement could cause a response to air movement rather than due to visual cue.)

Displays blink reflex in response to: ☐ Light ☐ Hand movement

Comments: _____

_____

_____

5

(continued on next page)

10. Pupillary Responses to Light

The pupil should constrict under bright light and dilate when light is dimmed. This is an indication of light perception in people with ocular visual impairments but may not necessarily indicate light perception in people with cortical visual impairment. In a room with moderate illumination, observe pupil response to light by directing a penlight into one eye at a time from a distance of 12 in. If necessary, increase the contrast by turning down the room lights. Note whether each pupil constricts, dilates, or stays the same when the bright light source is presented and removed. Any unusual responses should be evaluated by an eye care specialist (e.g., no pupil response, slow or sluggish response, different response patterns between the eyes to the same stimulus).

☐ Both pupils constrict equally and remain constricted when light is present and shone in either eye.

☐ Other _____

11. Unusual Visual Behaviors

☐ Presses eyes   ☐ Tilts head when viewing   ☐ Flicks fingers in front of face

☐ Pokes eyes   ☐ Twirls or spins objects   ☐ Shakes head side to side

                                                   ☐ Other

Comments: _____

_____

_____

12. Awareness of Stimuli

☐ Responds to any stimulus (auditory, olfactory, tactile, gustatory, visual)

☐ Orients visually to light source

☐ Reaches for light source

☐ Orients visually to stationary, nonilluminated object

☐ Reaches for stationary, nonilluminated object

☐ Orients visually to visually stimulating pattern

☐ Reaches for visually stimulating pattern

Comments: _____

_____

_____

13. Sustained Fixation

Fixates on light source or object: ☐ Yes   ☐ No

Comments: _____

_____

_____

14. Shift of Gaze

Present two lights or two objects to the student in the positions indicated below. Shine, blink, or shake one object, then pause and do the same with the second object. Additional response time may be needed for students who have motor coordination or motor planning difficulties.

Shifts gaze from one light source to another in the following positions:

☐ Left to right   ☐ Top left to lower right
☐ Right to left   ☐ Top right to lower left
☐ Top central to bottom central   ☐ Lower right to top left
☐ Bottom central to top central   ☐ Lower left to top right

Shifts gaze from one object to another in the following positions:

☐ Left to right   ☐ Top left to lower right
☐ Right to left   ☐ Top right to lower left
☐ Top central to bottom central   ☐ Lower right to top left
☐ Bottom central to top central   ☐ Lower left to top right

Comments: _____

_____

_____

15. Following (Tracking)

Use a small object or light source that holds the student's attention. Move object or light slowly while it is within the student's range of vision.: right, left, up, down, circularly, and obliquely (upper left to lower right, upper right to lower left).

Follows object or light source 12 in away: ☐ Left   ☐ Right   ☐ Up   ☐ Down
☐ Circularly   ☐ Obliquely

Follows a person's movement: ☐ Within 3 ft   ☐ Within 10 ft   ☐ Within 25 ft

Following is: ☐ Smooth   ☐ Jerky

Follows across midline: ☐ Yes   ☐ No

Follows with: ☐ Head   ☐ Head and eyes   ☐ Both eyes   ☐ Right eye only   ☐ Left eye only

Pour objects from a container or roll objects on table or floor directly in front of student. Use a piece of felt to decrease auditory cues. Suggested materials include marbles, styrofoam balls, ping pong balls.

Follows rolling toys: ☐ Left   ☐ Right   ☐ Up   ☐ Down   ☐ Obliquely

Following is: ☐ Smooth   ☐ Jerky

Follows across midline: ☐ Yes   ☐ No

Follows with: ☐ Head   ☐ Head and eyes   ☐ Both eyes   ☐ Right eye only   ☐ Left eye only

Comments: _____

_____

_____

(continued on next page)

16. Eye Preference for Near Work

If student consistently holds objects under one eye rather than the other or both, that eye is the preferred eye for near work.

Eye preference: ☐ Right eye ☐ Left eye ☐ None observed

Comments: _____

_____

_____

17. Peripheral Visual Fields (Confrontation Field Test)

As a functional measure, it is not necessary to test each eye individually. Sit directly in front of the student and encourage him or her to look at your nose or at a light source (penlight or other small light) held directly in front of him or her. It is important for the student to maintain steady, central fixation. Bring a second light source in slowly from above, below, left, and right. This is easier if another evaluator stands behind the student and moves the second light source into position. Note when the student first notices the moving light source entering his or her field of view. If the student does not attend to the light source, dimming the room lights may promote student's use of vision. Visual fields should generally be evaluated with eyeglasses removed, if possible, since the frames can restrict the visual field.

Note: If a person is monocular, then only the visual field of the seeing eye is being measured and there will be an expected reduction in visual field on the side of the nonseeing eye.

Record any modifications made to target or room illumination.

Confidence in findings: _____

The following are examples of right visual field measurements for the right eye:

90°   45°

Right field: ☐ Full 90 degrees to temporal side   ☐ About 45 degrees
              ☐ < 20 degrees   ☐ No response
Left field: ☐ Full 90 degrees to temporal side   ☐ About 45 degrees
              ☐ <20 degrees   ☐ No response
Upper field: ☐ Full 50 degrees   ☐ 25 degrees
              ☐ <20 degrees   ☐ No response
Lower field: ☐ Full 70 degrees   ☐ About 45 degrees
              ☐ <20 degrees   ☐ No response

8

When moving, often bumps into objects: ☐ To the left   ☐ To the right   ☐ Above   ☐ Below
Often fails to notice objects: ☐ To the left   ☐ To the right   ☐ Above   ☐ Below

Comments: _____

_____

_____

18. Attentional Visual Field

When student is looking directly ahead at a central vision task of interest (object, activity, light source), move a bright light source or a large, bold object in different locations in the periphery (right, left, above, below).

Is aware of major visual activity in the periphery: ☐ Yes   ☐ No

19. Preferred Area of Viewing

Observe the student's visual behaviors during usual activities for preferred areas of viewing. Pay attention to direction and distance. For students with physical impairments, it is important to determine if responses are due to physical or visual limitation, or both.

Responds and/or reaches for objects or people based on vision alone:
   ☐ To the right   ☐ To the left   ☐ Above   ☐ Below   ☐ Directly in front

Responds and/or moves to objects or people based on vision alone:
   ☐ Within arm's reach only   ☐ Up to 5 ft only   ☐ Up 10 ft only
   ☐ Up to 25 ft only   ☐ At any distance

Comments: _____

_____

_____

20. Preferred Modes of Viewing

Natural viewing distance for viewing up close _____

Natural viewing distance for viewing far away _____

Describe head tilts when viewing. (These postures may be adopted to achieve the null point for nystagmus, to compensate for a peripheral field loss, or to view eccentrically if there is a central scotoma.) _____

☐ Must first touch or hear object before using vision to investigate it. (Often associated with cortical visual impairment.)

Comments: _____

_____

_____

9

(continued on next page)

21. Distance Visual Acuity Using Symbols (Optotypes)

Test administered _____

☐ With correction   ☐ Without correction

☐ Both eyes viewing   ☐ Right eye only   ☐ Left eye only

☐ With directional lamp   ☐ Under usual room illumination

Distance presented _____   Symbol size read _____

Visual acuity (test distance/symbol size) _____

Converted to equivalent Snellen acuity _____

Difference in visual acuity with different illumination: ☐ Yes   ☐ No

Describe difference _____

Confidence in finding _____

Test administered _____

☐ With correction   ☐ Without correction

☐ Both eyes viewing   ☐ Right eye only   ☐ Left eye only

☐ With directional lamp   ☐ Under usual room illumination

Distance presented _____   Symbol size read _____

Visual acuity (test distance/symbol size) _____

Converted to equivalent Snellen acuity _____

Difference in visual acuity with different illumination: ☐ Yes   ☐ No

Describe difference _____

Confidence in finding _____

Test administered _____

☐ With correction   ☐ Without correction

☐ Both eyes viewing   ☐ Right eye only   ☐ Left eye only

☐ With directional lamp   ☐ Under usual room illumination

Distance presented _____   Symbol size read _____

Visual acuity (test distance/symbol size) _____

Converted to equivalent Snellen acuity _____

Difference in visual acuity with different illumination: ☐ Yes   ☐ No

Describe difference _____

Confidence in finding _____

Comments: _____

_____

_____

22. Distance Visual Acuity Using Gratings (Stripes)

Test administered _____

☐ With correction ☐ Without correction

☐ Both eyes viewing ☐ Right eye only ☐ Left eye only

☐ With directional lamp ☐ Under usual room illumination

Distance presented _____ Grating size _____

Difference in visual acuity with different illumination: ☐ Yes ☐ No

Describe difference _____

Confidence in finding _____

Test administered _____

☐ With correction ☐ Without correction

☐ Both eyes viewing ☐ Right eye only ☐ Left eye only

☐ With directional lamp ☐ Under usual room illumination

Distance presented _____ Grating size _____

Difference in visual acuity with different illumination: ☐ Yes ☐ No

Describe difference _____

Confidence in finding _____

Comments: _____

_____

_____

23. Near Visual Acuity Using Symbols (Optoypes)

Test administered _____

☐ With correction ☐ Without correction

☐ Both eyes viewing ☐ Right eye only ☐ Left eye only

☐ With directional lamp ☐ Under usual room illumination

Distance naturally used _____   Smallest symbol size read at that distance:
(M units or point size) _____

Closest working distance _____   Smallest symbol size read at that distance:
(M units or point size) _____

Distance presented for test protocol _____   Smallest symbol size read (M units or
point size) _____

Confidence in finding _____

11

(continued on next page)

Test administered _____

☐ With correction   ☐ Without correction

☐ Both eyes viewing   ☐ Right eye only   ☐ Left eye only

☐ With directional lamp   ☐ Under usual room illumination

Distance naturally used _____   Smallest symbol size read at that distance:
(M units or point size) _____

Closest working distance _____   Smallest symbol size read at that distance:
(M units or point size) _____

Distance presented for test protocol _____   Smallest symbol size read (M units or
point size) _____

Confidence in finding _____

Comments: _____

_____

_____

24. Contrast Sensitivity

Normal Michelson contrast is 0.5 percent. A student with 3.0 percent Michelson contrast, for example, requires contrast to be six times greater than normal for optimal viewing. Normal Weber contrast is 1.0 percent to 2.0 percent.

Test administered _____

☐ With correction   ☐ Without correction

☐ Both eyes viewing

☐ With directional lamp   ☐ Under usual room illumination

Distance presented _____   Lowest percent contrast noted _____

How many times greater than normal contrast required _____

☐ Relatively normal contrast sensitivity (up to 1.5 percent Michelson contrast or 3 percent Weber contrast)

☐ Moderately reduced contrast sensitivity (2.0 percent to 4.5 percent Michelson contrast or 3.5 percent to 9 percent Weber contrast)

☐ Severely reduced contrast sensitivity (over 4.5 percent Michelson contrast or over 9 percent Weber contrast)

Confidence in finding _____

Test administered _____

☐ With correction   ☐ Without correction

☐ Both eyes viewing

☐ With directional lamp   ☐ Under usual room illumination

Distance presented _____   Lowest percent contrast noted _____

How many times greater than normal contrast required _____

☐ Relatively normal contrast sensitivity (up to 1.5 percent Michelson contrast or 3 percent Weber contrast)

☐ Moderately reduced contrast sensitivity (2.0 percent to 4.5 percent Michelson contrast or 3.5 percent to 9 percent Weber contrast)

☐ Severely reduced contrast sensitivity (over 4.5 percent Michelson contrast or over 9 percent Weber contrast)

Confidence in finding _____

Comments: _____

_____

_____

25. Stereopsis

This is of importance for fine near tasks such as threading needles, pouring liquids, or reaching for objects within arm's reach. For activities such as walking, climbing stairs, and stepping down from curbs, the major cause of reported difficulties is poor contrast sensitivity rather than poor stereopsis. Commercially available tests include the Stereo Smile or the Frisby Test.

Test administered _____

Test results indicate reduced stereopsis: ☐ Yes   ☐ No

Comments: _____

_____

_____

26. Light Sensitivity

Light sensitivity is best determined through observation and by comparing performance with and without a directional lamp. A test of visual acuity is a good way to assess for possible performance differences. Be sure to observe lighting needs of students who must lie on their backs in the classroom; in some cases, overhead lights may be uncomfortable for them.

General lighting requirements: ☐ Very bright   ☐ Normal   ☐ Dim

Outdoors, student prefers to use: ☐ Baseball cap   ☐ Visor   ☐ Sunglasses

☐ Requires tinted lenses indoors

☐ Squints in bright light   ☐ Avoids looking toward bright light

☐ Visually disoriented for _____ minutes when going from indoors to outdoors

☐ Visually disoriented for _____ minutes when going from outdoors to indoors

☐ Orients using bright light source (window, lamp, sun)

☐ Performs near tasks more accurately or easily with directional light on tasks (based on information from observation or tests of visual acuity)

13

(continued on next page)

Comments: _____
_____
_____

27. Color Vision

If results of formal tests are not available, observe the student in free play to determine if he or she demonstrates any color preferences and if he or she can select, match, verbally identify, or sort items according to color. The latter tasks are not sensitive enough to detect color vision disorders.

Test administered _____

☐ With correction ☐ Without correction

☐ Both eyes viewing

☐ With directional lamp ☐ Under usual room illumination

☐ Red-green deficiency ☐ Blue-yellow deficiency

Confidence in finding _____

☐ Selects or points to named primary colors _____

☐ Matches primary colors _____

☐ Sorts red and green (make certain color saturation of test objects is equivalent)

☐ Sorts blue and yellow (make certain color saturation of test objects is equivalent)

☐ Demonstrates color preferences (specify colors) _____

Comments: _____
_____
_____

28. Visually Guided Reach

Using manipulative activities such as stacking cones, pounding benches, or beads, observe student's visually guided reach. Objects must be visually motivating for the student.

Visual reach for objects at midline:

    ☐ Curved motion when reaching

    ☐ Hand brought in from side then moved straight ahead

    ☐ Other _____

Accuracy of visually guided reach:

    ☐ Usually direct reach

    ☐ Usually overreach

    ☐ Usually underreach

Comments: _____
_____
_____

29. Sensory Preference

Using manipulative activities such as stacking cones, pounding benches, or beads, observe student's exploration and manipulation methods.

Explores using the following method(s): ☐ Vision ☐ Touch ☐ Hearing

Primary method is: ☐ Vision ☐ Touch ☐ Hearing ☐ Combination _____

Comments: _____

_____

_____

30. Visual Matching

If student has not matched objects during observation, present student with a single object to one side and a group of four objects slightly separated from the single object. Three of the four objects should be very different from the single object and one should be exactly the same as the single object. Ask the student to match the single object, or demonstrate the task and have the student imitate your action. Repeat this with different sets of objects.

Student matches objects using vision: ☐ Yes ☐ No

Describe objects matched most accurately. _____

_____

Attributes used for matching: ☐ Color ☐ Size ☐ Shape ☐ Texture ☐ Other

Comments: _____

_____

_____

31. Eye-Hand Coordination

Using a black felt-tip marker, make large lines on a white surface. This should be done in front of the student. Give the marker to the student and note if he or she makes any attempt to draw. If the student attempts to imitate you, make intersecting lines, circles, and various shapes of increasing complexity as models for the student. Consider student's grade level in evaluating him or her.

☐ Draws lines   ☐ Requires prompt (specify) _____

☐ Draws intersecting lines   ☐ Requires prompt (specify) _____

☐ Draws shapes (specify) _____   ☐ Requires prompt (specify) _____

☐ Colors within lines   ☐ Requires prompt (specify) _____

☐ Cuts along lines   ☐ Requires prompt (specify) _____

☐ Pastes within lines   ☐ Requires prompt (specify) _____

Comments: _____

_____

_____

15

(continued on next page)

32. Picture Recognition

☐ Recognizes simple pictures: smallest size _____

☐ Recognizes complex pictures: smallest size _____

☐ Recognizes black and white photos of people: smallest size _____

☐ Recognizes color photos of people: smallest size _____

Describe how student communicates awareness or recognition (e.g., touches picture, vocalizes, becomes excited, etc.). _____

_____

Comments: _____

_____

_____

33. Visual Perceptual Skills

If the student does not respond to pictures in order to complete a commercially-available test of visual perception (e.g., Motor-Free Visual Perception Test, Visual Functioning Assessment Tool, Test of Visual-Perceptual Skills, Frostig Test of Visual Perception), observe the following activities:

<u>Visual identification or discrimination:</u> Student can match identical objects.

<u>Visual closure:</u> Student can identify favorite objects when only a part is visible.

<u>Figure ground:</u> Student can locate favorite objects when they are placed among other objects against a busy background.

<u>Visual memory:</u> On viewing an object (viewing time depends upon student), the student can locate it among an easily visible group of objects.

<u>Object constancy:</u> When asked to find a specific shape or object in a group of objects, the student can identify the shape or object no matter what size is presented and no matter in which orientation the object is presented (right side up, upside down, etc.).

Test administered _____

Error pattern, test scores, and interpretation _____

_____

The student finds the following areas challenging:

☐ Visual identification/discrimination

☐ Visual closure

☐ Figure-ground

☐ Visual memory

☐ Object constancy

Comments: _____

_____

_____

16

Sample Functional Vision Evaluation Report: Juanita

Student: Juanita Brown **Age:** 8 years

Program: Misty Hills Elementary School

History

A report from an ophthalmological evaluation three years ago by Frederick Smith, M.D., indicated that Juanita has severe bilateral optic atrophy (i.e., degeneration of the optic nerve in both eyes) and cortical visual impairment (i.e., decreased visual function due to brain damage). The report indicated that Juanita fixates on a light with either eye but does not fixate on a grating test that uses stripes (i.e., Teller Acuity cards) to determine visual acuity (ability to see details). She had bilateral conjugate nystagmus (involuntary side-to-side, up-and-down, and/or rotary eye movements in both eyes). No significant refractive error was reported. Juanita has also been diagnosed with cerebral palsy and uses a wheelchair to get around, but her hand use has not been affected. Juanita has basic receptive language skills (understanding and responding to simple requests and directions) and some expressive language.

A functional vision evaluation report dated two years previously by Michael Ricassi, teacher of students who are visually impaired, indicated that Juanita always turned her head to place items in her central field of vision and rarely picked up visual cues if they were not presented at midline. Juanita rarely sought items removed from view or touch, and a verbal prompt was necessary to initiate a search that was often tactile rather than visual in nature. Juanita's viewing distance was 2 to 3 inches away and of short duration. Juanita would gaze briefly at new materials placed in front of her during tasks that required manual manipulation. Mr. Ricassi was concerned that Juanita might not have vision in her right eye.

A report from a functional vision evaluation dated 1 year previously, by another teacher of students who are visually impaired, Maria Rodriguez, indicated that Juanita inconsistently responded to the 200-ft symbol at 3 ft on the Lighthouse Symbols Test for Children. Juanita chose a working distance of 6 to 8 in on the Lighthouse Apple, House, and Umbrella Near Vision Tests and tended to position items on her left side. She viewed items as small as 1-1/2 inches in size. Juanita named green items with accuracy. Juanita was noted to fixate visually on objects, but this was rarely observed. Juanita consistently showed better responses for items presented centrally and slightly to the left of center.

Evaluation

The current assessment was a 1-year reevaluation of Juanita's vision needs in the educational setting for programming purposes. Juanita was observed during her school day in her school setting, with her vision teacher in attendance throughout the evaluation. Her classroom teacher observed portions of the evaluation in the classroom and her physical therapist observed an evaluation segment in the physical therapy room. Several tests of visual functioning were also administered.

(continued on next page)

Distance Visual Acuity

The *Bailey-Hall Cereal Test* was administered with both eyes viewing with no correction at 1 ft. While seated in her wheelchair, Juanita was presented with two cards: one was a picture of a piece of round cereal that was called an "O," and the other was a picture of a square. The task was presented at close range (1 ft) in order to maintain Juanita's attention. Juanita was asked to point to or touch the "O" and was rewarded with praise whenever she complied with the request. Juanita appeared to comprehend the request to touch or point to the "O," but followed task directions inconsistently. When Juanita was rewarded by "giving five" to the examiner (i.e., slapping the examiner's palm with her palm) for every response, her interest in the task increased. Juanita's interest in the task increased even more when she was asked to "give five" to the "O." Juanita consistently tapped the picture of the "O" on request down to the 10 ft symbol card but not the 5-ft symbol card when presented at 1 ft (1/10). This indicates an estimated equivalent Snellen visual acuity of at least 20/200. Juanita may have better visual acuity than was measured, since her attention to the task decreased with increased task difficulty (i.e., as the pictures decreased in size). Even when motivated to "give five" to the "O," Juanita had to be prompted verbally to look at the cards before she touched one. As the symbols decreased in size and the task became more visually difficult, Juanita required more verbal prompting.

Visual Fields

The *Confrontation Field* test was administered with both eyes viewing with no correction. The target was about 1 ft away. In a dimly lit room a penlight with a colored translucent toy monster cap was brought in from above, below, and from the right and left sides. A second penlight monster was held directly in front of Juanita in an attempt to encourage steady, central fixation, but she would look at it for 1 or 2 sec only, and its use was discontinued. Juanita was asked to find the single penlight monster as it was brought into her visual field from various directions as she moved her head and eyes. (Juanita would not tolerate a teacher gently holding her head still.) At times, her classroom teacher stood behind Juanita and moved the penlight monster into Juanita's field of gaze while the examiner was positioned in front of Juanita to observe her behavior. Juanita followed the penlight sporadically and did not appear to show consistent interest in it. She appeared to note it more readily when it was brought in from below and from the left. When she followed the request to "find the monster," Juanita consistently turned her head all the way to the right when searching to her right. She did not turn her head all the way to the left when she appeared to search in that direction.

Later in the therapy room, Juanita was in a prone position in a large sling, and a favorite yellow ball was rolled toward her. Juanita did not respond to the ball when it was rolled toward her from her right but appeared to anticipate the ball rolling to her from her left. Her vision teacher made a game of covering Juanita's left eye with her hand. She was only able to do this for a few seconds at a time. As a result, it was unclear whether or not the left eye was completely covered during the game, and information comparing left and right eye functioning could not be obtained with any reliability.

Contrast Sensitivity

The *Mr. Happy Contrast Sensitivity Test* was conducted with both eyes viewing with no correction at 1 ft. Contrast sensitivity examines the ability to see subtle shades of gray that can affect the ability to see facial features, detect stairs, curbs, or drop-offs. Juanita was presented picture pairs of Mr. Happy (a large face) and a blank card. The Mr. Happy picture was first presented at 100 percent contrast (black on white); the contrast was then gradually reduced. When Juanita touched the Mr. Happy picture, Mr. Happy "gave" Juanita a very loud kiss, which seemed to involve Juanita in the task. Juanita quickly and consistently touched the Mr. Happy picture down to the 1.2 percent Michelson contrast card in seven of eight trials, the lowest contrast on this test (normal Michelson contrast is 0.5 percent).

Color Vision Observation

Juanita was randomly presented with squares of four colors: red, green, yellow, blue. Juanita identified squares by color name upon request. She once confused red and green but corrected her response when asked again. She also said the yellow square was green on one trial but when asked again, she named it correctly and continued to name it correctly in subsequent trials. A red square and a green square were then placed on the table in front of Juanita. She was handed a red or green square and was asked to put the square down on the matching square. She was used to matching objects in her class and appeared to understand the task directions clearly. Juanita matched the squares with only one error, placing a red square on a green one in the first match in six. This was repeated with the blue and yellow squares, and Juanita matched six squares with no errors. This indicates that Juanita has some understanding of color, but a more specific test of color vision is required to determine any color vision deficiencies.

Visual Behaviors

Juanita was constantly moving her head from side to side throughout the evaluation. When searching for objects on her right, Juanita turned her head to the right. When she appeared to fixate carefully on objects that were held to her left, Juanita appeared to turn her head slightly to the right and move her eyes to the left. When Juanita was reaching for objects to her left in the therapy room, she appeared to turn her head away (i.e., to the right) as she reached. She did not want objects placed on or near her eyes (e.g., scarf, patch, hand). Juanita occasionally brought objects fairly close (about 3 in) to her left eye to view them and flicked her hand in front of her left eye.

When Juanita was being pushed through the school's hall in her wheelchair and children were walking on her left, Juanita reached out with her left hand as though trying to touch them. As she approached the classroom in her wheelchair, Juanita made a direct reach for the doorknob to her classroom door, which was to her left. Juanita identified large, colored pictures against a white background that she had seen before, often naming the color of the object as well as the picture (e.g., red shoe, yellow ball, green sock, blue shirt). Juanita did not appear interested in coloring with a crayon or marker or in looking at crayon or marker strokes on paper. Her teacher reported that she cannot visually identify her name when it is written in large letters. Juanita matched squares with various objects pasted on them (such as beans and pieces of sponge) or with colored raised glue designs on them. She protested when a textured sticker picture was placed on her hand but appeared very interested in feeling an unfamiliar, velvety headband.

(continued on next page)

Summary

Juanita appears to have limited vision. Her distance visual acuity is difficult to determine since her visual interest in tasks appears to vary with the visual and cognitive complexity of the task as well as with the other types of sensory input provided by it. Juanita is able to see isolated symbols and her visual attention to tasks seems to be longer when symbols are simple, large, and familiar. Detecting subtle shades of gray in simple tasks does not appear to be a problem for Juanita. She appears to detect objects on her left more readily than on her right. This type of behavior was also noted during previous evaluations of functional vision. Whether this is due to a right visual field loss or to diminished vision in her right eye needs to be determined by Juanita's eye care specialist. Juanita can name red, green, yellow, and blue and performs simple matching tasks with those colors. She seemed to be visually interested in her surroundings when moving down the hallway in her wheelchair.

During the evaluation sessions, Juanita displayed a number of behaviors that have been noted in children with cortical visual impairment: inconsistent visual interest in stationary tasks, increased interest in moving objects, interest in brightly colored objects, turning the head away when reaching, use of unusual head postures when viewing specific objects, and the need for verbal or tactile cues to encourage her use of vision for specific tasks.

Recommendations

1. Juanita appears to qualify as a student with exceptional educational need in the area of vision.
2. Juanita's eye care specialist should be consulted to provide as much information as possible about Juanita's field of vision and the use of her right eye for viewing. The eye care specialist may be able to help answer these questions: Does Juanita have usable vision in her right eye? Does she have reduced visual fields?
3. Information regarding general instructional strategies to promote visual functioning in children with cortical visual impairment was given to Juanita's teacher and caregivers at the time of this evaluation.
4. Visual material for Juanita should be presented within arm's reach, as this seemed to be her preferred area of visual attention.
5. Until more information is available from Juanita's eye care specialist, Juanita should be positioned in the classroom so that activities she is to be following visually occur from her midline to her left to make viewing easier for her. School staff should be aware that Juanita may turn her head in unusual postures to view material.
6. Since Juanita may not be able to follow fast-moving activities visually, it is recommended that she sit close to group activities and that all activities be explained to her verbally whenever possible. This will allow her to participate more fully and help her to develop listening skills.
7. Objects or pictures presented to Juanita should be quite large, of high contrast (e.g., black on white is higher contrast than black on dark red), and without distracting background designs or colors. While Juanita may be able to detect symbols that are as small as 1 inch in height from 1 ft away, she may not be interested in examining them visually because of their small size and cognitive complexity.
8. Juanita may prefer to look at colored objects and symbols rather than those presented as black on white. There was not sufficient time to determine this during the evaluation, but her teachers can experiment with this possibility when presenting symbols or letters. If colored symbols

are used, they should first be printed against a white background to increase contrast. Juanita's teachers should continue to use color to interest Juanita in her various activities.

9. When Juanita does not appear to look at objects, she can be encouraged to touch them first, or she can be prompted verbally to look at them. Then she can be asked to work with them visually. For many children with cortical visual impairment, a verbal or tactile cue is often required to encourage the use of vision.

10. Since Juanita often prefers to attend to modes of input (auditory, tactile) that are not visual, it is recommended that during any intensive visual instruction sessions Juanita be given breaks to use other input modes in favored activities. She can then return to the vision training with renewed vigor.

11. In children with cortical visual impairment, visual functioning can vary dramatically when they are hungry, tired, or ill, for example. Those working with Juanita should be made aware of this variable functioning, since Juanita may be able to see things at some times but not at others. Juanita's visual behaviors could be recorded at different times to determine if there is variation and if there is a pattern to her variable visual behaviors. Those working with Juanita must be prepared to be flexible and accommodate any variation in her visual behavior.

12. It has been reported in the literature that children with cortical visual impairment may not be interested in exploring plastic toys or objects since they are often difficult to differentiate from each other by smell or touch. It is recommended that a variety of real objects be incorporated into Juanita's instructional program for exploration, play, and learning.

13. Juanita can be encouraged to use her vision during functional tasks at school and home. For example, Juanita can be asked to identify objects visually before touching them (cup, spoon, bowl), choose between two shirts, or reach for a favored toy across her midline.

14. Since she appeared to use her vision when moving in her wheelchair, this can be incorporated into her usual routines at school. For example, she can be asked to find the doorknob to open the door, find the light switch (which can be outlined with high-contrast colored masking tape) to turn on the room lights, or locate different large landmarks outside various rooms at school that Juanita uses.

15. Juanita can be given special jobs in her classroom that require vision. For example, she can be asked to hand certain items to students and staff. This can be made into a pleasant game. Juanita can be asked to locate and point to a specific person, and she can then be assisted to move toward him or her in the wheelchair to hand that person his or her item.

16. Juanita might enjoy working independently with a simple computer program using a touch screen to learn cause and effect. When she presses a key or touches the screen, there would be movement on the screen and many changes of color (like a fireworks display). The images on the screen must be large, moving, and of high contrast to attract Juanita's attention. The touch screen overlay reduces the contrast on the computer screen somewhat. If the contrast reduction is too much for Juanita, the touch screen should not be used and keyboard alternatives can be considered (e.g., hitting one key instead of the touch screen).

17. Based on previous reports and observations during the evaluation, Juanita appears to be wary of touching certain textures, especially on or near her face. An occupational therapist can be consulted to assist in the development of a program to encourage Juanita to examine various textures, since touch is a primary learning channel for her.

(continued on next page)

18. Juanita should be encouraged to use her auditory skills for learning since auditory input is also a primary learning channel for her. Listening to stories, relating the facts, retelling the stories, and answering simple inferential questions might prove helpful for Juanita.

19. Juanita's teachers have tried introducing braille and print labels when working with Juanita to identify letters and her name. While it was reported that Juanita may not yet demonstrate sufficient sequencing skills to understand the composition of braille words, it might be worthwhile to introduce some braille to Juanita as a new texture for her to feel and to determine if she can associate a tactile symbolic label with an object. If possible, the braille words should vary in length (e.g., shoe, banana) so that they are clearly different. Braille labels could be printed on cards that Juanita can match to real objects. This exercise could be attempted with large print words and corresponding real objects also to see if Juanita performs differently with tactile or visual symbols. The goal would be to determine how Juanita associates the use of braille and visual symbols with the objects they represent. Another alternative to encourage object-symbol association for Juanita would be to use less demanding tactile symbols than braille that are matched to real objects, for example, matching a card with a piece of sock material glued onto it to an actual sock.

Evaluation Methods and Functional Implications: Children and Adults with Visual Impairments

ROBERT GREER

This chapter will provide the necessary background for assessing the functional implications of low vision in individuals from children to adults. Although the educational and rehabilitation concerns facing children and adults may differ in specific content, their functional capabilities to perform everyday activities using vision can be determined, in part, using many of the same assessment tools with appropriate modifications (National Research Council, 2002). Among the topics to be covered in this chapter are assessments using tests of visual functions, including distance and near visual acuity, visual fields, contrast sensitivity, light sensitivity, color vision, oculomotor control, and accommodation and the functional implications of assessment findings. In addition, the chapter covers evaluation of functional vision as it is used in tasks that are critical in daily living, such as reading, computer use, work, travel, and leisure. The chapter prepares the reader to administer various tests, to interpret test findings, and, most important, to understand the functional implications of test results. Once the test results are available, practitioners should be able to answer the question, "How do I best make use of these test results when caring and planning for this person?"

In order to perform an assessment of vision, some basic equipment is needed. In the Resources section at the end of this book are listings of information about sources of eye charts for distance and near testing, contrast sensitivity and color vision tests, as well as miscellaneous equipment such as penlights, occluders, and finger puppets. The examiner does not need to use all the items listed, but should expect to use a range of methods and materials to obtain comprehensive results. As noted, some tests are better suited to children, adults, or non-English speakers. Before focusing on specific evaluation methods, gathering of preliminary information through interviews and observation is discussed.

OBTAINING PRELIMINARY INFORMATION

Since vision loss can affect a variety of functional capabilities that are rarely amenable to one solution, there is a need for an array of tests for individuals with low vision. Individuals with impaired vision tend to have one solution for their visual problems (e.g., eyeglasses or contact lenses), until they reach their forties and then need an additional solution for near tasks (e.g., reading glasses or bifocals). Individuals with low vision, however, nearly always require many solutions to best meet their specific functional needs. For near tasks, for example, the possible alternatives range from increasing contrast to electronic magnification. To correctly determine which devices, environmental modifications, or training might be most pertinent requires interpretation of results from many tests.

Interview Guide

The interview (called the case history in medicine) may be the most important assessment performed during an evaluation of children or adults (see the interview guides in Chapter 4). The interview is the examiner's opportunity to find out information about the child or adult and to form a bond. It may assist with the assessments that follow by helping to set priorities among the tests to be performed. For example, difficulties with mobility may be the person's main concern. From the answers to questions asked, it may be possible to obtain a sense of whether the difficulty is due to of an inability to see contrast (Do you have difficulty seeing stairs?) or due to visual field problems (Do you often bump into things when walking?). In either case, measurements of contrast sensitivity or visual fields should probably be performed first to help answer these questions. In addition to the information about interviews presented in Chapter 4, the points discussed in the following sections should be considered.

ESTABLISHING A TRUSTING RELATIONSHIP

One of the most important tasks of the interviewer is to bond with the person being assessed: to establish a relationship of trust and make the person feel comfortable in the examiner's presence. These are important factors if the rest of the evaluation is to be fruitful. Individuals must sense that the examiner cares about them. This can be conveyed most easily if examiners simply listen, make eye contact, and become engrossed in what the person being examined is saying. It is important to be engaged in and curious about what is being said, just as one would during a conversation with a friend. Being relaxed will make the interviewee relaxed as well. With children, the examiner should attempt to converse on their level and not be overly clinical in approach. Not rushing through this part of the assessment will give the person being assessed time to think about the questions and reflect on his or her responses.

DISCOVERING PERTINENT INFORMATION

The interview next needs to enlighten the examiner about pertinent aspects of the individual's history. First and foremost, why is this person in need of low vision services? What is the most prominent problem? (In medicine, this is referred to as the chief complaint or purpose of the visit.) What is the person (or caregivers) expecting or wanting? This needs to be well understood by the examiner. If the person states that reading is a significant concern, the assessor must establish the details. What does the person want to read: the newspaper? the Bible? bills arriving in the mail? For a child in school, the most important challenge is typically dealing with schoolwork, reading books, seeing the chalkboard, and attending to and completing the various tasks associated with learning. Once again, if the examiner can get specifics from the child (or, if necessary, a caregiver or teacher) about the tasks that are most difficult, the assessment gains meaning and the examiner can begin to set goals.

Observation Guide

Chapter 4 presents some information on the role of observation in the assessment process. In addition, when observing an individual, the following behaviors may provide clues to his or her level of vision:

➤ An individual may have difficulty getting around without assistance if his or her vision is very poor.

➤ Those with very poor vision often do not make eye contact because of unusual eye or head movements that allow them to use other than central vision.

➤ The use of peripheral vision to see straight ahead, called eccentric viewing, may reveal poor central vision. Some people are very adept at eccentric viewing, while others make large searching motions with their head or eyes in an attempt to locate the area of their best vision. Others with extremely severe vision loss may not use eccentric viewing because it does not help them. Instead they will look toward a person but not really focus on him or her. It is as if they are looking through or beyond the person they are viewing.

➤ The individual may seem unaware of objects in certain portions of his or her visual field. If you shake hands, did the person notice your hand being held out or did you have to touch his or her hand to make the person aware that your hand was there? If you point out things in the room, does the individual notice immediately what you are doing, or do you need to give verbal directions as well?

➤ The person may hesitate when walking from one visually different surface to another, for example, from a dark carpeted area to a lighter tiled floor. This hesitancy may indicate problems with visual acuity, depth perception, peripheral vision, or contrast sensitivity.

Observations can provide information about a person's acuity, peripheral vision, and possible contrast sensitivity and will allow the examiner to begin deciding on testing methods to be used and their sequence of administration. In general, areas deemed most important to assess should be tested near the beginning of the battery of assessment. This ensures that the person being tested is the freshest and may yield results that are more reliable than if the test is performed when the person is more fatigued.

USING TESTS OF VISUAL FUNCTION TO EVALUATE FUNCTIONAL VISION

The following sections examine the assessment of the visual functions generally included in a low vision evaluation, including distance and near visual acuity, visual fields, contrast sensitivity, light sensitivity, color vision, oculomotor control, and accommodation. Many of these procedures can also be used to examine visual skills and abilities when evaluating functional aspects of vision. Administration of specific tests and implications for visual functioning are discussed for each.

Distance Visual Acuity

Measurement of distance visual acuity is probably the most familiar assessment of vision. When someone says that he or she sees 20/20 most everyone knows that this is normal vision. In reality, normal acuity is better than 20/20: in a healthy eye with its best correction, it is around 20/15, even in those over age 75 (Elliott, Yang, & Whitaker, 1995; see Chap. 3 and Sidebar 6.1 for a full discussion of Snellen notation). Normal visual acuity requires that nothing be wrong with the eye or the visual pathways leading to the brain, beyond the need for spectacles. Distance visual acuity is simple to measure with the correct equipment and an understanding of the principles involved in the design of visual acuity charts.

To accurately measure the visual acuity of a person with low vision requires charts specifically designed for the task. (See the Resources section of this book for a list of charts commonly used to assess distance visual acuity.) Standard Snellen charts are not well designed for measuring visual acuity in persons with low vision (see Fig. 6.1). Snellen charts have very few letters on each row in the larger sizes, which is where the acuity of people with low vision is likely to be measured. This makes the task for the person being tested much different as each row of letters is read. Most people know that the largest letter on the chart is an "E," and that it is all by itself. Reading this solitary "E" is not the same task as reading the rows composed of six smaller letters, which is the required task for those with unimpaired vision. In addition, the letter sizes change at a different rate in the largest sizes. The "E" (labeled 400) is twice as large as the letters on the next row down (labeled 200), and that row of letters is twice as large as the next row down (labeled 100). The rows with the smaller letters change by about 1.25 times from row to row. For example, the row of letters labeled 25 is

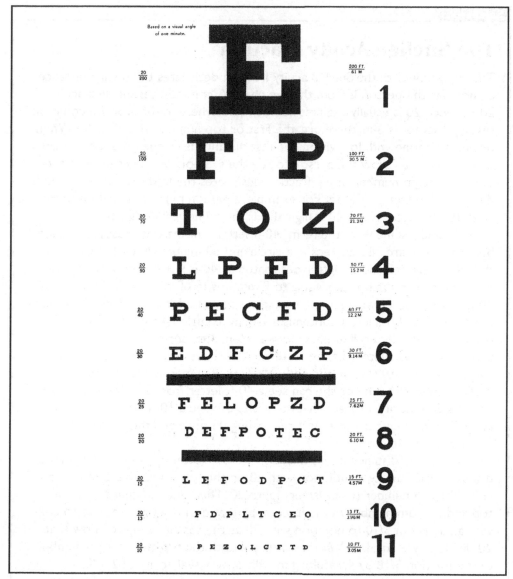

Figure 6.1. Snellen chart. *(National Eye Institute, National Institutes of Health)*

1.25 times larger than the row labeled 20. Because there are larger differences in letter size from row to row in the larger letters on a typical Snellen chart, one cannot measure acuity as finely in those with low vision who can only see these large-sized letters. These charts can vary in their design, and it is important to understand chart construction in order to select the one best suited to a particular person.

The Snellen Acuity Fraction

The top number of the Snellen acuity fraction designates the testing distance, or how far the person is from the eye chart. A common testing distance is 20 ft, hence 20 is usually the first number. (Elsewhere in the world, a common testing distance is 6 m; therefore, the first or top number would be 6.) When testing someone with low vision, the test distance is frequently shorter than 20 ft in order to allow the person to see the symbols on the chart. The second or bottom number of the fraction designates the letter size. Letter size is designated in feet or meters. For example, a person might read a 40-ft letter at 20 ft. The letter is not 40 ft high; this is the numerical designation.

To understand what the term "40-ft letter" means, one must first remember that there are 360 degrees in a circle and 60 minutes in each degree of that circle. By definition, a letter designated as 40-ft letter subtends an angle, from the top to the bottom, equal to 5 minutes (5/60 of a degree) when it is 40 ft away. In other words, the entire letter makes a 5-minute angle. Each horizontal stroke of the letter subtends a 1-minute angle (see Fig. 6.2 for an illustration). A 30-ft letter likewise subtends a 5-minute angle when it is 30 ft away and each stroke subtends a 1-minute angle. A 10-ft letter subtends a 5-minute angle when it is 10 ft away, and so forth. Thus, if someone has an acuity of 20/40, it means that he or she can see a 40-ft letter from 20 ft away. If a person has 5/10 acuity it means that he or she can see a 10-ft letter from 5 ft away. The top number represents the testing distance and the bottom number represents the letter size.

If the test distance is less than 20 ft, people often convert the reported distance visual acuity to notation with 20 on the top. To do this, one first divides the top number (test distance) into 20. Then one multiplies both the top and bottom number of the fraction by that quantity. For example, to convert an acuity of 5/10 to notation with 20 as the top number, we know that 20 divided by 5 equals 4. We then multiply both the top and bottom number of the fraction 5/10 by 4, resulting in a distance visual acuity of 20/40.

$$\frac{5}{10} \times \frac{4}{4} = \frac{20}{40}$$

CHANGES IN LETTER SIZE AND SPACING

Optotype is the original name Herman Snellen, a Dutch ophthalmologist, gave to the letters he used on his chart. The word optotype generally refers to the letters, symbols, and characters used on acuity charts. Acuity can also be measured using sine or square wave gratings, but gratings would not be considered to be optotypes. A square wave grating consists of alternating black and white stripes

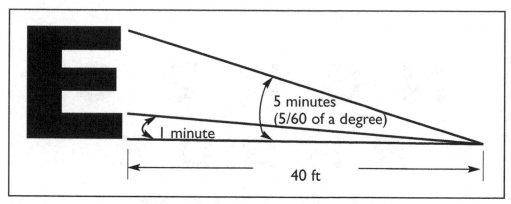

Figure 6.2. Angles used in the definition of Snellen letters. This is a "40-ft" letter.

with very sharp borders between them. A sine wave grating consists of black and white stripes that do not have sharp borders, but instead blend into each other. As already noted, typical Snellen charts seldom have enough letters in the larger sizes to obtain an accurate measurement of acuity for persons with visual impairments. If these charts are in a fixed position, as in most eye specialists' offices, the examiner cannot bring the chart closer to the patient if necessary.

A person's ability to resolve detail is affected by the presence of surrounding letters, symbols, or characters and is called contour interaction. Contour interaction was first investigated by Flom and co-workers in 1963 (Flom, Heath, & Takahashi, 1963). It can have a significant effect on acuity in persons with amblyopia and macular degeneration (Kitchin & Bailey, 1981). If an eye chart is constructed with more crowding of optotypes on some rows than on others (see the Snellen chart in Fig. 6.1), the visual tasks on these rows differ and affect the accuracy of the acuity measures. If the crowding is identical from row to row, then the contour interaction effect will be the same no matter where on a chart a person is reading.

Charts such as the Bailey-Lovie Chart, Early Treatment of Diabetic Retinopathy Study (ETDRS), or Distance Test Chart for the Partially Sighted (Feinbloom Chart) were designed for testing people with low vision and are reviewed later in this chapter. Some of the essentials for a chart to be used in the assessment of persons with low vision include portability and characters (i.e., letters, shapes, etc.) in a large range of sizes. The ideal chart will have the same number of symbols or characters in each row, so that as one goes from row to row the only variable is the size of the symbol. This requires that the spacing between symbols on a row and the spacing between rows of symbols change in proportion to the change in size of the symbols.

The Bailey-Lovie and ETDRS charts (see Fig. 6.3) are excellent examples of charts that have the same number of symbols in each row (five symbols), spacing that is proportional to symbol size (each row changes by a factor of about 1.25), and both very large letters and very small letters. Since symbol and spacing changes on these charts vary by a constant ratio (1.25 in the case of the Bailey-

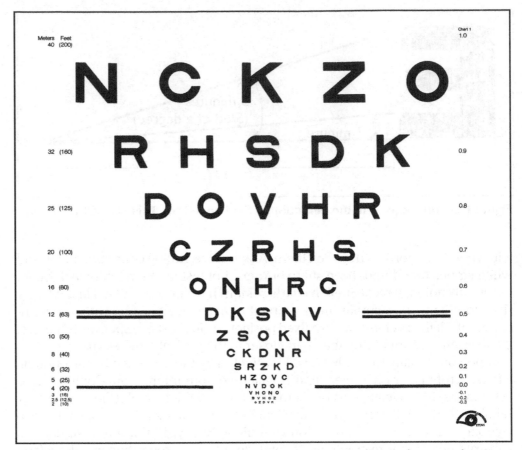

Figure 6.3. Early Treatment of Diabetic Retinopathy Study (ETDRS) chart. *(National Eye Institute, National Institutes of Health)*

Lovie and ETDRS), changes in acuity on different parts of these charts represent the same proportion of change. For example, on the Bailey-Lovie chart, moving three rows higher represents a doubling of the letter size and moving three rows lower represents halving of the letter size, no matter where you are on the chart. Bailey-Lovie and ETDRS charts are called logMAR charts (for logarithm of the minimum angle of resolution). The logMAR varies from row to row by 0.1. For more details on the construction of these charts, see Sidebar 6.2.

TEST ADMINISTRATION

A number of factors need to be considered in administering tests to evaluate distance visual acuity to persons with low vision. The chart should be placed at a known distance from the person. The distance is measured from the chart to the person, usually in feet in the United States (meters are used in most of the rest of the world).

The distance chosen for measuring acuity should allow the individual to read more than one row on the chart but not to be able to read all the rows on the

LogMAR Chart Construction

Minimum Angle of Resolution (MAR)

Visual acuity testing determines the smallest letters a person is able to read at a given distance. The size of the letter is not given in terms of its actual height but in terms of the angle the letter makes. If straight lines were drawn from the person to the bottom of the letter and to the top of the letter, one could calculate the angle created between the two lines. The smallest or minimum angle created by the letter is the one created by the details of the letter. For instance, the width of the black stroke that comprises the letter is a detail. If lines were drawn from the person to one side of a black stroke and one to the other side of the same black stroke, this would represent the smallest angle created by a feature or detail of the letter. This smallest or minimum angle is called the minimum angle of resolution (MAR): the smallest angle that letters can make and still be recognized by the person.

The MAR is the inverse of the acuity fraction. For example, the inverse of an acuity of 20/40 is 40/20. If you divide the top number by the bottom number you will get the MAR. In this example it is 2 minutes (40/20 = 2). A 40-ft letter makes a 5-minute angle when at 40 ft but a 10-minute angle when 20 feet away. In the same manner, the details of the letter also make twice as large an angle when twice as close (because the letter is twice as close to its designation). Therefore, if a person is able to read 20/40, his or her MAR is 2 minutes (40 ÷ 20 = 2). The MAR is always calculated by taking the reciprocal of the Snellen fraction and dividing it.

Logarithm

The log of a number is the power to which 10 must be raised in order to obtain that number. The log of 10 is 1, the log of 100 is 2 and the log of 1000 is 3 (10^1 = 10, 10^2 = 100, 10^3 = 1000). In our example of a MAR of 2, the log of 2 is 0.3 ($10^{0.3}$ = 2).

Log Scaling on logMAR Charts

The letter size and spacing on logMAR charts change by 0.1 log unit (about 1.25). The log scaling allows the letters to change size at a rate that is constant and proportional throughout the chart.

The largest letters on a Bailey-Lovie or ETDRS chart are often 200-ft letters. The progression of letter size follows this sequential scale: 200, 160, 125, 100, 80, 63, 50, 40, 32, 25, 20, 16, 12.5, 10, 8, 6.3, 5, 4, 3.2, 2.5, 2, and so forth. The numbers begin to repeat themselves, but with the decimal point moved.

The letter size differs from row to row by 0.1 log units, or approximately 1.25. Every three steps on the scale is a doubling or halving (depending on whether one goes up or down). For example, if one starts at 100 and goes three steps down the chart (step 1=100 to 80, step 2 = 80 to 63, Step 3= 63 to 50), one ends up at 50, which is one-half of 100. Three steps from 50 will result in 25 (50 to 40 to 32 to 25): 50/2 = 25.

chart. An appropriate test distance for measuring the distance acuity may be determined during the interview. If the person appears, based on observation and interview results, to have extremely poor vision, be sure to start with the chart very close, perhaps as close as 2 to 3 ft away. It can be discouraging to the individual if he or she is unable to recognize even the largest letters on the chart. The examiner is then forced to move the chart closer. This may have a negative effect on the person's ability to perform the test, since the person may lose enthusiasm for the test and be more pessimistic about his or her abilities. Conversely, if it becomes apparent that the individual has reasonably good vision, do not start with the chart so close that he or she can read even the smallest row of characters. This will not result in a measure of true visual acuity, because the person might have been able to read even smaller print when tested at that distance. Instead, increase the distance to the chart, perhaps doubling it, and continue asking the person to read down the chart. Because the chart is farther away, the individual will not be able to read all the available rows of characters and an accurate assessment of acuity will be obtained.

Charts need to be uniformly illuminated and without glare. Proper illumination may require auxiliary lighting such as a movable gooseneck lamp. In an ideal setting, the brightness of the illumination on the chart should be variable. This may be achieved by moving the gooseneck lamp closer to (brighter illumination) and farther away from (dimmer illumination) the chart. Some charts, such as the ETDRS, are available in back-illuminated versions but these require a special light box that renders the chart less portable. The advantages of back-illuminated charts are the uniformity of the illumination from edge to edge on the chart and variability of the brightness of illumination. If auxiliary lighting is used, care must be taken to direct the light only onto the chart and not into the person's eyes, which might create glare or discomfort and affect the test results negatively.

If, during the interview, the person mentions or it becomes apparent that his or her vision in one eye is poorer than in the other, measure the acuity in the better eye first. This also instills confidence in the individual, because his or her first exposure to the test is a positive experience. Acuity is typically measured one eye at a time. A measurement of binocular acuity may be of value when evaluating functional vision.

Because one eye must be occluded, some sort of device must be available to cover an eye. Handheld paddles, covers that clip onto eyeglasses, or conventional so-called pirate patches are all methods used for occluding an eye. Many eye conditions that affect central vision will cause the person to move his or her eyes or head in order to best make use of any remaining vision. When the person attains unusual eye positions or uses frequent head movements, a patch might be the preferred method of occlusion. The use of a patch eliminates the need for the examiner or person being tested to hold an occluder. For children, holding an occluder may be difficult and best done by the examiner. An occluder that clips to the eyeglasses or patches eliminate the need to worry whether occlusion is being maintained throughout the test.

Make certain that the person is wearing any spectacles appropriate for viewing at the distance used for administration of the test. If the person possesses more than one pair of spectacles, the examiner should ascertain which eyeglasses are for which distance during the interview. Without the proper eyeglasses in place, the measurement is meaningless when one is attempting to interpret the results.

Encourage the person to see the smallest letters possible. Encourage guessing. For the most accurate results, one wants to know the smallest possible letters the person is capable of reading at the chosen test distance.

Listen to how the individual reads the letters. Knowing that an individual is able to read efficiently if the letter size is large enough is helpful in anticipating what may happen when the person reads text or words. If the person was never able to read efficiently, even with letters well above threshold size (smallest size visible), it may predict that reading will be difficult, no matter what the letter size. Notice the following behaviors:

➤ Is the person moving along quickly from character to character or in a very slow and halting way?

➤ Does the person jump around in the row, rather than reading in order from left to right?

➤ If the person efficiently reads the larger letters but begins to slow down and become less efficient with smaller letters, make note of the size that he or she last recognized quickly and efficiently.

➤ Note if none of the letters is read with efficiency, regardless of size.

People with low vision will often read the eye chart very slowly. This may result in a great deal of fatigue. To prevent fatigue, have them read the first few letters in a row. If they read them rather easily, consider having them jump down to read the next row of letters. Continue to do this until the person is unable to read any smaller letters. Then return to the row where letters were last identified correctly and have the patient read across. Remember to encourage guessing; gently push the person being tested to continue reading until he or she truly cannot identify letters any smaller. This will be your endpoint and his or her true threshold.

The acuity measurement recorded is the row containing the smallest letters the person was able to read. If the person did not correctly identify all of the letters on that row, add a minus sign and the number of letters not correctly identified. If the person also identified letters on the next row, add a plus sign and the number of letters correctly identified. For example, the person was tested at 5 ft and successfully read all the 40-ft letters on the row. The acuity is written as 5/40. If the person read the 40-ft letters but missed two letters on the row, the acuity would be written as $5/40^{-2}$. If the person read the 40-ft letters and one letter on the next row down, the acuity would be written as $5/40^{+1}$.

If the examiner is using a gooseneck lamp to illuminate the chart, investigate what effect illumination has on the person's acuity. Bring the lamp closer to the chart to increase the illumination. Note whether the acuity is better, worse, or the same under those conditions. Move the lamp farther away from the chart, or turn the lamp off, and note the effect of that change on the person's acuity. Noting the effect of lighting will allow the examiner to advise the person better about his or her specific lighting needs.

Near Visual Acuity

Once the examiner has established the person's visual acuity at distance, it is important to measure his or her acuity at near. Near acuity is typically measured with word or text charts, if the person is able to read. If a child is too young or is unable to read, there are charts designed to measure near acuity that use characters, shapes, or numbers (these are discussed in Chap. 5). Distance acuity can yield some information about a person's ability to read, but near acuity measurements using text or words do it even better, because reading letters is a different task for the visual system than is reading a word or sentence. For people with macular problems, their word or text acuity is 1.5 to 2 times poorer than their letter acuity (Kitchin & Bailey, 1981). The effect of letter crowding in words makes the reading task more difficult than recognizing individual letters. Also, the person must be able to put together several letters to form the word: that requires precise eye movements and cognitive processing. Although it is accurate to give credit to a person for reading a certain row of letters on a chart, regardless of the order in which the letters were read, this is not true for reading words or sentences. The letters and words must be processed in the proper order for the individual to be able to make sense of what is written. It is, therefore, essential that reading acuity be measured and distance acuity not be used to infer too much about reading ability. (See the section on Reading Skills later in this chapter for more information on measuring reading ability.)

Specification of Print Size

Print size is specified in many more ways than distance letter sizes. Distance letters are always designed such that the letter makes a 5-minute angle when it is a specified distance away (see Sidebar 6.1 and Fig. 6.2). A 50-ft letter makes a 5-minute angle when 50 ft away or an 80-ft letter makes a 5-minute angle when 80 ft away. In order to make those angles, the letter has to be a very specific height. At near, the specifications are not as uniformly applied. Near print size is commonly specified in Jaeger (J), reduced Snellen, point, or meter (M) notation.

Jaeger notation defines the smallest print on this type of chart as J1, with J2 being the next largest and so on. Unfortunately, the fonts originally used are no longer available and the print size on Jaeger charts differs from manufacturer to manufacturer depending on the font style used (Law, 1951). Therefore, Jaeger charts should not be used to measure near acuity when accuracy is desired.

Reduced Snellen acuity charts have distance acuity fractions listed next to each row size. The charts are calibrated for use at a particular distance. When this is done, the near acuity is equivalent to the listed distance acuity. For example, if the chart is designed to be used at 16 inches and the person reads the letters labeled 20/20, the near acuity is equivalent to a distance acuity of 20/20. These types of charts are difficult to interpret when used at testing distances other than the designated one.

Meter (M) notation is the same size designation as used in distance charts but in a metric form. A 1M letter makes a 5-minute angle when it is 1 m away.

Point size refers to the block of metal once used by printers in a printing press. A point is 1/72 of an inch. An 8-point letter has a block that is 8/72 in height (Law, 1951). This does not actually tell you how tall the letter on the block is. It is common for lower case letters without ascenders or descenders such as "a", "c", "e", "m", "n" to occupy about half of the block. This results in 8-point print being equivalent to 1M print or 1.45 mm tall.

The letter size recorded will depend on the type of chart used: Jaeger, reduced Snellen, point, or M notation. Near acuity is written in the same way as distance acuity, with the test distance being the top number (numerator) and the letter size the bottom number (denominator). Another common way of recording near acuity is to state the letter size followed by the test distance: 14 point at 16 in., 20/80 at 20 cm, or 4M at 10 cm. It is typical to record M notation with the test distances also in meters but this is not required, although highly desirable (e.g., 0.4/1.2M). To convert between centimeters and inches, remember that there are 2.54 cm in an inch. To convert centimeters to inches, divide the number of centimeters by 2.54. To convert inches to centimeters, multiply the number of inches by 2.54. (For a quick estimate, use 2.5).

TEST ADMINISTRATION

Equipment for near acuity measurements includes charts with words or text. (See the Resources section of this book for a list of commonly used charts to assess near visual acuity.) If the individual does not read, then charts with numbers or others characters may be used. It is best if the charts include very large print (up to 10M or 80 point) and go down to very small print (0.25M or 2 point). If the chart is not composed of words or text, it should be constructed so that the numbers or characters are close enough together to simulate the crowding effects of words. A tape measure will also be required to measure test distances, and an auxiliary light should be available to illuminate the chart and assess the effects of illumination on an individual's reading ability.

Because reading or near acuity is a functional test, it is often only measured binocularly. If monocular acuity was measured at distance, it may not be necessary to measure monocular reading acuity, although it would not be improper to do so. It is possible for a person to prefer reading under conditions that are monocular and that should be noted. For the most part, individuals will read with both eyes open but possibly preferring one eye to the other. It is best to measure a near acuity under the same conditions that the person typically reads, whether binocularly or monocular. If the person does not know whether he or she reads with one or both eyes, then the examiner needs to ask him or her to read the chart and observe how the person uses his or her eyes.

For near acuity measurements, it is common practice to allow the person to hold the near visual acuity chart. Many examiners will simply ask the person to hold the chart at his or her usual reading distance. Be aware that the distance at which people hold charts can vary greatly. For young children and young adults, this is usually not a problem. They will typically exert some accommodation to bring the material into focus. Accommodation is an adjustment to the lens of the eye that allows people to focus at different distances. With age, people lose the ability to focus up close and thus begin to wear reading glasses (see Chap. 3 for a more detailed discussion of accommodation).

If the person uses reading glasses or bifocals, then the chart must be held at the distance appropriate for him or her when wearing glasses. This requires that the add power of the glasses be known. Add is short for addition and is the power, in diopters, that is in addition to their distance prescription (see Chap. 3 for more details). The more diopters a lens possesses, the more it will bend light. If the add power is equal to or greater than +2.50 diopters then the person should hold the near chart at the focal point of the add power to ensure that it is in good focus. The distance to the focal point, in centimeters, is 100 divided by the add power. For example, if the individual is wearing a +2.50 prescription, the chart should be placed at 40 cm ($100/2.50 = 40$ cm). A +4.00 add requires that the chart be held 25 cm from the individual ($100/4 = 25$ cm).

If the add is less than +2.50, it is not as straightforward. Adds of less than +2.50 are usually given to younger people who still have some residual accommodation. It means that the individual is going to contribute some accommodation. How much accommodation the person will contribute is not known, so it is best to have the person hold the material where it appears to be clearest and note the distance. (As a rule of thumb, the examiner can have the person hold the material at 40 cm or 16 in because this is a comfortable, natural distance for adults.) If a child is wearing bifocals or reading glasses with less than a +2.50 add, the child needs to hold the material where it is comfortable; this will vary depending on the age and size of the child.

As for distance acuity, one must measure the distance from the person to the chart. Most eye care specialists measure this distance in meters or centimeters, but measuring the distance in inches is also acceptable.

During near acuity measurements, it is extremely important to listen to the person as he or she reads. Make note of the smallest print he or she reads with good efficiency, as well as the smallest print size he or she could read. This allows the examiner to recommend print sizes that will make it easier for the person to read comfortably (see the discussion of the MN Read test later in this chapter).

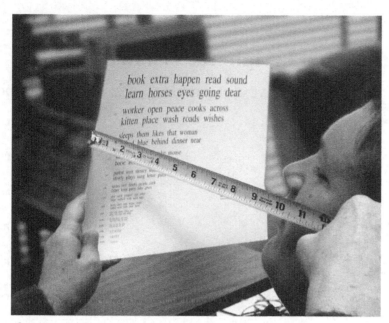

Measuring the test distance for near visual acuity assessment. *(Robert Barkaloff)*

FUNCTIONAL INFORMATION OBTAINED

The ability to see detail is determined by measuring a person's visual acuity. If 20/20 is considered to be normal vision, (usually erroneously, as previously discussed) the size of the denominator, relative to 20, provides information about the person's vision. If the denominator is five times larger than 20 (20/100) then the vision may be thought of as being reduced from normal by a factor of 5. A person with 20/20 acuity will be able to read from 100 ft away what the person with 20/100 acuity can read from 20 ft away. A person with 20/100 acuity will need things to be five times larger or to be five times closer than does a person with normal vision in order to recognize the details in objects or print. Those with reduced acuity will usually require magnification to allow them to see print of normal size. The amount of magnification necessary may be calculated from the acuity measurements (see Chap. 2).

Visual Fields

When evaluating an individual for visual field losses, the examiner should have a mental image of a normal visual field. Visual field size will vary depending on the ambient lighting conditions, the test targets used, the testing method, and various other conditions. The anatomy of the skull around the eye can limit peripheral vision. When the person is looking straight ahead, the measurement of the extent of peripheral vision from this straight ahead point out toward the person's ear is typically referred to as the temporal direction (toward the temple).

TABLE 6.1

Minimal Extent of Normal Peripheral Vision

DIRECTION OF GAZE	EXTENT IN DEGREES	EXTENT IN CLOCK HOURS*
Temporally (toward the ear)	85	About 3 clock hours
Down and temporally	85	About 3 clock hours
Down	65	About 2 clock hours
Down and nasal (toward the nose)	50	Just under 2 clock hours
Nasal	60	About 2 clock hours
Up and nasal	55	About 2 clock hours
Up	45	Just under 2 clock hours
Up and temporally	55	About 2 clock hours

*See Figure 6.4 for an explanation of clock hours.
Source: *Physicians Desk Reference for Ophthamology 2000,* 28th ed. (Montvale, NJ: Medical Economics Co., 1999).

When the person is looking straight ahead, the measurement of the extent of peripheral vision from this straight ahead point toward the person's nose is typically referred to as the nasal direction. People with unimpaired peripheral vision have a greater extent of vision toward their ear (temporally) than toward their nose (nasally). People also see much farther downward (inferiorly) than upward (superiorly). Table 6.1 shows the minimal extent of normal peripheral vision.

ASSESSMENT METHODS

Measuring the extent of an individual's peripheral vision can be done using a variety of methods. Commonly it is measured by an instrument called a perimeter. Computerized or automated perimeters have become the instrument of choice in most eye care offices not specializing in low vision due to the precision with which visual fields can be measured and because the accuracy is not affected by a lack of experience or expertise on the part of the examiner (American Academy of Ophthalmology, 1996.) Although useful when measuring the peripheral vision of unimpaired or minimally impaired vision, automated perimeters are often poor choices for people with low vision who are often unable to keep their eyes fixated on the appropriate light inside the instrument because of nystagmus or central scotomas (blind spots). This causes the findings to be unreliable.

Better methods of determining the extent of their peripheral vision include Goldmann perimeters, which are manual visual field instruments. Goldmann perimeters however, require significant training and practice on the part of the tester to obtain good results, are not portable, and are not found in many optometrist's or ophthalmologist's offices due to the more frequent use of automated perimeters. Commonly used methods of assessing visual fields in people with low vision include confrontation visual fields, tangent screen, and Amsler grids, which are described in the following sections.

CONFRONTATION VISUAL FIELDS. The term *confrontation visual field testing* derives from the fact that the field is assessed while the examiner is face-to-face with the person being evaluated. The methods and targets used are varied. Confrontation visual fields should be measured with the person's glasses off because there is the possibility that the eyeglass frame may create blind areas in the person's field of vision. Peripheral vision is not very sensitive to blur and removal of the glasses will have little or no effect on the results.

The confrontation visual field method requires that the person sit face-to-face with the examiner, looking at the examiner or some other target in line with the examiner, so that it is possible to monitor where the person is looking. While the person is looking at the examiner, and maintaining steady central fixation, a target of some sort is brought in from the side, beyond where the person can see it, toward the person's line of sight. The person signals either verbally or through hand or eye movements when he or she sees the target. The examiner then judges the extent of the visual field.

Visual fields are measured in degrees relative to the line of sight. For example, while looking at the examiner, the person is able to see the target when it is at right angles to his or her line of sight, which is 90 degrees. The examiner would record the number of degrees as 90, and this figure is always an estimate of the person's peripheral vision. The accuracy of this test depends on how accurately the examiner is able to estimate degrees. A handy method for estimating how far from the person's line of sight a target was detected requires that one imagine the person's eye to be the center of a clock. His or her line of sight extends from the center of the clock through the number 12, which is straight ahead. Each clock hour away from 12 represents 30 degrees. For example, if the target was observed at about 2 o'clock, then the number of degrees of field is 60 (see Fig. 6.4.). Visual fields should be assessed superiorly (upward), inferiorly (downward), to the person's left and right, up and to the person's left and right, and down and to the person's left and right.

Visual fields are usually measured monocularly, although they are measured binocularly for functional information, especially in young children or people with visual and multiple disabilities (see Chap. 5). The testing of visual fields can be time-consuming, and it may be difficult for young children or people with

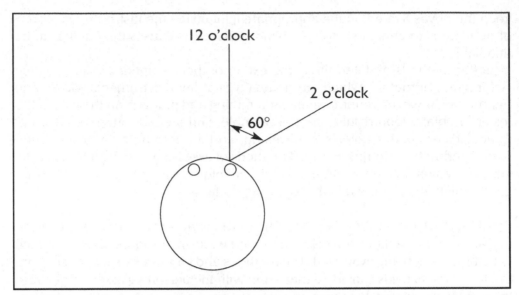

Figure 6.4. Measurement of visual field—degrees related to clock hours. Each clock hour away from 12 o'clock represents 30 degrees.

multiple disabilities to concentrate for long periods of time. The length of time required is greatly decreased if the test is only performed once, rather than twice (once for each eye), yet it can still yield a result that will be useful in determining functional deficits. If, in the tester's judgment, the person is likely to tolerate the length of the test and perform reliably for each eye, monocular measurements are preferred because they provide information about what each eye, by itself, is capable of seeing. Visual field loss in one eye may not show up when tested binocularly because the other eye without the field loss will be doing the detecting.

A patch is the easiest way to occlude an eye and ensure that the eye's peripheral vision is also occluded. Once an eye is occluded, the examiner should sit directly in front of the individual about 2 ft away (the distance is not critical). Have the person look into the examiner's eye that is opposite the nonoccluded eye.

If the person's vision is too poor to see the examiner's eye while maintaining steady, central fixation, the following adjustments may be helpful:

➤ The examiner can either move closer or ask the person to look toward the middle of the examiner's face.

➤ If that is still too difficult because of the person's vision deficits, a dim light can be provided as a fixation target.

➤ For children, it may be preferable to use a rubber finger puppet "monster" mounted on a penlight. The finger puppet will glow with light and provide a more interesting target for them to look at.

Whatever fixation target is used, it should be held up by the examiner's face so that it is possible to make judgments easily as to whether the person is still looking straight ahead or the eyes are wandering. The object the person is attempting to detect during confrontation visual fields can vary in size, shape, color, and brightness. If the person's vision is very poor, a large object or very bright object is preferred. Objects commonly used for testing are stationary or wriggling fingers, hands, penlights, finger puppets mounted on penlights, and pieces of white paper.

The technique requires beginning with the object in a location beyond the person's peripheral vision: 1 to 2 ft away. It is brought slowly toward the person's line of sight, using a slight arc to the target's path, until the person signals that he or she can see it. Always move the object from where the person cannot see it to where he or she can see it. This will result in more reliable results. If the object is moved from where the person sees it to a position where the person no longer sees it, he or she will have a much more difficult time judging when that happens.

TANGENT SCREEN. The tangent screen method of assessing visual fields is less convenient, takes more practice to become skilled, is not possible to do in every setting (unlike confrontation methods), but is more sensitive to field loss than other methods. The tangent screen is typically a black piece of felt mounted on a wall. The felt has a white object in the center that the person will look at throughout the test (called the fixation target). Sometimes white tape or string will be placed over the tangent screen to form an "X" with the crossover point directly over the fixation target. This marking will enhance a person's ability to fixate accurately if he or she has a central scotoma. Often the tangent screen has circles of black thread stitched into it that delineate the number of degrees from the center and the location of the physiological blind spot (which everyone has, regardless of vision status). The tangent screen is only useful for mapping the central portion of the visual field (about 30 degrees out from fixation) and will not yield information about the extent of the person's peripheral vision.

Tangent screen testing is very useful when assessing possible reasons for reading difficulties. For example, blind spots (scotomas) to the right of fixation may cause reading to be difficult because the person will always be reading into their scotoma. Tangent screen testing can also be useful for evaluating visual fields in a person when it has already been established, via other means, that the only remaining vision is the central portion.

The standard stimuli or test targets consist of circular white dots of various diameters, ranging from 1 to 10 mm, mounted on the tip of wooden rods that are painted flat black. Tangent screen testing is nearly always performed using one eye at a time. The person being tested should be seated facing the tangent screen and at eye level with the central fixation target at the standard test distance of 1 m. The person should be wearing his or her glasses or contact lenses appropriate for the test distance (usually their distance correction).

It is customary, but not required, to begin testing by starting on the temporal field of the person's right eye (to the person's right side). The examiner switches

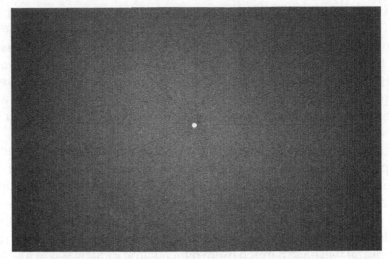

Tangent screen with black stitching demarcating the meridians and degrees from fixation. *(Robert Greer)*

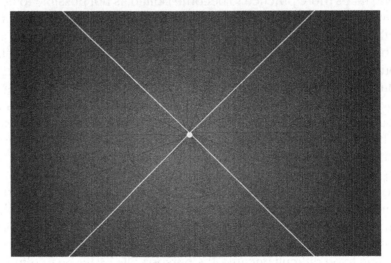

Tangent screen with white string to assist with fixation. *(Robert Greer)*

location to the person's other side to test the nasal field of the right eye (to the person's left side). This sequence is then repeated for the left eye. As with other field tests, the examiner explains that the target on the wooden rod will be moved by the examiner from a position where it is not visible to a position where it is visible. The examiner needs to show the person what the test target looks like prior to testing.

If the person's vision is very poor, choose a large target; if his or her vision is relatively good, choose a small target. The target should be moved at a medium speed, neither too fast nor too slow, toward the central fixation target. The indi-

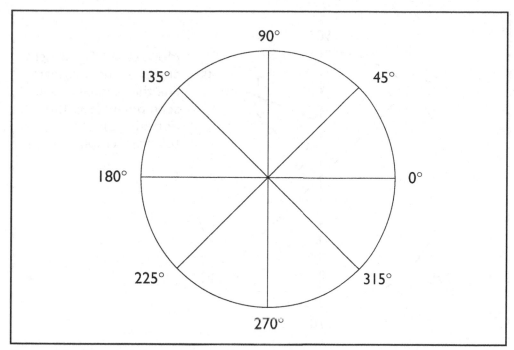

Figure 6.5. The meridians measured during tangent screen testing. Each meridian is 45 degrees apart from the next.

vidual signals, by voice or hand motion, when he or she first notices the white test target on the rod.

At a minimum, the field should be investigated along the meridians (lines going from the center out to the edge of the circle) labeled 0, 45, 90, 135, 180, 225, 270, and 315 degrees in Figure 6.5 (the person would be looking at the center of the circle in the diagram). Each meridian is labeled in degrees (there are 360 degrees in a circle) and there are 45 degrees between each meridian in this example.

To keep the person from being able to anticipate where the target will next be located, the examiner needs to attempt to be random with the testing. For example, the examiner can test superiorly, then inferiorly, and then go back to superiorly. As the person signals that the target is seen, the examiner may mentally keep track of where the test target was first noticed, or use pins pushed into the felt, or write an "X" in the appropriate location on recording paper. No matter how the examiner chooses to keep track of the results, eventually these should be transferred to paper.

The examiner needs to be aware that everybody, even people with completely unimpaired vision, has a blind spot in each eye where the optic nerve connects to the back of the eye. This normal blind spot is often referred to as the physiological blind spot. The position of the physiological blind spot in the right eye is about 15 degrees to the right of the fixation target, and it is about 15 degrees to

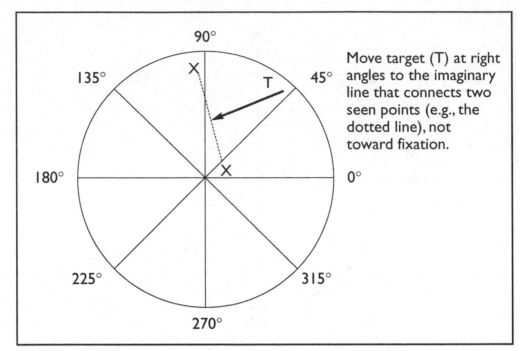

Figure 6.6. Measuring an area of visual field loss with a tangent screen.

the left of the fixation target in the left eye. The physiological blind spot is about 5 degrees in size, is typically slightly taller than wide, and its middle is usually slightly below the fixation target. If the person is unable to hold his or her eyes very still, an examiner may not be able to find the physiological blind spot.

If a particular portion of the visual field is found to be reduced, the examiner can investigate further the shape of the reduced section of peripheral vision. This may require that the test target no longer be moved toward the central fixation point. Instead, the target can be moved at right angles to an imaginary line that connects two visible points on either side of the reduced area of visual field (see Fig. 6.6).

AMSLER GRID. The central portion of a person's visual field may be more finely assessed with a device called the Amsler grid, after Dr. Marc Amsler, a Swiss ophthalmologist. The Amsler grid (see Fig. 6.7) is a series of squares measuring 5 mm by 5 mm. The entire grid is 20 squares by 20 squares. Thus each side of the grid measures 10 cm. When the grid is held 28 to 30 cm away, each square corresponds to an angle of 1 degree, thus allowing testing of the central 10 degrees of vision. There is a central fixation point. By having the person fixate on this central point, the grid will be seen with his or her peripheral vision.

The Amsler grid test is performed on one eye at a time. An occluder or eye patch works well to permit this. The examiner instructs the person to look at the center of the grid and describe what he or she can see. The individual needs to

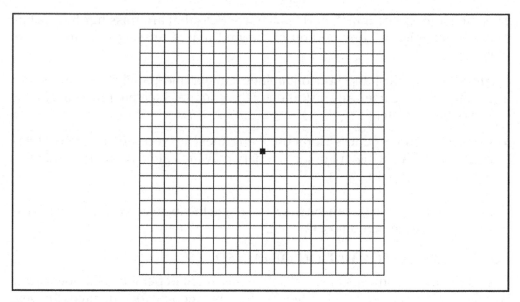

Figure 6.7. The Amsler grid.

be looking through the appropriate spectacle prescription for the 28- to 30-cm testing distance. It is extremely important for the examiner to remind the person being tested always to look at the central fixation point, thus ensuring that peripheral vision is being assessed.

The Amsler grid is not very sensitive when assessing an individual with long-standing visual field loss (Ariyasu, et al., 1996; Schuchard, 1993). This lack of sensitivity may be due to the person filling in the grid so that it appears to be completely normal. This filling in is not conscious, but is a subconscious result that can occur after loss of vision (Achard et al., 1995). Because of this insensitivity and filling in, if the grid is perceived as being normal in appearance, the examiner has learned little or nothing about the person's central visual field. The person may have nothing wrong with the central portion of his or her peripheral vision and therefore describe the grid as looking fine. However, the person may also describe the grid as looking fine despite deficits in the central portion of his or her peripheral vision, which is possible because of the unconscious act of filling in.

The following questions should be asked of the person undergoing Amsler grid testing (Amsler, 1950):

1. Do you see the spot in the center of the square? If the person does not see the central fixation point, this may indicate a central scotoma.

2. Do you see the corners and sides of the large square; in other words, do you see the entire large square? Any portion of the grid that is missing may indicate a scotoma.

3. Is the large square intact, or does it have areas that are missing? If so, what areas are missing? Any portion of the grid that is missing may indicate a scotoma.

4. Are all the vertical and horizontal lines straight and parallel? Are the small squares all the same? Any distortion of the grid may indicate problems in the eye or visual system.

5. Do you see movement or vibration of any lines? Do you see any areas of different color? Anything out of the ordinary may indicate a problem within the eye or visual system.

Instruct the person to draw on the Amsler grid the location of any defects, distortions, or missing portions of the grid.

FUNCTIONAL INFORMATION OBTAINED

One of the main purposes of visual field assessment in persons with low vision is to determine if any loss of peripheral vision may account for difficulties the person is having. Confrontation visual fields, it has been mentioned, are not very sensitive and will miss subtle peripheral vision loss. Tangent screen, although more sensitive, will only test about 30 degrees away from fixation and does not yield information about the full extent of peripheral vision. If peripheral vision is being assessed as it relates to a person's mobility, it may be best to limit the testing to confrontation visual fields because this will provide information about the total extent of peripheral vision. If peripheral vision is being assessed to provide information pertaining to a person's reading, tangent screen and/or Amsler grid testing is likely to provide better information. It is not necessary to use all possible peripheral vision tests on any given person. Depending on the problems presented by the person being examined, more than one peripheral vision test may be needed.

If the individual is missing a large portion of his or her inferior (downward) visual field, he or she might have difficulties with mobility. For a child, books and other learning tools should not be presented low in his or her vision. If a large portion of the superior field is missing, the individual may bump into objects that are up high, such as kitchen cabinet doors. If visual fields are missing to the person's right or left, he or she may bump into objects located on that side. Children sitting in classrooms might benefit from being placed in the room on the same side as their field loss. In this way, they will have the majority of the classroom on the side of their remaining vision. An individual with a scotoma to the right of straight ahead may have difficulty reading fluently because he or she is reading into the scotoma. The same person will be able to return easily to the beginning of the line because the peripheral vision is functioning to the left. If an individual has a scotoma to the left of fixation, he or she may be able to read fluently but may have difficulty returning to the beginning of the next line because the blind spot is in the way.

Contrast Sensitivity

Contrast sensitivity is a measure of the eye's ability to detect shades of gray or differences in brightness. Unlike visual acuity charts that are composed of black letters on a white background (100 percent contrast), contrast sensitivity tests use letters, stripes, or other shapes of varying contrast. These tests provide a sense of how much difficulty a person will have with typical tasks of daily living. Very little of our world is in high contrast. Even reading, which we think of as most often involving black letters on white paper, is often more likely to be grayish letters on yellowish paper. This is especially true of documents such as bills, which may be gray letters on a blue or other colored background.

Contrast sensitivity is often measured binocularly in people with low vision for functional purposes but can be measured monocularly. Numerous tests are used for measuring contrast sensitivity and some are described in the following sections. The normal contrast value will vary depending on the test used. Such tests usually report their findings in Michelson contrast units (normal contrast is 0.5 percent to 1.0 percent) or Weber contrast units (normal contrast is 1.0 to 2.0 percent). (See Chap. 5 for more information on contrast measures.) If the test does not use repeating patterns (for example, letters), then Weber contrast is typically used to specify the contrast. Michelson contrast describes the difference between the darkest and lightest parts of a pattern and is typically used when stripes (gratings) are the test target. Weber contrast describes the difference between the object (e.g., a letter) and the background on which it sits. See the Resources section of this book for a list of commonly used tests to assess contrast sensitivity. Most tests mentioned in this chapter are in one of two major categories: tests in which the contrast is constant but the symbol size changes, and tests in which the symbol size is constant and the contrast changes.

TEST ADMINISTRATION

In the Cambridge Low Contrast Gratings, Hiding Heidi, and Mr. Happy tests, two panels are shown to the individual; one of the panels contains stripes (Cambridge) or a face (Hiding Heidi, Mr. Happy) while the other panel is blank gray matched in brightness to the first panel. The person is asked to point to or indicate verbally which panel contains the stripes or face. In typical situations, the test proceeds to less and less contrast until the person is no longer able to identify which panel contains the stripes or face. The panel with the least amount of contrast that was correctly identified determines the person's contrast sensitivity.

CAMBRIDGE LOW CONTRAST GRATINGS. The Cambridge Low Contrast Gratings test is frequently used for persons with normal vision (adapted from Wilkins & Robson, 1988) and is designed for a test distance of 6 m (20 ft). Test takers wear their usual spectacle or contact lens correction.

The following steps are recommended by the manufacturer for test administration. Each test page is shown in sequence (from highest to lowest contrast), until the person makes an error (there are 10 test pages plus a demonstration page). After an error is made, the test administrator goes back four test pages from where the error was incurred (or to the demonstration test page if the error occurred in the first three test pages) and performs the test a second time. The tester presents the test pages in sequence, as before, until an error occurs, and repeats a third and fourth time, going back four test pages each time from where the error occurred. To arrive at a score, the tester notes the number of the test pages where the errors occurred and adds together the page numbers. The table on the score sheet then allows one to convert the total into a score for contrast sensitivity.

Some modification may be necessary for people with low vision. Although the test distance for individuals without visual impairment is 20 ft, the test can be administered at much closer distances for people with low vision. The distance must be far enough away that the person is unable to see individual dots. Therefore, the test is often administered as close as 2 feet for those with low vision. For a functional measure of contrast, it is possible to ask a person with low vision to identify the plate containing stripes when both eyes are viewing at the closer distance. The plates are presented from high to low contrast and the last plate the person can discriminate is recorded. The evaluator can then find the Michelson contrast of that plate in the test manual to determine the person's ability to detect low contrast targets.

PELLI-ROBSON TEST. This test requires individuals to read letters on the Pelli-Robson Contrast Sensitivity Chart, starting with letters of the highest contrast and proceeding to letters with less and less contrast, until no letters can be identified. The letters with the least amount of contrast correctly identified provide the contrast sensitivity for the individual. The normative range of contrast for the Pelli-Robson chart for individuals without visual impairment is 1.1 to 1.7 percent for young people and 1.23 to 2.0 percent for older people (Elliott & Bullimore, 1993). The lower the percentage of contrast, the higher (or better) the contrast sensitivity.

BAILEY-LOVIE HIGH AND LOW CONTRAST CHARTS. The Bailey-Lovie test requires that two visual acuity measurements be made: one using the typical high-contrast Bailey-Lovie chart and one using a low-contrast version of the chart, located on the back of the high-contrast chart. The low-contrast chart has letters at 10 percent Weber contrast. The two acuities are then compared. Individuals without visual impairment will have a low-contrast acuity that is about two lines poorer than their high-contrast acuity (Lovie-Kitchin & Brown, 2000). The greater the loss of low-contrast acuity beyond two lines, the greater the person's loss of contrast sensitivity.

VCTS 6500. The VCTS 6500, test commonly used in clinical settings, may be encountered when reading low vision evaluation reports, is made up of sine wave gratings (stripes with fuzzy edges) presented in several widths and contrast levels.

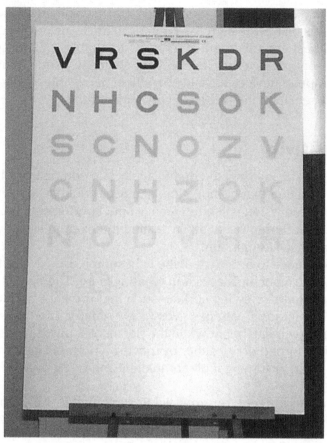

Pelli-Robson Contrast Sensitivity Chart. *(Ohio State University College of Optometry Instructional Media Center)*

The test requires the individual to make judgments as to the direction in which the stripes are leaning, at all the stripe widths. The least amount of contrast that still allows the individual to judge the direction of the stripes correctly is noted for each stripe width. The results are plotted on paper provided by the test manufacturer. The VCTS 6500 recording sheet has normative data on the paper that allow a rapid comparison to be made.

FUNCTIONAL INFORMATION OBTAINED

No special glasses, contact lenses, or filters will improve an individual's contrast sensitivity, although yellow filters may give people the impression that their contrast has been improved, especially when used outdoors. This may occur because there is a fair amount of blue light outdoors that yellow filters can block. This results in many objects appearing darker and hence the perception that items seen have increased contrast.

Although there are no optical treatments to improve contrast sensitivity, there are many ways to increase the contrast of objects and tasks around the home, school, or office. If a person has reduced contrast sensitivity, then advice and recommendations on how to increase contrast in the living environment can be provided. If contrast enhancement is required to enable the individual to read efficiently, electronic devices are an excellent choice. Closed-circuit televisions (CCTV) and computer devices have the benefit of being able to take print of low contrast and present it on the screen in very high contrast.

Light Sensitivity

Light sensitivity can be investigated during acuity and contrast sensitivity testing. Changes in illumination that do not affect acuity or contrast sensitivity in a person without impaired vision will often greatly affect performance by an individual with low vision. During visual acuity testing the examiner can easily assess the effect of changing illumination.

The examiner needs to be sure that the light source used in this testing is not shining directly into a person's eyes and creating glare. The light source should shine at an angle to the viewing surface such that the light bounces off at an angle, not directly into the patient's eyes (see Fig. 6.8). The test should begin with the illumination being bright when the person's acuity is measured. The illumination is then turned down either by moving a portable light source farther away from the chart or turning it off completely and using only the room lights for illumination.

If the person does not require strong lighting to function, he or she will still be able to read, or almost read, the smallest characters that he or she could read

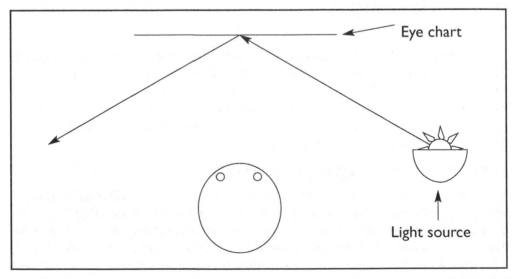

Figure 6.8. Proper illumination for assessing light sensitivity. Arrange lighting so that the chart does not become a source of glare; nor should the light shine directly into the person's eyes.

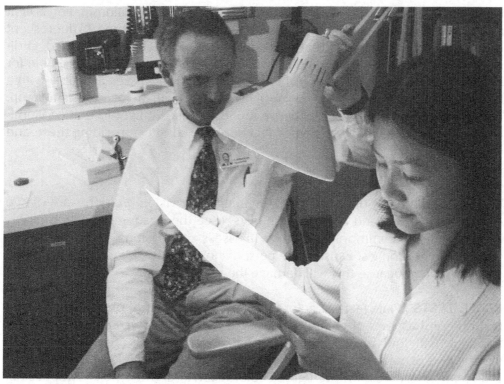

Assessing light sensitivity. *(Robert Barkaloff)*

previously. If strong lighting is necessary for good function, then acuity will range from slightly to extremely reduced compared to the acuity measured under ideal lighting conditions. Less frequently, a person's vision will be such that the dimmer lighting is more conducive to good visual function. The examiner can make note of what lighting conditions appear to maximize performance and provide recommendations for optimal lighting.

The same type of investigation can be used during contrast sensitivity testing. The person's contrast sensitivity needs to be compared under bright and dim lighting conditions. This will provide a clearer sense of the person's functional vision capabilities and his or her need for light.

Color Vision

Color vision is often tested in children and adults because defects in color vision can be inherited as well as acquired due to eye disease. As with contrast sensitivity, there is no treatment for color vision problems, but one can provide information, advice, and recommendations. The most reliable results will be obtained when color vision is tested using an illuminant "C" lamp, also known as a "daylight" lamp (illuminant C mimics standard daylight). The color of objects will be perceived differently depending on the color of light used to view them. If an illuminant "C" or daylight lamp is not available, the next best illumination is light from a northern window (in the northern hemisphere), a Chroma 75 fluorescent bulb (General Electric), or Color Classer 75 fluorescent (Duro-Test Corp). Ordinary incandescent lamps and cool white fluorescent bulbs are undesirable for such testing. (Hovis & Neumann, 1995). There are also glasses available with a bluish tint, called Daylight Glasses, designed for use with an incandescent lamp. The Daylight Glasses effectively cause the incandescent light to imitate illuminant "C" (see Resources section of this book for sources providing these and other lights).

ASSESSMENT METHODS

The most commonly used tests for screening color vision problems are of two designs: plate tests and arrangement tests. (See the Resources section of this book for a list of commonly used tests to assess color vision). No matter which type of color vision test is used, the person should not be allowed to touch the colored paper because this will damage the test.

PLATE TESTS. Plate tests of color vision are comprised of plates (pages) that test different aspects of color vision. These tests are not usually administered to people with low vision because reasonably good vision is required in order to see the dots of color that comprise the tests' various figures. Also, the more common plate tests assess only red/green color vision loss. One type is composed of pseudoisochromatic plates (ones with different colors that appear alike to those with color vision problems) in a book format that require the individual to identify what he or she sees on each page. These tests offer several advantages: they are rapidly and easily administered; no training is required; they are readily available; they are relatively inexpensive; and they can be used to test most people, from children to adults. Plate tests also have certain disadvantages: The type of light illuminating the plates affects the visibility of the figures; and it is difficult, if not impossible, to classify accurately the person's color vision defect based on his or her test performance. Pseudoisochromatic tests should be used primarily as screening tests to identify individuals who have problems with color vision.

Each page or plate tests a different aspect of color vision. The administration of plate color vision tests may be done binocularly or monocularly. For testing functional color vision, binocular testing is sufficient. If there is a need to document asymmetry between the eyes or to evaluate the progress of a disease, the testing should be performed monocularly. If an eye is to be occluded, a pirate patch can be used to eliminate the need for the person or examiner to hold something over an eye during the entire testing procedure. The examiner should locate the most appropriate lighting available and proceed with the testing. For the plate tests, the examiner simply asks the person to identify what he or she sees on each page. The person should be given about 3 sec to answer before moving to the next plate. If the person is unable to identify what is on the page in a reasonable amount of time, the examiner can assume that he or she has made an incorrect identification. If a person cannot read numbers, then some plate tests, such as the Series of Plates Designed as a Test for Colour-Blindness by Dr. Shinobu Ishihara (commonly referred to as the Ishihara test), have plates that ask the person to trace a path (preferably with a brush rather than his or her finger, so as to not ruin the color). If the person does not correctly identify the figures on the plates, he or she is assumed to have a color vision defect. A confirmation of the color vision defect, its type, and severity would require further testing.

ARRANGEMENT TESTS. Another test design uses colored caps (plastic pieces with colored paper embedded in the top) that are arranged in a particular order by the individual being tested. Arrangement tests have the advantage of being easy to administer, but require manual dexterity, patience, concentration, and the understanding of abstract ordering. They are therefore less suitable for use by young children.

To administer an arrangement color vision test such as the Farnsworth D-15, one needs a table or counter for the tray and caps to rest on. The loose caps are mixed up so that they are in no particular order and are placed near the tray. The first cap is typically glued into place in the tray or it is the first cap presented. The person is given instructions to choose from among the loose caps the one that most closely matches the color of the cap in the tray. The person is forewarned that none of the caps exactly match the color of the first one, but he or she is to pick the one that most closely matches it. Once the person has chosen the cap, he or she is to place it into the tray next to the first one. From among the remaining caps, the individual is to choose the one that most closely matches the color of the second cap. This proceeds until all the caps have been placed in the tray. The examiner then closes the tray, flips it over, and opens it. The caps will be upside down but the examiner will now see numbers on the underside of each cap. The order the person placed the caps needs to be written down. If the person's color vision is good, he or she will have placed the caps in order from 1 to 15.

If the person has a color vision problem, the caps will not have been placed in order. The more out of order the caps are placed, the greater the person's the color vision defect. If more detail is required concerning the severity and type of color vision defect, it would be best to consult with an optometrist or ophthalmologist.

FUNCTIONAL INFORMATION OBTAINED

It is extremely rare, (approximately 1 in 33,000) for an individual to be completely color-blind and see things in shades of gray (Sharpe et al., 2000). It is not uncommon for a person to have defective or deficient color vision; (about 8 percent of males have some form of color blindness) (Pokorny et al., 1979).

If someone has reduced color vision (other than those with complete color-blindness) then vibrant, primary colors should be emphasized when asking them to recognize colors. For school age children whose color vision is poor, dark colors such as navy and black may be indistinguishable. Pastels may also be quite difficult to tell apart. Adults may have difficulty with sock colors (differentiating among dark brown, navy, or black) and will need to use other methods for matching their clothing. Career counseling may be necessary because certain jobs will exclude those with serious color vision defects, including jobs requiring the identification, coding, or wiring of electronic equipment, or in areas of transportation such as airline pilots, railroad engineers, and maritime pilots.

Oculomotor Control

The assessment of oculomotor control (i.e., eye position and movement) involves discerning whether the eyes are straight and are able to move fully in all directions. Oculomotor control problems may be noticed by educators, rehabilitation specialists, and low vision therapists, but it is essential that persons with suspected problems be carefully assessed by an optometrist or ophthalmologist. If an eye is not straight but turns inward, outward, upward, or downward relative to the other eye, this is also known as strabismus, squint, or heterotropia (sometimes shortened to tropia). A strabismus implies that the individual is not binocular at times. The person may compensate for not being binocular by paying attention to one eye's image or the other. Which eye is attended to may even change with viewing conditions such as distance. An eye turn in a person with low vision is rarely treated, because binocularity is more difficult to attain when vision is poor. Strabismus, which is common in persons with low vision, should be assessed by an optometrist or ophthalmologist.

ASSESSMENT METHODS

The cover test enables the examiner to detect eye turns; the extraocular motility test (sometimes called versions or version testing) assesses the ability of the eyes to move in all directions. The necessary equipment includes an occluder in the form of a paddle (cover paddle), letters or symbols for both distance and near, and a penlight. These tests are screening procedures, and if any new unusual findings are noted, the person should be referred to his or her eye care practitioner for additional testing.

COVER TEST. The cover test should be performed twice: first while the person is looking at distance and then, when the person is looking up close. This is because some people will have an eye turn that is only manifested when they look at certain distances. The test is done after distance and near visual acuities have been measured. The lighting in the room should allow the examiner to see the person's eyes easily.

The individual is asked to look at a letter or symbol that is two to four rows larger than the smallest he or she was able to see during acuity measurements. The examiner asks the person to keep the letter as clear as possible and always to look at the center of the letter. The examiner places the cover paddle in front of one of the person's eyes while observing the other eye. If the other eye does not move it will have been pointing at the letter. The examiner uncovers the eye and then covers the eye again or switches to covering the opposite eye. If neither eye moves when its counterpart is covered, then each eye, in turn, will have been pointing straight at the letter and no eye turn exists. If one of the eyes moves when the other is covered, then an eye turn exists.

EXTRAOCULAR MOTILITY SCREENING TEST. The ability to move the eyes in all directions is evaluated with the extraocular motility test, using a penlight or some other easily seen target. The examiner places himself or herself opposite the person being assessed and explains that he or she needs to look at the target (penlight, etc.) as the examiner moves it around. The person is to use his or her eyes only and keep the head still. The examiner moves the penlight to the person's far left, up and left, up and right, down and right, and down and left, tracing a box shape using the penlight. It is important to make the person move his or her eyes in to extreme gaze in order to ensure that the eye movements are full.

If the person's eye movements are not full in all directions, once again, it would be best to obtain further assessment by an optometrist or ophthalmologist to determine the cause of the incomplete eye movement. An eye may not move fully in all directions due to congenital or acquired neurological deficits or structural problems with the muscle itself. The possible courses of treatment range from surgical to eye exercises to no treatment. An optometrist or ophthalmologist should be consulted if an eye turn is detected because of the many reasons for an eye turn, especially if the eye turn is new: this may indicate problems that require immediate attention. Eye turns can result from low vision but they can also indicate neurological problems. Uncovering the proper diagnosis and treatment is often difficult and best left to those more familiar with eye turns.

Accommodation

No normal values for have been established for accommodation in people with low vision (Leat & Gargon, 1995). If a person is holding material 10 cm away but is only able to accommodate to 20 cm, then his or her vision is not being maximized. In order to maximize vision when accommodation is deficient, spectacles are prescribed for reading. The spectacles supplement the eye's accommodative system, allowing near tasks to be in better focus. Accommodation is not easily assessed without special instruments and testing procedures and will likely require examination by an optometrist or ophthalmologist. However, the screening methods described here may be attempted and if any new, unusual findings are noted, the person should be referred to his or her eye care practitioner for additional testing.

NEAR POINT OF ACCOMMODATION TEST

One method used for individuals without visual impairment is the near point of accommodation test (NPA). It may, however, have limited value when testing persons with low vision. It requires the person to recognize when something becomes blurry. Individuals with low vision never truly see things clearly and may not be able to make that judgment accurately.

With the person sitting opposite the examiner, a symbol, character, or letter that is small and has some detail to it is held at a distance that allows the individual to recognize the symbol but not easily. The examiner instructs the person to keep the symbol clear as the examiner slowly brings it closer. The symbol is kept at eye level and on the midline between the two eyes. The person is instructed to tell the examiner when the symbol first becomes blurry. The examiner then measures how far from the person's face the symbol was when it was just starting to look blurry. This is the person's near point of accommodation and is recorded in diopters. If the distance is measured in centimeters, divide 100 by the number of centimeters to yield diopters. For example, a symbol became blurry when it was 10 cm from the person's face: $100 \div 10 = 10$ diopters (see Chap. 3 for a fuller explanation of optical measurement).

MAR EQUIVALENCY

The MAR equivalency test takes advantage of the fact that acuity (or the MAR) remains the same regardless of test distance, as long as the chart remains in focus. Once focus is not maintained (insufficient accommodation) then acuity (or MAR) becomes poorer. It requires the use of a near chart that has equal size changes in the symbol size from row to row, such as the Bailey-Lovie Word Reading Chart. The meter size (M notation) range is 10, 8, 6.3, 5, 4, 3.2, 2.5, 2, 1.6, 1.25, 1, 0.8, 0.63, 0.5, 0.4, 0.32, and 0.25. If a person is able to read 3.2M when the chart is 20 cm away, then he or she will read 2.5M if the chart is 16 cm away (if accommodation is maintained).

Using the scale of the chart, the examiner measures what size print the person can read at a given distance. For each step closer on the scale, the person will be able to read one line smaller on the chart (i.e., acuity will be maintained). As the examiner moves the chart closer to the person, there will come a point when the person is unable to read one line smaller. This will signal an inability to accommodate any further. As with the NPA test described above, the distance can be converted into diopters of accommodation.

EVALUATION OF VISION USE IN CRITICAL TASKS

In addition to evaluating performance on tasks of visual functions that combine to define an individual's functional vision, it is crucial to assess his or her visual functioning in the context of important everyday tasks. However, evaluation of visual skills related to tasks that a person usually performs can involve a complex array of measures and observations that must be taken into account in order to understand the effect of various visual skills and behaviors on his or her task performance. Because literacy is so crucial for both education and everyday living, evaluation of visual skills related to reading has received the most attention in the literature. It will be discussed first, followed by a review of visual skills for specific work, daily living, travel, and leisure tasks, as well as those required for computer use.

Reading Skills

If reading is currently difficult for the person being assessed, and improving his or her ability to read is an important goal, a more thorough evaluation of reading skills may be important. Several aspects of vision have been found to affect a person's ability to read with ease and fluidity. These factors (Whitakker & Lovie-Kitchin, 1993) are summarized in Sidebar 6.3 and discussed in detail in the following sections.

SIDEBAR 6.3

Characteristics of Vision and Print That Affect Reading Efficiency

CHARACTERISTICS	EFFECT ON READING EFFICIENCY

Characteristics of Vision

Acuity reserve	Print should be 3 to 5 times larger than threshold.
Contrast reserve	Print should have 10 to 20 times more contrast than threshold, preferably black on white or white on black.
Field of view	Four to six characters should be visible simultaneously, which may necessitate holding any handheld optical devices close to the eye.
Size of central scotoma	For optimal reading, a central scotoma should be less than 22 degrees in diameter, although even small absolute central scotomas will likely have a deleterious effect on reading.
Working distance	This will be highly dependent on a person's ability to accommodate or the power of the devices used for near tasks.

Characteristics of Print

Character size	This will depend on the individual's reading acuity. Characters should be three to five times larger than threshold.
Polarity	For individuals with no media opacities (cataracts, etc.), black on white or white on black tends to be equally easy to read. Those with media opacities frequently prefer white on black for reading.
Contrast	The higher the contrast of the reading material the better. This will maximize contrast reserve.
Color contrast	Adding color to print and its background has not been found to be of benefit.

ACUITY RESERVE

Acuity reserve refers to the necessity of having print significantly larger than the minimum that can be seen for reading to be comfortable (see Chap. 2). The size of print that is recommended for sustained comfort and performance during reading is often two to five times larger than the smallest print the person is capable of reading. Cheong, Lovie-Kitchin, and Bowers (2002) suggest that print that is two times larger than the smallest print a person is able to read is sufficient to ensure ease of reading, but the exact amount that results in fluid reading varies from person to person. Another recommendation is that print size be the smallest size that the person is able to read with good efficiency. If the individual is not able to read any size of print with efficiency, the examiner may recommend the print be two to five times larger than the smallest the individual can read. However, if reading is extraordinarily difficult, laborious, or slow for an individual, then visual reading may not be the best method. Other methods, such as auditory reading (e.g., tapes or computer speech output) or braille, may need to be considered.

CONTRAST RESERVE

For maximum reading rates and accuracy, the print should have 10 to 20 times more contrast than the least amount of contrast the person is capable of detecting (contrast reserve). Because of the reduced contrast sensitivity that results from many eye conditions, even pure black and white print is seldom 20 times greater in contrast than what many with low vision people can detect. This factor alone will result in slower, less accurate reading by individuals with low vision. Contrast of reading material is highly variable, and many of the printed materials in daily life are far from pure black and white. Notoriously poor contrast is found in newspapers and phonebooks. If contrast sensitivity is significantly reduced, a CCTV may provide improved contrast for reading material, and may possibly improve the user's reading efficiency.

FIELD OF VIEW

The number of characters that a person is able to see simultaneously defines his or her field of view. Most research has found that when the field of view is increased beyond six characters there is no further improvement in reading rate (Whitakker & Lovie-Kitchin, 1993). For that reason, low vision devices, if held close to the eye, do not limit the field of view to less than six characters and are not likely to contribute to inefficient reading. To maximize an individual's reading ability, however, still requires practice on the part of people with low vision, especially if they are not already familiar with using magnifiers or other optical aids. Getting the eye closer to any optical device or using the least amount of magnification necessary to accomplish the desired task will also result in a larger field of view.

SIZE OF CENTRAL SCOTOMA

Many diseases that cause low vision also result in central scotomas. Even relatively small central scotomas result in significant decreases in reading rates. A person with a central scotoma must use another portion of the retina for reading and other recognition tasks. When peripheral retina is used to perform visual tasks normally performed by the macula, this is called eccentric viewing. The more eccentric the viewing, the slower the person's reading rates become. Research suggests that for reading to be fluent the central scotoma should be smaller than 22 degrees in diameter (Whitakker & Lovie-Kitchin, 1993). The size of a central scotoma may be assessed with an Amsler grid or a tangent screen (see the previous section on Visual Fields).

To optimize reading performance, one needs to optimize illumination, character size (correlated with working distance), polarity (black letters on a white background or white letters on a black background), contrast, and the use of assistive devices and techniques. An examination of vision skills for reading must consolidate information about a number of these variables. Some of the factors may be evaluated as part of the near visual acuity measurement while others may require additional testing.

CHARACTER SIZE

Advice concerning the size of print a person can read at different distances to optimize reading ability is of great value. Charts that measure near visual acuity should have a large range of character sizes, at minimum from 5M (40 point) down to 0.25 M (2 point) and perhaps up to 10M (80 point). (A list of near vision charts can be found in the Resources section of this book.)

WORKING DISTANCE

Working distance describes how far away a person is from reading material or other near tasks. The appropriate working distance will also result in a reasonable field of view as well as promoting optimal reading performance. If the person has a tendency to use a magnifier a long distance from the eye, then field of view constraints may hinder reading performance.

ACCOMMODATION

Working distance and accommodation are closely related. A rule of thumb for working distance is that, as print size increases, working distance can increase proportionally. In older adults who have less ability to accommodate, working distance cannot vary greatly with print size. Younger children, however, can read at a greater range of reading distances due to their greater range of accommodation.

READING FLUENCY

Even though a person may be able to see print of a certain size under optimal conditions, he or she may not be able to read smoothly and quickly. The types of reading errors that a person makes can be documented during tests of near acuity and when performing additional reading testing. If a pattern of reading errors cannot be overcome by training or assistive techniques or devices, then alternative reading modes (audiotapes, braille) might be more appropriate than print.

READING SPEED

Reading speed is most conspicuously affected in persons with low vision who have an absolute scotoma covering the central 5 degrees of the visual field (Legge et al., 1985). Under optimal reading conditions (size, contrast, polarity) reading rates of adults with low vision with no field loss have been shown to approach those of subjects with no visual impairments (Legge et al., 1985). This was not the case for persons with central field loss. Reading speed is an important issue for school aged children learning to read and for students who are visually impaired who must maintain reading loads equivalent to the peers without visual impairment. It has been estimated that for spot reading (e.g., price tags) a reading rate of 40 words per minute (wpm) is adequate, while fluent reading, at a second grade level, requires a minimal reading rate of 80 wpm (Whittaker & Lovie-Kitchin, 1993).

READING DURATION

It is also important to evaluate an individual's ability to read for extended periods of time. Low vision can result in a decreased ability to perform reading or other near tasks for more than a few minutes at a time. This decreased ability may be due to the greater concentration required by those with low vision. When assessing the effects of extended reading, the individual is best evaluated after reading silently for 5 to 10 minutes. Often reading speed and efficiency will slow down, which suggests that other methods for reading (e.g., braille, audiotapes) will be needed to supplement print when the person's reading demands are high.

COMPREHENSION

If people are having difficulty seeing and deciphering text, then their reading comprehension will likely be reduced. Little research has been done to examine the reading comprehension of persons with low vision (Watson, Wright, & De l'Aune, 1992; Watson, Wright, Long, 1996). However, it is clear, for example, that students in educational settings with large reading loads must understand what they read in order to extract information for learning. The Morgan Low Vision Reading Comprehension Assessment (Watson, Wright, & Long, 1996) can be used to determine reading level and improvement of reading comprehension skills of adults over time in a training program.

POLARITY OF READING MATERIAL

Some individuals read white letters on a black background (negative polarity) more easily or comfortably than black letters on a white background (positive or reversed polarity). This becomes important when determining use of a CCTV magnifier or large print screen displays for computers. In some experiments, persons with cloudy media (the cornea and/or lens of the eye is not perfectly clear) read white on black better than black on white, while there was no difference for persons with low vision with clear media (Legge, Rubin, & Schleske, 1987). This preference must be examined carefully for each person by having the person read using positive and negative polarities, examining their reading performance, and asking about their personal preference.

CONTRAST AND COLOR OF READING MATERIAL

Black print on white or white on black will maximize contrast and therefore increase contrast reserve better than other color combinations. It has been shown that adding color to print has no practical benefit for reading for aduls with low vision (Knoblach, Arditi, & Szlyk, 1991; Legge, Parish, Luebker, & Wurm, 1990; Legge & Rubin, 1986). Therefore, it is preferred that reading material be of high contrast and be black on white or white on black to ensure the most contrast reserve.

ASSISTIVE DEVICES AND TECHNIQUES

In addition to traditional testing described previously, the effect of typoscopes (a reading window made from black card stock) or other line marking devices should be assessed. Typoscopes may improve a person's ability to scan across a page and keep his or her place when returning to the beginning of a line. The black typoscope may also offer enhanced comfort by eliminating some of the glare that white paper produces. Some people may benefit from using their fingers as place keepers or to trace along a line of print. It is important to document these techniques and to address them in a training program. Reading stands may promote increased reading duration by increasing comfort and control during reading.

Evaluation of Reading Skills During Near Visual Acuity Testing

Assessing reading skills can begin when listening to the person perform the reading or near acuity evaluation tasks. The examiner can note these factors as the person reads as well as listening to the efficiency with which the person reads and his or her reading style. The assessment of reading skills during reading acuity tests will only take 5 to 10 minutes. The examiner can consider the following questions:

➤ Does the person read easily or in a halting, labored manner?

➤ Does the print size make any difference to the person's reading fluency? Does he or she read large print easily and then begin to labor as the print reaches smaller sizes? Does he or she read with great difficulty regardless of print size?

➤ Does the person often need to backtrack, reread, or search when reading a sentence?

➤ Does the person need to spell the words, letter by letter, or does he or she read word by word?

➤ Does the person use line markers, fingers as place keepers, or other aids for following lines of print?

➤ Does use of a reading stand promote efficiency and comfort and improve a person's reading performance over time?

MN READ

Thie MN Read test (Legge, Ross, & Luebker, 1989) contains continuous text reading charts suitable for measuring the near acuity of persons both with and without low vision. Charts are composed of sentences with words commonly found in second and third grade reading material. Each sentence contains the same number of characters and spaces. The size progression of the sentences uses a log scale. In addition to measuring acuity, the charts may be used to measure maximum reading speed and what is termed critical print size. Critical print size is the smallest print the person can read at maximum speed, and knowing it is of benefit when attempting to provide the appropriate size of print for reading. This test provides an excellent platform for the evaluation of other factors that affect reading performance, including reading fluency, error patterns, and effects of illumination.

PEPPER VISUAL SKILLS FOR READING TEST (PVSRT)

The Pepper Visual Skills for Reading Test (PVSRT) (Baldasare, Watson, Whittaker, & Miller-Shaffer, 1986) is not designed to measure visual acuity but to assess the "visual components of the reading process in low vision individuals" (Whittaker, Watson, & Steciw, 1983). Each test form consists of 13 rows of unrelated letters and/or words, which eliminate any contextual clues while reading. The spacing between lines and words becomes progressively smaller while the length of the words becomes progressively longer. This arrangement is designed to "assess the visual skill of guiding eye movements" (Baldasare et al., 1986). The PVSRT has been found to predict continuous text reading rates with reasonable accuracy (r [36] = 0.82, $p \leq 0.05$) (Watson, Baldasare, & Whittaker, 1990).

There are three forms of the PVSRT, each with different word and letter items and all of which are sixth grade level or lower. Each form is available in five sizes of print: 1M, 1.5M, 2M, 3M, and 4M. The test is conducted with the individual reading the letter size corresponding to next size larger than his or her threshold. Thus, if a person's threshold print size is 0.8M, then the 1M form would be used for testing. The person is timed while reading the form aloud and his or her reading errors are recorded. The person is allowed to use any reading distance that is comfortable and any optical device. Testing is complete if the entire form is read or the person fatigues, fails to recognize a word within 20 seconds, twice fails to find the beginning of a new line, or makes 10 consecutive errors (Baldasare et al., 1986). The error and reading rates allow the examiner to place the reader in one of three categories and thus guide training strategies: "readers who are inaccurate and slow, readers who are accurate but slow, and readers who are both relatively accurate and quick" (Baldasare et al., 1986).

Visual Perceptual Skills

During the assessment, if the examiner becomes suspicious that the person being assessed is not reading well due to factors other than acuity, then perceptual skills testing may provide information as to why the person has difficulty reading.

Just as with individuals without visual impairment, people with low vision can be limited in their ability to read by factors other than their vision.

The visual perceptual skills of people with low vision may be related to more complex educational, vocational, or daily living tasks, such as reading, and these skills may improve with training. The Frostig Figure Ground Test for adults with low vision, for example, has been shown to assess performance factors other than visual acuity when looking at predictors of reading performance (Quillman, Mehr, & Goodrich, 1981). A relationship between figure-ground discrimination and certain reading tasks for people with low vision has also been demonstrated (Quillman et al., 1981; Overbury, Goodrich, Quillman, & Faubert, 1989). Figure-ground performance has also been shown to improve with training in adults who have acquired visual impairments (Trudeau, Overbury, & Conrod, 1990).

Although research related to performance of individuals with low vision has not been conducted for all skills assessed on tests of visual perceptual skills, information from these tests may provide valuable functional information (Overbury et al., 1990). The following areas are often included in tests of visual perceptual skills:

➤ Visual identification or discrimination (matches identical forms)

➤ Visual closure (identifies a form when presented with an incomplete picture of that form)

➤ Figure-ground (differentiates a form from its background)

➤ Visual memory (remembers dominant form features or recalls an exact sequence of forms)

➤ Form constancy (identifies forms regardless of size, orientation, or embedded in other forms)

Tests may also include copying and eye-hand coordination tasks that have a visual-motor component.

Further research is needed to delineate more precisely the visual perceptual skills that are related to more complex performance tasks and the effects of training on such skills. Until such research becomes available, assessing visual perceptual skills in schoolchildren and adults with low vision can provide useful information about this area of visual performance. Several commercially available tests assess visual perceptual skills: the Motor-Free Visual Perception Test, the Gardner Test of Visual Perceptual Skills, and the Developmental Test of Visual Perception (which is the current edition of the *Frostig Test of Visual Perception*) (see the Resources section of this book for sources of these tests). Although these tests have been developed for use with young children, their use by older students and adults can provide information related to visual performance. Since these tests have not been specifically standardized for people with low vision at different age ranges, it is recommended that the scores not be reported. The test results will provide a sense of what areas may be deficient in a person with low vision, but the examiner will not be able to compare results with normative values. In addition, if the test protocols are adapted to meet the needs of older schoolchildren or adults, the scores cannot be reported with accuracy since testing methods have been altered. In administering the Frostig Test of Visual Perception, for example, Quillman et al., (1981) did not strictly adhere to test administration protocols but carefully monitored individual performance styles, which included response accuracy, visual examining approaches, and persistence in task completion. Information about a person's error patterns, performance differences on motor-free tasks compared to visual-motor tasks, and task persistence can be documented to provide a descriptive picture of that person's capabilities across a variety of visual perceptual tasks.

Visual Skills for Everyday Tasks

Visual skills for everyday tasks are often best assessed using usual tasks performed in the actual home, work, school, vocational, or leisure environment. As mentioned in Chapter 4, it is important to complete an environmental analysis, in which critical tasks a person wishes to perform are analyzed for their visual demands. The person is then assessed to determine if vision or other methods can be used to meet these identified task demands. Critical or meaningful tasks can be determined through interviews or direct observation. Performance requirements of critical tasks should be analyzed, and visual demands listed. The best methods to meet each task demands may vary.

DAILY LIVING SKILLS

The visual skills necessary for daily living involve a variety of visual functions including visual acuity, contrast sensitivity, peripheral vision, and color vision. Typical daily living tasks include the following:

➤ Dial a telephone

➤ See the television

➤ Set stove dials

➤ Discern when a cup is full

➤ Match clothing

➤ Read mail

➤ Set thermostat

➤ Do laundry

➤ Read the telephone book

➤ Pay bills

➤ Read labels on cans, jars, medicine bottles

➤ Prepare food from recipes

➤ Locate household items in various parts of the house

It is important that persons with low vision be able to complete these tasks or others that they consider important to maintain their quality of life. Through careful interviews and evaluations of their ability to accomplish real life tasks, one can assess the visual skills used. Observation of an individual in his or her living environment may provide further information about difficulties with visual tasks. Samples of bills, phonebooks, medication bottles, packaged food, or telephones can be kept at hand to assess the person's abilities to complete daily living tasks.

TRAVEL SKILLS

Independent travel or mobility depends on adequate contrast sensitivity, visual fields, and, to a lesser extent, visual acuity (Marron & Bailey, 1982). For a person with limited visual fields, independent mobility will require him or her to perform more scanning with the eyes in order to detect obstacles. For persons with poor contrast sensitivity (unable to detect 10 percent contrast or less), travel and mobility become extremely difficult, due to difficulty detecting doorways, steps, stairs, the junction between walls and floors, and most objects in their path. Improved scanning techniques or higher magnification do not allow them to see objects better. Other skills will be required, such as long cane travel. If the person's chief problem is reduced acuity, magnification through monocular or binocular telescopes will often be beneficial for reading signs, traffic signals, and bus numbers.

LEISURE ACTIVITIES

Leisure activities can be addressed using the information from visual acuity, contrast, visual field, and color vision testing. Depending on the activity, different aspects of the visual system may play a greater role. If pleasure reading is the goal, magnifiers, both handheld and stand, and strong reading glasses may not accomplish this goal. Closed-circuit televisions and auditory reading may allow an individual to read more comfortably and for longer periods of time than do other methods (Goodrich, Mehr, & Darling, 1980).

Computer Use

If an individual is to work at a computer, his or her visual needs and abilities while at the computer should be evaluated, including the following:

➤ Identify aspects of the computer screen the individual can see: cursor, icons, pull-down menus, text and numbers, toolbars.

➤ Can the individual see the hard copy used for data entry?

➤ How large do the characters on the computer screen need to be and what is an appropriate working distance? If visual acuity is decreased, then the characters on the computer monitor will need to be larger than typical or the individual will need to get closer to the monitor or a combination of both. Remember that the font size chosen for the text only reflects the size that will be printed. It does not indicate the size of font on the screen itself.

➤ The size of the letters on the monitor is a function of font size, monitor size, and pixel density (or resolution). For a given font size and pixel density, a larger monitor will have larger characters (letters, icons, etc.) than a smaller monitor. For a given font and screen size, a lower pixel density (lower resolution) will result in larger letters and icons on the monitor. Without special software, the size of the letters, icons, and other elements can be maximized by choosing a large monitor and the lowest pixel density (typically 640 × 480).

➤ As noted earlier in this chapter, maximizing contrast will maximize contrast reserve, resulting in improved reading efficiency. Maximum contrast will be most easily attained using black print on white or white on black. Although it has been shown that adding color to print has no practical benefit for reading (Knoblach et al., 1991; Legge et al., 1990; Legge & Rubin, 1986), reading comfort may be improved using different colors for text and background than the typical black or white.

➤ Ergonomics: The computer screen should be at the person's preferred distance, which may be very close, while allowing the neck and head to be in a natural position to allow prolonged reading performed at the computer.

➤ Lighting and glare at the workstation will also be important issues to address for maximum comfort.

FUNCTIONAL VISION EVALUATION REPORT

Once the functional vision evaluation is completed, a functional vision report needs to be prepared to summarize the evaluation information. The summary form presented in Appendix 6.1 serves as an aid for organizing and summarizing evaluation data. The form is comprehensive, covering a wide range of assessment areas. Not all items need be completed for every person. The information included in the form can also be used as the basis for creating the more extensive and complete written version of the assessment findings. (See Chapter 4 for more information about writing a full report.) Three sample reports are provided in Appendix 6.2. Each report emphasizes different elements because different activities of daily life need to be addressed for each of the individuals with low vision who were evaluated.

CONCLUSION

Evaluation—evaluation of the individual's visual capabilities, ability to function in various settings, needs, goals, and desired activities—forms the basis for planned service delivery and individualized, effective instructional programs. The preceding chapters have described the importance of evaluation, the key considerations involved in working with clients of various ages and capabilities, and the appropriate techniques that result in effective evaluation of diverse clientele. In the section that follows, intervention and programming, which flow from and are based on comprehensive assessment, are explored. Together, these critical activities form the continuum of services for persons with low vision seeking to maximize their functional abilities and capacity for independently performing the activities of life.

REFERENCES

Achard, O. A., Safran, A. B., Duret, F. C., & Ragama, E. (1995). Role of the completion phenomenon in the evaluation of Amsler grid results. *American Journal of Ophthalmology, 120,* 322–329.

American Academy of Ophthalmology. (1996). Automated perimetry. *Ophthalmology, 103,* 1144–1151.

Amsler, M. (1950). Quantitative and qualitative vision. *Transactions of the Ophthalmological Society of the United Kingdom, 69,* 397–410.

Ariyasu, R. G., Lee, P. P., Linton, K. P., LaBree, L. D., Azen, S. P., & Siu, A. L. (1996). Sensitivity, specificity, and predictive values of screening tests for eye conditions in a clinic-based population. *Ophthalmology. 103,* 1751–1760.

Balsadare, J., Watson, G. R., Whittaker, S. G., & Miller-Shaffer, H. (1986). The development and evaluation of a reading test for low vision individuals with macular loss. *Journal of Visual Impairment & Blindness, 80,* 785–789.

Cheong, A. C., Lovie-Kitchin, J. E., & Bowers, A. R. (2002). Determining magnification for reading with low vision. *Clinical & Experimental Optometry, 85,* 229–237.

Elliott, D. B., & Bullimore, M. A. (1993). Assessing the reliability, discriminative ability, and validity of disability glare test. *Investigative Ophthalmology & Visual Science, 34,* 108–119.

Elliott, D. B., Yang, K. C. H., & Whitaker, D. (1995). Visual acuity changes throughout adulthood in normal, healthy eyes: Seeing beyond 6/6. *Optometry & Vision Science, 72,* 186–191.

Flom, M. C., Heath, G. G., & Takahashi, E. (1963). Contour interaction and visual resolution: Contralateral effects. *Science, 142,* 979–980.

Goodrich, G. L., Mehr, E. B., & Darling, N. C. (1980). Parameters in the use of CCTV's and optical aids. *American Journal of Optometry & Physiological Optics, 57,* 881–892.

Hovis, J. K., & Neumann, P. (1995). Colorimetric analyses of various light sources for the D-15 color vision test. *Optometry & Vision Science, L72,* 667–678.

Kitchin, J. E., & Bailey, I. L. (1981). Task complexity and visual acuity in senile macular degeneration. *Australian Journal of Optometry, 64,* 235–242.

Knoblauch, K., Arditi, A., & Szlyk, J. (1991). Effects of chromatic and luminance contrast on reading. *Journal of the Optical Society of America, A8,* 428–439.

Koenig, A. J., & Holbrook, M. C. (1993). *Learning media assessment of students with visual impairments.* Austin, TX: Texas School for the Blind and Visually Impaired.

Law, F. W. (1951). Standardization of reading types. *British Journal of Ophthalmology, 35,* 765–773.

Leat, S. J., & Gargon, J. L. (1995). Accommodative response in children and young adults using dynamic retinoscopy. *Ophthalmic & Physiological Optics, 16,* 375–384.

Legge, G. E., Parish, D. H., Luebker, A., & Wurm, L. H. (1990). Psychophysics of reading: XI. Comparing color contrast and luminanced contrast. *Journal of the Optical Society of America, A7,* 2002–2010.

Legge, G. E., Ross, J. A., & Luebker, A. (1989). Psychophysics of reading: VIII. The Minnesota low-vision reading test. *Optometry & Visual Science, 66,* 843–851.

Legge, G. E., & Rubin, G. S. (1986). Psychophysics of reading: IV. Wavelength effects in normal and low vision. *Journal of the Optical Society of America, A3,* 40–51.

Legge, G. E., Rubin, G. S., Pelli, D. G., & Schleske, M. M. (1985). Psychophysics of reading: II. Low vision. *Vision Research, 25,* 253–266.

Legge, G. E., Rubin, G. S., & Schleske, M. M. (1987). Contrast polarity effects in low vision reading. In G. Woo (Ed.), *Low vision: Principles applications* (pp. 288–307). New York: Springer-Verlag.

Lovie-Kitchin, J. E., & Brown, B. (2000). Repeatability and intercorrelations of standard vision tests as a function of age. *Optometry & Vision Science, 77,* 412–420.

Marron, J. A, & Bailey, I. L. (1982). Visual factors and orientation-mobility performance. *American Journal of Optometry & Physiological Optics, 59,* 413–426.

National Research Council (2002). *Visual impairments: Determining eligibility for social security benefits.* Washington, DC: National Academy Press.

Overbury, O., Goodrich, G. L., Quillman, R. D., & Faubert, J. (1989). Perceptual assessment in low vision: Evidence for a hierarchy of skills? *Journal of Visual Impairment & Blindness. 75,* 109–113.

Pokorny J., Smith V. C., Verriest G., Pinckers, & A. J. L. G. (1979). *Congenital and acquired color vision defects.* New York: Grune & Stratton.

Quillman, R. D., Mehr, E. B., & Goodrich, G. L. (1981). Uses of the Frostig Figure Ground in evaluation of adults with low vision. *American Journal of Optometry, 58*(11), 910–918.

Schuchard, R. A. (1993). Validity and interpretation of Amsler grid reports. *Archives of Ophthalmology, 111,* 776–780.

Sharpe, L. T., Stockman, A., Jägle, H., & Nathans, J. (2000). Opsin genes, cone photopigments and colorblindness. In K. Gegenfurtner & L. T. Sharpe (Eds.), *Color vision: From genes to perception* (pp. 3–52). New York: Cambridge University Press.

Trudeau, M., Overbury, O., & Conrod, B. (1990). Perceptual training and figure-ground performance in low vision. *Journal of Visual Impairment & Blindness, 84,* 204–206.

Watson, G. R., Baldasare, J., & Whittaker, S. (1990). The validity and clinical uses of the Pepper visual skills for reading test. *Journal of Visual Impairment & Blindness, 84,* 119–123.

Watson, G. R., Wright, V., & De l'Aune, W. (1992). The efficacy of comprehension training and reading practice for print readers with macular loss. *Journal of Visual Impairment & Blindness, 86,* 37–43.

Watson, G. R., Wright, V., & Long, S. (1996). *The Morgan low vision reading comprehension assessment.* Lilburn, GA: Bear Consultants, Inc.

Watson, G. R., Wright, V., Long, S., & De l'Aune, W. (1996). A low vision reading comprehension test. *Journal of Visual Impairment & Blindness, 90,* 489–494.

Whittaker S. G., & Lovie-Kitchin J. (1993). Visual requirements for reading. *Optometry & Vision Science, 70,* 54–65,

Whittaker, S., Watson, G., & Steciw, M. (1983). The development and evaluation of functional assessment instruments. *Low Vision Research and Training Center final report.* National Institute of Handicapped Research, part 2, 19–38.

Wilkins, A. J., & Robson, J. G. (1988). *Cambridge Low Contrast Gratings. Instructions for use.* Essex, UK: Clement Clarke International, Ltd.

Functional Vision Evaluation Report:
Children and Adults

Assessor _____   Assessment date _____

Student or client's name _____   Birth date _____

Address _____

School or work location _____

Type of employment or school program information _____

Visual diagnosis _____

Visual prognosis ☐ Stable   ☐ Deteriorating   ☐ Capable of improvement   ☐ Unknown

Eye Care Specialist: Name _____   Phone _____

                     Address _____

                     Date of most recent evaluation _____

Visual acuity without correction from specialist's report: Right eye ____ Left eye ____ Both eyes ____

Visual acuity with correction from specialist's report: Right eye ____ Left eye ____ Both eyes ____

Visual field from specialist's report _____

Eye care specialist's recommended activity limitations _____

Summary and Recommendations (based on information gathered for this evaluation)

_____

_____

_____

_____

_____

_____

_____

_____

_____

_____

_____

_____

Conclusion:

For schoolchildren: Student has a visual impairment that adversely affects educational performance in expanded core curricular areas (daily living, career, academics etc.).   Yes ☐ No ☐

For adults: Client has a visual impairment that adversely affects work, daily living, other.   Yes ☐ No ☐

Other Evaluations Recommended

☐ Low vision evaluation   Reason _____

☐ Ophthalmological evaluation   Reason _____

☐ Orientation & mobility evaluation   Reason _____

☐ Other _____

Suggested Viewing Distances

☐ Chalkboard: _____   Prefers: ☐ Blackboard   ☐ White dry-erase board

☐ Television (screen size _____) _____

☐ Computer (screen size _____) _____

☐ CCTV (screen size _____) _____

☐ Lectures/demonstrations _____

☐ Overhead projector _____

☐ Wall clock _____

☐ Faces _____

☐ Sign language _____

☐ Movies _____

☐ Wall menus _____

☐ Vocational tasks (specify) _____

☐ Other (specify) _____

2

(continued on next page)

Contents

Checklist of Evaluation Findings

1. Optical Correction Information

Wears: ☐ Distance glasses When prescribed? _____ Improves performance: ☐ Yes ☐ No
                        Wears regularly ☐ Yes ☐ No

        ☐ Contact lenses When prescribed? _____ Improves performance: ☐ Yes ☐ No
                        Wears regularly ☐ Yes ☐ No

        ☐ Reading glasses When prescribed? _____ Improves performance: ☐ Yes ☐ No
                        Wears regularly ☐ Yes ☐ No

        ☐ Bifocals   When prescribed? _____ Improves performance: ☐ Yes ☐ No
                        Wears regularly ☐ Yes ☐ No

        Condition of eyeglasses? _____ Adequate? ☐ Yes ☐ No

2. Other Relevant Health/Medical/Educational Information

_____

_____

_____

3. Main Concerns of Student or Client

☐ Reading ☐ Writing ☐ Inclusion in school or community activities ☐ Socialization
☐ Prevocational or vocational activities ☐ Hobbies ☐ Recreation/leisure activities
☐ Academic pursuits (specify) _____ ☐ Safety or health issues (specify) _____
☐ Daily living activities ☐ Mobility ☐ Driving ☐ Other _____

Comments: _____

_____

_____

4. Knowledge of Eye Condition

☐ Understands visual condition and prognosis

Describes eye condition information as follows: _____

_____

☐ Orients materials appropriately for visual needs
☐ Expresses visual needs appropriately for environmental modifications
☐ Devises own environmental modifications (specify): _____

_____

4

(continued on next page)

Comments: _____
_____
_____

5. Social Behaviors Dependent on Vision Cues

☐ Identifies people from distance (specify distance) _____

☐ Identifies facial expressions (specify distance) _____

☐ Maintains appropriate social distance when talking (specify distance) _____

☐ Uses appropriate gestures (for school age students) _____

☐ Recognizes gestures of others _____

☐ Uses eye contact appropriately _____

☐ Other (specify) _____

6. Use of Assistive Devices Involving Vision

Check only those devices currently being used. Report print size in M (meter) or Pt (point) notation unless specified otherwise.

Optical Devices

☐ Hand magnifier   ☐ Formal training   ☐ Uses regularly   ☐ Rarely uses

Independent use ☐ Yes   ☐ No

Independent care ☐ Yes   ☐ No

Manufacturer _____ Catalog number _____ Power _____

Prescribed by _____ Date prescribed _____

Usual print size read _____ Words per minute read _____

Number of characters seen with magnifier/usual print size _____

Specify uses _____

☐ Stand magnifier   ☐ Formal training   ☐ Uses regularly   ☐ Rarely uses

Independent use ☐ Yes   ☐ No

Independent care ☐ Yes   ☐ No

Manufacturer _____ Catalog number _____ Power _____

Prescribed by _____ Date prescribed _____

Usual print size read _____ Words per minute read _____

Number of characters seen with magnifier/usual print size _____

Specify uses _____

☐ Telescope   ☐ Formal training   ☐ Uses regularly   ☐ Rarely uses
Independent use ☐ Yes   ☐ No
Independent care ☐ Yes   ☐ No
Manufacturer _____   Catalog number _____   Power _____
Prescribed by _____   Date prescribed _____
Specify uses _____

☐ Other Optical   ☐ Formal training   ☐ Uses regularly   ☐ Rarely uses
Device (specify) Independent use ☐ Yes   ☐ No
_____   Independent care ☐ Yes   ☐ No
Manufacturer _____   Catalog number _____   Power _____
Prescribed by _____   Date prescribed _____
Usual print size read _____   Words per minute read _____
Number of characters seen with magnifier/usual print size __   _____
Specify uses _____

Illumination Control

☐ Sunglasses outdoors   ☐ Wears regularly   ☐ Rarely uses
☐ Requires filters indoors   ☐ Wears regularly   ☐ Rarely uses
☐ Visor   ☐ Wears regularly   ☐ Rarely uses
☐ Sun hat (baseball cap)   ☐ Wears regularly   ☐ Rarely uses
☐ Directional lighting: near tasks   ☐ Uses regularly   ☐ Rarely uses

Electronic Devices

☐ Closed circuit   ☐ Formal training   ☐ Uses regularly   ☐ Rarely uses
television   Independent use ☐ Yes   ☐ No
Independent care ☐ Yes   ☐ No
Manufacturer _____   Screen size _____
Print size read (actual measure, in or cm) _____
Working distance _____   Words per minute read _____
Specify uses _____
Prefers ☐ Black on white   ☐ White on black
☐ Colors (specify) _____

6

(continued on next page)

☐ Computer   ☐ Formal training   ☐ Uses regularly   ☐ Rarely uses

Independent use ☐ Yes   ☐ No

Independent care ☐ Yes   ☐ No

Manufacturer _____   Screen size _____

Print size read (actual measure, in or cm) _____

Working distance _____   Words per minute read _____

Preferred font style _____   Pixel density _____

Lighting requirements _____

Screen items seen: ☐ Cursor   ☐ Icons   ☐ Pull-down menu
                  ☐ Text and numbers   ☐ Toolbars

☐ Sees hard copy for data entry

Special ergonomic concerns _____

Preferred polarity _____   Preferred colors _____

Specify uses _____

☐ Large print computer software   ☐ Formal training   ☐ Uses regularly   ☐ Rarely uses

Independent use ☐ Yes   ☐ No

Independent care ☐ Yes   ☐ No

Manufacturer _____   Preferred print size _____

Specify uses _____

☐ Other (specify) _____   ☐ Formal training   ☐ Uses regularly   ☐ Rarely uses

Independent use ☐ Yes   ☐ No

Independent care ☐ Yes   ☐ No

Provide details of device use _____

Specify uses _____

Other Reading Devices

☐ Large print   ☐ Uses regularly   ☐ Rarely uses

                 Preferred print size _____   Preferred working distance _____

☐ Typoscope   ☐ Uses regularly   ☐ Rarely uses

☐ Line guide   ☐ Uses regularly   ☐ Rarely uses

☐ Plastic overlays   ☐ Uses regularly   ☐ Rarely uses

                 Specify color _____

☐ Reading stand   ☐ Uses regularly   ☐ Rarely uses

☐ Other (specify)   ☐ Uses regularly   ☐ Rarely uses

_____

Writing Devices

☐ Fiber-tip pen   ☐ Uses regularly   ☐ Rarely uses

☐ Bold-line paper   ☐ Uses regularly   ☐ Rarely uses

☐ Other line guide   ☐ Uses regularly   ☐ Rarely uses
    (specify) _____

☐ Other (specify)   ☐ Uses regularly   ☐ Rarely uses

_____

Devices Tried and No Longer Used: _____

_____

_____

7. Appearance of Eyes

List any unusual appearance of the eyes that should be evaluated by an eye care specialist.

_____

_____

8. Oculomotor Control

List any unusual muscle imbalance (eye turn). This can include esotropia (eye turn inward) or exotropia (eye turn outward). Muscle imbalances must be evaluated by the eye doctor.

Right eye _____   Left eye _____

Test used: ☐ Cover test   ☐ Extraocular motility test

9. Sensory Nystagmus

☐ Present   ☐ Not present   Increases under stress: ☐ Yes   ☐ No

Naturally uses null point: ☐ Yes   ☐ No

Describe head position for null point. _____

_____

10. Preferred Modes of Viewing

Natural viewing distance for viewing up close _____

Natural viewing distance for viewing far away _____

Describe head tilts when viewing. (These postures may be adopted to achieve the null point for nystagmus, to compensate for a peripheral field loss, or to view eccentrically if there is a central scotoma.)

☐ Must first touch or hear object before vision is used to investigate it. (Often associated with cortical visual impairment.)

8

(continued on next page)

Comments: _____

_____

_____

11. Eye Preference for Near Work

If the person consistently holds objects or reading material under one eye rather than the other or both, that eye is the preferred eye for near work.

Eye preference: ☐ Right eye   ☐ Left eye   ☐ None observed

Comments: _____

_____

_____

12. Peripheral Visual Fields (Confrontation Field Test)

As a functional measure, it is not necessary to test each eye individually. Sit directly in front of the person and encourage him or her to look at your nose or at a light source (penlight) held directly in front of him or her. It is important for the person to maintain steady, central fixation. Hold a second light source 2 ft away and bring it in slowly from above, below, left, and right. This is easier if another evaluator stands behind and moves the second light source into position. Note when the person first notices the moving light source entering his or her field of view. If the person does not attend to the light source, dimming the room lights may promote his or her use of vision. Visual fields should be evaluated with eyeglasses removed since the frames can restrict the visual field.

Note: If a person is monocular, then only the visual field of the seeing eye is being measured and there will be an expected reduction in visual field on the side of the nonseeing eye.

Record any modifications made to target, target size, target distance, or room illumination.

_____

Confidence in findings: _____

The following are some examples of right visual field measurements for the right eye:

Right field: ☐ Full 90 degrees to temporal side ☐ About 45 degrees
              ☐ <20 degrees ☐ No response

Left field: ☐ Full 90 degrees to temporal side ☐ About 45 degrees
              ☐ <20 degrees ☐ No response

Upper field: ☐ Full 50 degrees ☐ 25 degrees
              ☐ <20 degrees ☐ No response

Lower field: ☐ Full 70 degrees ☐ About 45 degrees
              ☐ <20 degrees ☐ No response

Often bumps into objects: ☐ To the left ☐ To the right ☐ Above ☐ Below
Often fails to notice objects: ☐ To the left ☐ To the right ☐ Above ☐ Below

Comments: _____

_____

_____

13. Central Visual Field
Amsler Grid Test (near point 10 degrees)

Distance tested: _____

          Left eye   Right eye

10

(continued on next page)

Tangent Screen Test (central 30 degrees)

Left eye

Right eye

List any behavioral indicators of central visual field loss. _____

_____

_____

Comments: _____

_____

_____

14. Distance Visual Acuity (Letter or Symbol Optotypes)

Test administered _____

☐ With correction ☐ Without correction

☐ Both eyes viewing ☐ Right eye only ☐ Left eye only

☐ With directional lamp ☐ Under usual room illumination

Distance presented _____ Symbol size read _____

Visual acuity (test distance/symbol size) _____

Converted to equivalent Snellen acuity _____

Difference in visual acuity with different illumination: ☐ Yes ☐ No

Describe any difference _____

Confidence in finding: _____

Test administered _____

☐ With correction   ☐ Without correction

☐ Both eyes viewing   ☐ Right eye only   ☐ Left eye only

☐ With directional lamp   ☐ Under usual room illumination

Distance presented _____   Symbol size read _____

Visual acuity (test distance/symbol size) _____

Converted to equivalent Snellen acuity _____

Difference in visual acuity with different illumination: ☐ Yes   ☐ No

Describe any difference _____

Confidence in finding: _____

Test administered _____

☐ With correction   ☐ Without correction

☐ Both eyes viewing   ☐ Right eye only   ☐ Left eye only

☐ With directional lamp   ☐ Under usual room illumination

Distance presented _____   Symbol size read _____

Visual acuity (test distance/symbol size) _____

Converted to equivalent Snellen acuity _____

Difference in visual acuity with different illumination: ☐ Yes   ☐ No

Describe any difference _____

Confidence in finding: _____

Comments: _____

_____

_____

15. Accommodation

Near point of accommodation _____   Test used: ☐ Near point of accommodation
                                                            ☐ MAR equivalency

12

(continued on next page)

16. Near Visual Acuity (Letter or Symbol Optoypes)

Test administered _____

☐ With correction ☐ Without correction

☐ Both eyes viewing ☐ Right eye only ☐ Left eye only

☐ With directional lamp ☐ Under usual room illumination

Distance naturally used _____

Symbol size read most efficiently at this distance: M units or point size _____

Smallest symbol size read at this distance: M units or point size _____

(At a specified working distance, the ratio of the symbol size read most efficiently to the smallest symbol size read is the optimal visual reserve.)

Closest working distance _____   Smallest symbol size read at that distance: M units or point size _____

Distance presented for test protocol _____   Smallest symbol size read: M units or point size _____

Confidence in findings: _____

Test administered _____

☐ With correction ☐ Without correction

☐ Both eyes viewing ☐ Right eye only ☐ Left eye only

☐ With directional lamp ☐ Under usual room illumination

Distance naturally used _____

Symbol size read most efficiently at this distance: M units or point size _____

Smallest symbol size read at this distance: M units or point size _____

(At a specified working distance, the ratio of the symbol size read most efficiently to the smallest symbol size read is the optimal visual reserve.)

Closest working distance _____   Smallest symbol size read at that distance: M units or point size _____

Distance presented for test protocol _____   Smallest symbol size read: M units or point size _____

Confidence in findings: _____

Comments: _____

_____

_____

17. Contrast Sensitivity

(Normal Michelson contrast is 0.5 percent. A person with 3.0 percent Michelson contrast, for example, requires contrast to be six times greater than normal for optimal viewing. Normal Weber contrast is 1.0 to 2.0 percent.)

Test administered _____

☐ With correction   ☐ Without correction

☐ Both eyes viewing

☐ With directional lamp   ☐ Under usual room illumination

Distance presented _____   Lowest percentage contrast noted _____

How many times greater than normal contrast required _____

☐ Relatively normal contrast sensitivity (up to 1.5 percent Michelson contrast; up to 3 percent Weber contrast)

☐ Moderately reduced contrast sensitivity (2.0 to 4.5 percent Michelson contrast or 3.5 to 9 percent Weber contrast)

☐ Severely reduced contrast sensitivity (over 4.5 percent Michelson contrast or over 9 percent Weber contrast)

Confidence in finding: _____

Test administered _____

☐ With correction   ☐ Without correction

☐ Both eyes viewing

☐ With directional lamp   ☐ Under usual room illumination

Distance presented _____   Lowest percentage contrast noted _____

How many times greater than normal contrast required _____

☐ Relatively normal contrast sensitivity (up to 1.5 percent Michelson contrast; up to 3 percent Weber contrast)

☐ Moderately reduced contrast sensitivity (2.0 to 4.5 percent Michelson contrast or 3.5 to 9 percent Weber contrast)

☐ Severely reduced contrast sensitivity (over 4.5 percent Michelson contrast or over 9 percent Weber contrast)

Confidence in finding: _____

Comments: _____

_____

_____

(continued on next page)

18. Light Sensitivity

Light sensitivity is best determined through observation and by comparing performance with and without a directional lamp. A test of visual acuity is a good way to assess for possible performance differences.

General lighting requirements: ☐ Very bright ☐ Normal ☐ Dim

Outdoors, prefers to use: ☐ Baseball cap ☐ Visor ☐ Sunglasses

☐ Squints in bright light ☐ Avoids looking toward bright light

☐ Visually disoriented for _____ minutes when going from indoors to outdoors

☐ Visually disoriented for _____ minutes when going from outdoors to indoors

☐ Orients using bright light source (window, lamp, sun)

☐ Performs near tasks more accurately or easily with directional light on tasks (based on information from observation and/or tests of visual acuity)

Comments: _____

_____

_____

19. Color Vision

If results of formal tests are not available, use observation or interview to determine if there are any color preferences and if the person can select, match, verbally identify, or sort items according to color. Socks and clothes are items that are matched by adults, for example. The latter tasks are not sensitive enough to detect color vision disorders.

Test administered _____

☐ With directional lamp ☐ Under usual room illumination

☐ Red-green deficiency ☐ Blue-yellow deficiency

☐ Reduced overall color discrimination

Confidence in finding: _____

Observation or Interview

☐ Identifies primary colors

☐ Matches similar dark colors, such as socks

☐ Sorts red and green (make certain color saturation of objects presented is equivalent)

☐ Sorts blue and yellow (make certain color saturation of objects presented is equivalent)

☐ Demonstrates color preferences (specify colors) _____

Comments: _____

_____

_____

20. Reading

Many of these factors can be measured in conjunction with formal reading tests (i.e., MN Read, reading level inventories) or using the subject's own reading material.

Check only those items that apply.

Reading Tasks

Current reading activities: _____

_____

Desired reading tasks person is currently unable to perform:

☐ Usual reading material (specify grade level if in school and type of material) _____

_____

☐ Paperback books	☐ Dictionary	☐ Labels and price tags
☐ Sheet music	☐ Bills, letters	☐ Maps, charts, graphs
☐ Newspaper text	☐ Newspaper headlines	☐ Wall menus
☐ Menus	☐ Stove, radio, television dials	☐ Food and medicine labels
☐ Cookbooks	☐ Other _____	☐ Other _____

Speed, Duration, Working Distance

☐ Reads regular print: Distance read _____   Reading speed _____

   Reading duration _____

☐ Reads large print (size ____): Distance read _____   Reading speed _____

   Reading duration _____

☐ Reads with magnifier (power ____): ☐ Handheld   ☐ Stand Reading speed _____

   Reading duration _____

Reading Fluency

Describe flow of reading: _____

_____

Reading Comprehension

Test used and results: _____

_____

_____

16

(continued on next page)

Reading Methods

☐ Moves only eyes   ☐ Moves only head   ☐ Moves head and eyes   ☐ Moves reading material

☐ Eccentric viewing used   ☐ Eccentric viewing training required

☐ Special positioning of reading material required to accommodate reading posture (specify)

_____

☐ Uses finger as line guide while reading

☐ Uses finger to hold place at beginning of line

☐ Often loses place on line

☐ Often skips a line

☐ Often skips words on a line when reading

☐ Often misses small words on a line when reading

☐ Reads letter by letter   ☐ Reads word by word   ☐ Reads two or three word phrases

☐ Sees whole words

Comments: _____

_____

_____

21. Writing

☐ Handwriting is legible

☐ Reads own handwriting (size _____)

☐ Reads manuscript writing

☐ Reads cursive writing

☐ Uses optical or electronic device to assist with handwriting (describe) _____

Prefers to read: ☐ Manuscript letters   ☐ Cursive letters

Prefers to write: ☐ Manuscript letters   ☐ Cursive letters

Comments: _____

_____

_____

22. Copying and Location Skills
Locating Items while Reading

☐ Locates page numbers in a book easily _____

☐ Locates words in dictionary easily _____

☐ Locates items on maps, charts, graphs easily _____

☐ Can follow unusual formats (e.g., columns, sidebars, descriptions under pictures, card catalog,

  bills) _____

Copying Skills

☐ Copies from chalkboard with few errors _____

☐ Copies from books with few errors _____

☐ Shifts gaze when copying easily _____

_____

Locating Items in the Environment

☐ Locates personal possessions easily _____

☐ Locates known items in familiar environments easily _____

☐ Locates items in unfamiliar environments easily _____

☐ Organizes environment to facilitate item location _____

☐ Uses systematic visual search strategies _____

List items in environment person needs to locate regularly and is having difficulty locating

_____

_____

Comments: _____

_____

_____

23. Visual Perceptual Skills

Complete a commercially available test of visual perception (e.g., Motor-Free Visual Perception Test, Visual Functioning Assessment Tool, Test of Visual-Perceptual Skills, Frostig Test of Visual Perception). Most of these tests have not been standardized for students with visual impairments; therefore test scores may not be valid. A report of the error pattern, however, can be helpful when determining intervention strategies.

Assessment Method _____

Error pattern, test scores, and interpretation: _____

_____

_____

The following visual perception areas were noted as challenging:

☐ Visual identification or discrimination (matches identical forms)

☐ Visual closure (identifies form when presented with an incomplete picture of that form)

☐ Figure ground (distinguishes a form from its background)

☐ Visual memory (remembers dominant form features or recalls an exact sequence of forms)

☐ Form constancy (identifies forms regardless of size, orientation, or embedded in other forms)

18

(continued on next page)

Comments: _____

_____

_____

24. Picture and Photograph Recognition

☐ Recognizes simple pictures: smallest size _____

☐ Recognizes complex pictures: smallest size _____

☐ Recognizes black/white photos of people: smallest size _____

☐ Recognizes color photos of people: smallest size _____

Comments: _____

_____

_____

25. Preferred Sensory Mode for Learning

Observe the person's exploration and manipulation methods. For school age children, use *Learning Media Assessment,* 2nd ed., by A. J. Koenig & M. C. Holbrook (Austin: Texas School for the Blind and Visually Impaired, 1995).

Explores using the following method(s): ☐ Vision ☐ Touch ☐ Hearing

Primary learning mode is: ☐ Visual ☐ Tactile ☐ Auditory ☐ Combination _____

Comments: _____

_____

_____

26. Eye-Hand Coordination (for students in primary grades)

Consider student's grade level in evaluating him or her.

☐ Draws lines

☐ Draws intersecting lines

☐ Draws shapes (specify) _____

☐ Colors within lines

☐ Cuts along lines

☐ Pastes within lines

☐ Accurate reach for objects

☐ Accurate placement of objects

Comments: _____

_____

_____

Sample Functional Vision Evaluation Reports

Sample Functional Vision Evaluation Report: Mrs. Leonides

This interdisciplinary report came from a clinic setting that included low vision optometrists, assistive technology specialists, and vision rehabilitation specialists on staff. It was written for a referring ophthalmologist.

Patient: Stella Leonides   **Age:** 80 years

History

Mrs. Leonides was accompanied by her daughter to the evaluation session at the low vision clinic. She lives with her daughter and son-in-law and leads an active, independent life. Mrs. Leonides attends activities at a local senior center, and travels there independently on public transportation. She walks to the local shopping mall where she meets with friends regularly, and she actively maintains a large collection of antique dolls.

According to her medical records, Mrs. Leonides's low vision is attributed to myopic maculopathy. Her reduced vision of the right eye was attributed to leakage from a choroidal neovascular membrane secondary to her myopic maculopathy. Her vision in the left eye has been reduced secondary to myopic atrophy of the macular pigment epithelium.

Mrs. Leonides came to our low vision clinic because she was having difficulty with near tasks such as reading and writing, as well as general household tasks involving near vision such as reading the dials on the stove, dishwasher, and radio.

Evaluation

Distance Visual Acuity

With her current glasses Mrs. Leonides's distance visual acuities, as measured with the Bailey-Lovie chart, were as follows:

O.D.:	+0.75 −3.00 × 080	8/25	(20/63 Snellen equivalent)
O.S.:	+0.25 −0.75 × 080	3.2/25	(20/160 Snellen equivalent with extreme difficulty)

Near Visual Acuity

Near visual acuities through a + 4.00D add with her distance prescription in place, measured with the Bailey-Lovie near chart, were O.U. 2.0M at 25 cm.

Retinoscopy and subjective refraction revealed the following refractive error and corrected visual acuities:

O.D.:	+0.50-0.50×180 over refraction	8/25 (20/63 equivalent)
O.S.:	no change	

Compiled by Amanda Hall Lueck and Geoff Perel, Senior Rehabilitation Counselor for the Blind

(continued on next page)

Contrast Sensitivity

Contrast sensitivity was found to be moderately reduced. With the Bailey Border Contrast Sensitivity test her contrast sensitivity was 1.4 log units (4 percent contrast). Normal contrast sensitivity is 2.0 to 2.3 log units (1 to 0.5 percent). With her level of impairment, she may have difficulty seeing shadows and textures. Mobility tasks such as seeing steps and stairs may also be difficult for Mrs. Leonides.

Visual Fields

Amsler Grid testing showed little distortion in the right eye, and metamorphopsia and loss of nasal and central vision in the left eye. The central scotoma in the left eye helps to explain her difficulty with using that eye to see. Confrontational fields testing showed restricted superior field and mild nasal and temporal field loss in both eyes.

Reading and Close Work

Due to Mrs. Leonides' problems with near vision, we tested her performance with several optical devices for close work. The Eschenbach 1584-3 illuminated stand magnifier enabled her to read 0.63M comfortably. We also showed Mrs. Leonides the Magnicam, a portable CCTV, the VERA reading machine with speech output, and enlarging software for computer use.

Summary

Mrs. Leonides has low vision due to myopic maculopathy. Our vision rehabilitation specialist demonstrated and provided Mrs. Leonides with information about various nonoptical adaptive devices such as large print address books, calendars, and kitchen gadgets as well as ways to mark dials and important items around the house. Mrs. Leonides was also given catalogs from which to obtain items that may be of use to her. Mrs. Leonides was referred to services that provide large print checks and registers from banks, and she was given information about assistance with local transportation. Techniques for improving contrast in daily tasks, labeling, and organizing methods were also discussed. Finally, Mrs. Leonides was referred for an orientation and mobility evaluation through a local agency, Special Services for the Blind and Visually Impaired. Mrs. Leonides was informed that the agency also provides home visits by rehabilitation teachers who can provide suggestions about organization of the home environment for easier access. Mrs. Leonides was not certain she needed such service at this time.

Recommendations

To allow the most efficient use of her vision for reading, we recommend the Eschenbach 1584-3 illuminated stand magnifier. This device has been ordered and will be funded through her health insurance. Mrs. Leonides is returning to our clinic once a week for 5 weeks to complete a training program in the use of the magnifier, which includes weekly homework assignments that will be monitored by her daughter. Information about adaptive devices Mrs. Leonides can use at home will be reinforced at that time. In addition, during those visits to our clinic, she will complete additional assessments with our assistive technology specialist to determine other electronic devices that may help with her reading and household tasks. We will also set up a instructional program to train Mrs. Leonides in the use of any devices she has upon selected completion of the technology evaluation.

We did not conduct a complete ocular health examination because she is under an ophthalmologist's care.

Functional Vision Evaluation Report: Margaret Tam

Student: Margaret Tam   **Age:** 18

A functional vision evaluation was conducted for this student in preparation for an individual transition plan meeting. Information for this report was obtained from medical records, from an interview, and from assessment data gathered at the school site. This evaluation was conducted by a teacher of students with visual impairments with a rehabilitation counselor in attendance.

History

Margaret is an 18-year-old "second year" senior who will be graduating this year and then plans to enroll in college. Her favorite subjects include English, drama, and theater arts. Her hobbies include art and sewing; she also enjoys swimming. She performs volunteer work in the community.

Until this year, Margaret went to local schools in her home community and was one of four students with visual impairments in the area. She is currently enrolled in a residential school for students who are visually impaired to expand her educational skills related to visual impairments before she transitions to college. She is receiving instruction in daily living skills in a special apartment living situation on her school campus, orientation and mobility (O&M) instruction, and organizational skills instruction in addition to her regular high school curriculum. She attends classes at the local high school with educational support services from a teacher of students who are visually impaired from the residential school. Margaret has no additional disabilities and is a capable student.

Margaret's medical records indicate that she was first diagnosed by her ophthalmologist, at age 3, with bilateral optic nerve atrophy (a degeneration of the optic nerve, which transmits electrical signals from the eye to the brain) and received her first pair of glasses at that time. She has been followed regularly by the eye care specialist, who indicated in a later report that her vision was stable. Her last eye examination by him was 6 months ago, and it indicated that Margaret was nearsighted. She received a pair of eyeglasses for the following prescription:

Right eye: $-3.25 + 0.75 \times 130$
Left eye: $-3.25 + 0.50 \times 45$

She reportedly had a distance visual acuity of 20/200 in the right eye and 20/400 in the left eye. The specialist's last report also indicated that Margaret demonstrated color vision deficits (mild red-green color deficit), sensitivity to light, and exotropia (outward eye turn) in her right eye. The report noted no nystagmus (rapid horizontal eye movement), and peripheral visual fields (area of side vision) were reported to be normal. She had been prescribed an 8× monocular telescope and a 12-diopter hand held magnifier.

Evaluation

Margaret's interview, observations, and formal assessment were conducted in a special assessment classroom in the residential school. Margaret was a willing participant throughout the functional vision evaluation. She worked very hard to complete all of the assessments. She was approachable regarding very sensitive issues about her vision, demonstrating maturity and insight.

(continued on next page)

Overview from Interview

Margaret clearly understood the diagnosis of her visual disorder as optic nerve atrophy. She expressed concern that, even though she was told that her condition was stable, she had recently noticed a significant change in her ability to identify colors but had not returned to her eye care specialist for assistance. Margaret indicated some specific goals during the initial interview: finding out if she could drive, wanting to see the chalkboard, and not wanting to bump into things so much while traveling. She expressed an interest in wanting to help other persons with visual impairments. Margaret noted that her residential school experience has taught her advocacy skills as a person with a visual impairment. On more than one occasion she mentioned how, in the past, peer pressure often affected her decisions about revealing to others that she was a person with a visual impairment. This had made her reluctant to learn special skills in some of her activities for daily living, especially mobility.

Distance Visual Acuity

Margaret reported difficulty noticing hazards such as sidewalk cracks while walking. She reported that she was not able to see details in faces, especially eye colors, eyebrows, and blemishes. She has an 8× monocular telescope, first obtained in the sixth grade, and uses it for distance spotting at the airport, viewing street signs while traveling, and for grocery shopping.

The Bailey-Lovie Distance Visual Acuity Chart was used with spectacle correction in place and with both eyes viewing unless otherwise noted. With no illumination, at 5 ft, Margaret read the 80-ft line with no errors. Equivalent Snellen acuity is 20/230. With illumination (directional lamp), at 5 ft, Margaret read the 50 ft line with no errors. Equivalent Snellen acuity is 20/200. With illumination (directional lamp) at 5 ft and using her 8× monocular with her right eye, Margaret read all the 12.5-ft letters with no errors. Equivalent Snellen acuity is 20/50.

Margaret's ability to see details at a distance is affected by differences in illumination. She appears to see details more clearly under brighter illumination. When proper lighting is provided, Margaret must move 10 times closer to see things than people with a visual acuity of 20/20. When lighting is not optimal, she must move even closer (16 times). Margaret is able to see smaller details using her monocular telescope under good lighting conditions than she can see without it.

Near Visual Acuity

Margaret reported she "doesn't read as much as she used to." Near tasks Margaret reported participating in included reading books and computer text, writing poetry, and engaging in hobbies such as artwork and sewing. She also noted that lighting significantly determines the size print she can read and that glare makes reading more difficult. Finally, Margaret reportedly "loves" her magnifier (12-diopter handheld magnifier), especially for sewing. Margaret noted that she benefits from a typoscope (black card with a reading window) to keep herself on track on a written page. Line markers are also reportedly helpful. Using a CCTV for enlarging print/objects for near acuity tasks has not been especially helpful according to Margaret (except for painting her nails) since extended reading makes her "seasick." While using a computer for school work, Margaret was observed to enlarge the font size to 1 inch letters on a 15-inch screen. She sat about 1 ft from the screen. Margaret reported that computer software magnification programs have not been beneficial, again creating a feeling of nausea. Furthermore, speech output has not been helpful because she reportedly prefers to "read rather than listen."

The MN Read Chart presents sentences of different print sizes. Margaret was tested with her glasses and with a directional lamp. When asked to hold the chart at a comfortable distance, Margaret's preferred natural viewing distance was 8 inches (20 cm), and she read print comfortably to the 2.5 M size (approximately the size of newspaper subheadlines) with no errors at this distance.

When Margaret held the reading card at the recommended test distance of 16 inches (40 cm) she read print down to 3.2 M in height with no errors (approximately newspaper headline size). At the 16-inch test distance, Margaret's reading speed increased when she read 5M print and stayed at this speed at the next print size, 6.3M. The 5M print at 16 inches provides the same angular print size as the one Margaret demonstrated earlier as her preference (2.5M print at 8 inches).

Margaret's best reading performance on the MN Read Chart indicates that she requires print to be 2.5M (2.5 times the size of newsprint, or 20-point) at her preferred reading distance of 8 inches to maximize her reading speed and accuracy. We did not evaluate Margaret's reading without directional lighting, and it is possible that this will affect her performance.

Visual Fields

The Confrontation Field Test was performed with a penlight with a colored cap as target in a dimly lit room with both eyes viewing. Margaret was asked to look directly at the examiner to maintain steady central fixation. Then a pen light was brought in from above, below, and the sides by one person standing behind Margaret, while another person directly in front of Margaret noted when she first saw the penlight. Margaret's left, right, and lower visual fields appeared full. Margaret did not notice the penlight when brought in from above until it reached her eye level. This finding needs to be checked by Margaret's eye care specialist.

Margaret's central visual field was not tested during this evaluation. This requires additional assessment by her eye care specialist.

Contrast and Illumination

Margaret reported a number of concerns related to her ability to manage contrast in various settings. As it relates to mobility, she indicated that she has difficulty negotiating the white lines of a crosswalk. She prefers, on sunny days, to find shade to remove herself from daylight glare; on cloudy days, she uses a cane while traveling, as things tend to "bleed together." She reports that she trips while traveling unless she concentrates on looking downward, attributing this to being unable to note contrast changes in the terrain.

Margaret's contrast sensitivity was assessed with the Cambridge Contrast Sensitivity Test, which assesses the ability to discern shades of gray or differences in brightness. At a distance of 5 ft, with correction, and viewing with both eyes under normal room illumination, Margaret identified stripes on the plates down 2.7 percent Michelson contrast. Normal Michelson contrast is 0.5 percent. This finding needs to be checked by Margaret's eye care specialist.

Color Vision

Color vision appeared to be important to Margaret because she strongly identifies art as an important part of her life. She reported that she had recently experienced an unexpected loss in color vision: specifically locating and identifying "warm" colors. She indicated having difficulty with color outside in full light, and with humor, told a story of looking for a friend's maroon car in a parking lot and being unable to identify it by its distinctive color.

(continued on next page)

The Quantitative Color Vision Test PV-16 was utilized to measure Margaret's ability to detect colors by requiring her to place a series of colored caps in sequence. She performed the test under normal room illumination and with her glasses. She was able to select the proper color progression sequence without error. This test detects major color vision difficulties. Since Margaret had reported color difficulties, she was also asked to complete a color vision test sensitive to milder color vision difficulties. The F-2 Plate is a color test in which one is asked to find a colored square located within a larger square. She was able complete this test accurately.

The reason for Margaret's report of loss of color vision needs to be carefully checked by her eye care specialist, especially since she completed the formal color vision tests in this evaluation accurately.

Visual Perception

The Motor-Free Visual Perception Test was performed to determine if visual perception is an area that affects Margaret's visual functioning. She successfully completed all the visual perception items without difficulty.

Summary

Margaret demonstrated decreased visual performance detecting details at a distance and at near. Margaret's performed best with high contrast materials. She requires reading material that is enlarged through size, optical, or electronic magnification and further evaluation is required to determine optimal methods for her to use for different tasks. More assessments need to be completed to determine the effects of illumination on Margaret's performance on near and distance tasks, but it is likely that illumination without glare may improve her performance on selected critical tasks.

Recommendations

The following recommendations were made based on results of an interview and the testing detailed in this report:

1. Areas of Margaret's vision that require further examination by her eye care specialist include color vision, contrast sensitivity, and peripheral and central visual fields. It will be important to clarify the underlying reason for Margaret's report of a decrease in her ability to detect color, since tests of color vision showed normal functioning. There is no information in the record regarding Margaret's central visual field, and this also needs to be evaluated by her eye care specialist.
2. It is also recommended that Margaret's eye care specialist determine any additional low vision optical devices that might help Margaret with her reading and distance tasks, now that Margaret reports that she is more receptive to using such devices.
3. Margaret expressed a desire to drive, and this topic needs to be addressed by Margaret's eye care specialist as well.
4. Margaret can be encouraged to use her monocular telescope in the classroom to view the chalkboard. Assessment of her telescope use is recommended to determine if additional instruction would improve her facility with it.
5. An evaluation of Margaret's school and daily living tasks would be beneficial so that methods to improve size, color, contrast, illumination, and positioning of specific tasks can be recommended.

6. Margaret discussed a number of concerns related to traveling. Margaret is currently receiving O&M instruction. Further assessment of alternative ways to reduce glare while traveling, such as the use of a visor or tinted glasses outdoors, might be beneficial. Margaret's eye care specialist can also be asked for input in determining if the use of tinted glasses for outdoor travel is warranted and, if so, the optimal tint for Margaret.

7. A thorough assessment of the most appropriate learning media for Margaret is recommended, examining the use of optical devices, electronic magnification, large print, and speech output. These methods can be assessed within critical near vision tasks that Margaret has identified: reading, sewing, art. This will be particularly important to address prior to Margaret's transition to college, where her reading demands will increase.

8. Margaret reported that she felt "seasick" when she used CCTV systems for reading. Margaret's use of CCTVs should be carefully evaluated to be certain that she has used newer devices and has explored various options such as reversed polarity (white on black), different options for print and background colors, and the use of some newer models for distance viewing.

9. The assessment of learning media and reading media alternatives will give Margaret the information she will need to make decisions about the best solutions. Since she is an adult, every effort must be made to demonstrate clearly the strengths and weaknesses of various methods to Margaret so that she can make informed decisions about them.

10. A reading media assessment for Margaret should consider her reading speed using alternative solutions so that she can determine the most effective methods for completing the large amount of reading required for college classes. Methods for efficient notetaking in college should also be evaluated for Margaret including the use of portable electronic notetakers, laptop computers, and tape recorders.

11. Margaret reported little interest in learning braille. This may be partially due to a lack of exposure to its potential to enhance her literacy, especially as she contemplates higher education. Margaret may benefit from a re-evaluation of her assumptions about braille's potential, especially given recent enhancements in the capacity of braille to be accessed both by notetaking devices and computer technologies and Margaret's change in receptivity to the use of adaptations. While braille is not recommended at this point, it should be evaluated along with other literacy alternatives for Margaret.

12. Margaret also reported that she does not care to use speech output devices for reading. Some instruction to facilitate improved listening skills may help Margaret to understand the applications for this reading method, which can be very valuable for college-level work.

13. Margaret might benefit from participating in a peer discussion group, since she reports that she has only recently learned to advocate for her vision needs and that, in the past, she felt pressure to appear fully sighted.

14. Margaret will begin to receive services from the Department of Rehabilitation when her Individual Transition Plan is developed. Additional services can be recommended at that time related to assistance with career and independent living services from both a rehabilitation counselor and a rehabilitation teacher. Evaluation of vision requirements in activities identified in her plan needs to be considered along with the best methods for Margaret to optimize her vision while pursuing them.

(continued on next page)

Functional Vision Evaluation Report: Richard Crown

Student: Richard Crown   **Age:** 8 years

Richard has recently moved to a new school district and is seeking the services of a teacher of students with visual impairments. This report was prepared by a teacher of students with visual impairments.

History

School records indicate that Richard was evaluated by his ophthalmologist 10 months ago. In his report, the ophthalmologist indicated that Richard had the hereditary condition ocular albinism, which is lack of pigment in certain parts of the eye. It is usually accompanied by reduced visual acuity, light sensitivity, and involuntary oscillating eye movements (nystagmus). He recorded Richard's visual acuity as 20/160 in the right eye, 20/100 in the left eye, and 20/100 for both eyes. Richard wears eyeglasses, but the prescription was not in the school records. Richard had been receiving services from a teacher of students who are visually impaired in his previous school district and is now attending a regular second grade program. He has been identified as gifted. Richard stated that he regularly goes for eye examinations every summer.

Evaluation

Richard was examined in the school library.

Distance Visual Acuity
On the Lea Symbol Chart (9 line) chart, viewing with spectacle correction, Richard gave the following results:

Right eye:	10/100	Snellen equivalent 20/200
Left eye:	10/80	Snellen equivalent 20/160
Both eyes:	10/80[+1]	Snellen equivalent 20/160[+1]

Richard's distance visual acuity tested in the school environment was measured as slightly lower than his distance visual acuity measured in the clinical setting, where the controlled lighting was likely to promote optimal responses.

Near Visual Acuity
Lea Symbols: Near Vision Card with Noncrowded Symbols
With both eyes viewing with correction, Richard read the 2M spaced symbols with no difficulty at 16 inches (40 cm), which is the standard testing distance. To read smaller print, Richard preferred to hold the card at 6 inches where he read 1M print with one error. Richard's nystagmus seemed to be less pronounced when he was looking at near symbols than at distant symbols.

Lea Symbols: Near Vision Card with Crowded Symbols
With both eyes viewing with correction on this test that simulates a reading task, Richard read 3.2M symbols fluidly and with no errors and 2M symbols more slowly and with one error at 16 inches (40 cm). When Richard held the card at his preferred viewing distance of 6 inches, he read down to 1M print with one error.

Lighthouse Continuous Text Card for Children

With both eyes viewing with correction, Richard read down to the 1M line with no difficulty, holding the card at 4.5 to 5 inches. He held the card at 5 inches to read the 0.8M and 0.6M lines with difficulty.

Using reading cards with high contrast, clear print (black on white), Richard can read continuous text down to the size of newsprint (1M) when the print was held 4.5 to 6 inches away from his eyes. It is possible that Richard had less difficulty with the continuous text reading cards than the simulated reading cards with symbols since he was able to use contextual cues to determine words on the actual reading task. It was not possible to determine Richard's ability to read for long duration at this close reading distance during this initial assessment or to determine the effect of illumination on his reading. This should be explored in further testing.

Color

Richard made no errors on the Quantitative Color Vision Test PV-16 (similar to the Farnsworth Panel D-15), indicating no severe color vision problems. This test does not detect mild color disorders.

Contrast Sensitivity

Contrast sensitivity involves the ability to detect differences in subtle shades of gray, which can relate to the ability to detect stairs and faces, for example. On the Cambridge Low Contrast Gratings with both eyes viewing with correction at 6 ft, Richard made correct responses down to plate 7 (but not plate 8), which has a Michelson contrast of 0.37 percent. Normal Michelson contrast is 0.5 percent. Richard does not appear to have difficulty in this area.

Visual Fields

The test of confrontation field in a dimly lit room (with both eyes viewing with correction) gave a gross estimate of Richard's area of vision when looking straight ahead. He looked straight ahead at a penlight while a second was brought in from above, below, and from the sides. Richard quickly noted the second penlight as it was brought in from all fields of gaze. Richard does not appear to have limitations of his peripheral visual fields, but this finding should be corroborated by his eye care specialist.

Writing

Richard was asked to write simple words on bold-lined and regular paper using a black, fiber-tipped pen and a number 2 pencil. Richard seemed to have less difficulty forming the letters when his printing was smaller (1/4 inches high rather than 1/2 inches high). He stated that he was able to make his strokes better with the smaller size. The paper was about 6.5 inches from his eyes when Richard wrote the 1/2-inch letters, and he came closer to write the 1/4-inch letters. When asked if he preferred the dark pen or the pencil, Richard said that the pen slowed down his writing and he thought the pencil was better. He reported that he had not used a fiber-tipped pen before for writing. He did not indicate whether the higher contrast of the pen helped him. Further investigation of Richard's print writing to determine the best writing size and best writing implements (pencil, erasable pen, black fiber-tipped pens of various widths) should be undertaken.

(continued on next page)

Optical Devices for Reading/Distance

Richard was asked to find words on a map from a school textbook that he will be using during the school year. He located many words on the map, but had more difficulty with lower contrast words. When he was given a 3× pocket magnifier to try out, he located the lower contrast words on the map with no difficulty. He used the pocket magnifier easily with no training and appeared to enjoy it. Richard drew a picture of a flashlight-type stand magnifier that he uses at home. There was no report of this magnifier in his records, and he does not bring this magnifier to school. Richard reported that he regularly uses a monocular telescope to see the time on the clock in his classroom, but he did not have it with him on the day of this initial assessment. This optical device also was not mentioned in his school records.

Summary

Richard has reduced distance visual acuity and needs to be closer to see details at a distance for his school work. He also has difficulty seeing very small symbols (smaller than newsprint) and, in some instances, may require large print or magnifiers or a CCTV for reading assignments, especially for dictionaries, maps, footnotes, and encyclopedias. Richard can detect material of low contrast, although he had difficulty identifying lower contrast writing on a complex map from one of his textbooks. He does not appear to have a problem with his area of vision (peripheral or side vision), but this should be corroborated by his ophthalmologist. Richard indicated that he has less difficulty printing smaller rather than larger letters, and this requires further investigation by school staff to determine the best writing methods for Richard. Richard reported that he regularly uses a stand magnifier at home for near tasks, and he showed no resistance and abundant dexterity in using a trial pocket magnifier presented during the evaluation. If Richard does acquire and use magnification devices (optical or electronic) for some reading tasks at school, this may decrease his need for large print materials. It is likely that Richard will require some adaptations for school reading tasks. The possible use of optical and electronic magnification devices for school tasks will be discussed with Richard's parents, with the suggestion that Richard return to his ophthalmologist for further evaluation in this area.

Recommendations

1. Richard appears to qualify as a student with exceptional educational needs in the area of vision.
2. Richard's eye care specialists can be consulted during his next yearly eye examination scheduled in 2 months to consider Richard's use of optical magnification devices for reading small print in the classroom.
3. Richard's eye care specialist should be consulted about his peripheral visual fields to be certain that he has no problems in this area.
4. Richard's teacher of students who are visually impaired can continue to experiment with alternative methods to facilitate Richard's handwriting skills, which may include smaller writing size and pens with erasable ink, for example.
5. Richard can read letters the size of newsprint if the contrast is high. The print in Richard's school textbooks will be larger than newsprint. Richard's teacher of students who are visually impaired should carefully monitor Richard's reading duration with the regular print in his textbooks to see if it poses a problem for him. If so, alternative reading methods can be considered

for longer reading tasks: larger print, magnifiers, or a CCTV. At this point, Richard should have access to both regular sized and large print textbooks until optical devices or a CCTV system are available. He will likely need large print textbooks or magnifiers for increased facility with map reading, dictionary work, and other tasks involving very small print. If Richard does obtain a magnifier and/or a CCTV system for school reading tasks, his need to use large print for these tasks may decrease.

6. Richard should receive additional evaluations of the use of his monocular telescope for distance tasks. His eye care specialist should be consulted to determine the most appropriate monocular for Richard at this time.

7. This initial evaluation considered immediate reading and writing tasks related to Richard's school work. Further evaluations should examine the use of vision in tasks of daily living.

Part 3

INTERVENTION METHODS

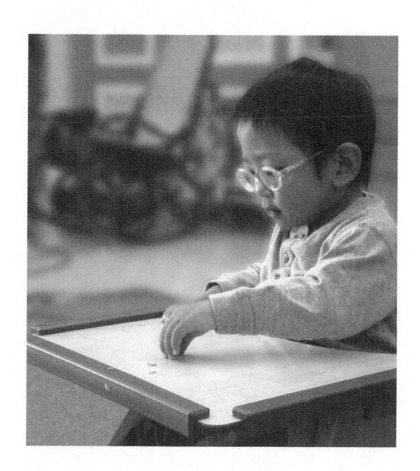

7

Overview of Intervention Methods

AMANDA HALL LUECK

The term *intervention* encompasses the delivery of appropriate services planned in response to the assessed needs and capabilities of an individual with low vision. As such, intervention is the other half of the continuum of low vision services that begins with evaluation and whose goal is the optimization of a person's functional vision, which can in turn contribute to a satisfying and independent life. Evaluation findings are one of the most important sources of information used to guide the decision making needed to plan instruction and select intervention approaches for the person with low vision. This information, which includes personal and family preferences, is vital in determining what goals to stress, what objectives to teach, and how to teach the selected objectives (Salvia & Yssledyke, 1991). The third section of this book focuses on intervention approaches and presents methods by which functional vision interventions can be considered within the context of broader goals and objectives designed for children and adults who have low vision.

PLANNING INSTRUCTION AND INTERVENTION

Major goals and objectives in instructional plans include the successful completion of critical tasks at school, at work, at home, or in the community to increase an individual's independence in those areas and improve his or her quality of life. Information compiled from interviews, observations, and other assessment methods can help to define the tasks that a person wishes to complete among his or her activities of daily living (e.g., taking photographs, cooking on a stove top, playing a violin) or that he or she needs to master to meet school or work requirements (e.g., reading a math textbook, operating a piece of machinery). Instructional strategies to help that person perform those activities are determined

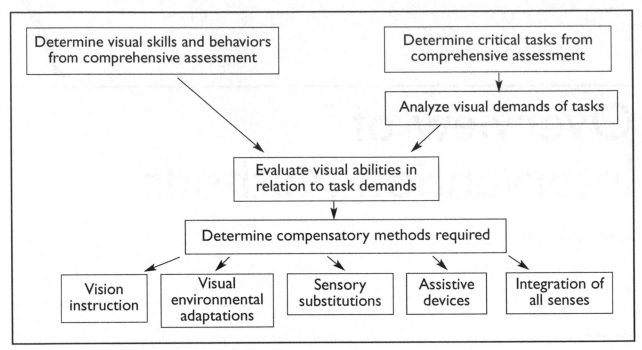

Figure 7.1. The planning process for intervention methods

from an analysis of his or her functional abilities in light of the visual, cognitive, social, and performance demands the tasks. Input is solicited from the team of specialists, the person with low vision, and, often, his or her family. For a person with low vision, a functional vision evaluation provides information about how he or she can use vision to perform critical tasks, whether instruction in vision use or visual adaptations would be beneficial and contribute to his or her efficient and effective task performance, and whether assistive devices or methods that do not rely on vision are warranted for a particular task. This planning process is outlined in Figure 7.1 and is discussed in more detail throughout this chapter.

This chapter discusses, in general terms, methods used by children and adults to compensate for impaired vision in the performance of school, work, leisure, and community activities. Later chapters present in more detail the specific ways in which these methods can be infused into broader instructional goals and objectives for children and adults with low vision.

COMPENSATORY METHODS

The compensatory or instructional methods used in intervention with individuals who have low vision fall into five main categories, which are depicted in Figure 7.1:

➤ Instruction to encourage vision skills and use. This includes:

- Visual environmental management instruction (e.g., placing an infant in a play area that encourages the child to use his or her vision in many ways)

- Visual skills instruction (e.g., teaching for a person who has an acquired visual field loss to scan efficiently for street signs visually)

- visually dependent task instruction (e.g., teaching an individual to search visually for a high-contrast coat hook that is large enough to be seen, rather than searching for it tactilely)

➤ Instruction in the selection and use of visual environmental adaptations—modifying elements in the environment to facilitate the use of vision—for example, using black, fiber-tip pens on white paper for writing

➤ Instruction in the selection and use of sensory substitutions—learning to use other senses in place of vision—for example, putting braille labels on medicine bottles or using a finger to identify when a glass of cold water is nearly full

➤ Instruction in the application of assistive devices to maximize vision use—for example, using a pocket magnifier to read labels in a grocery store

➤ Instruction in using and integrating information from all sensory systems—for example, teaching a student to begin a visual search for the door to the school cafeteria when the smell of food and sound of children reaches a certain level of intensity

Each of these compensatory methods is discussed in this chapter.

ANALYSIS OF VISUAL DEMANDS OF TASKS

When designing methods to compensate for impaired vision, these methods need to be considered in the context of tasks that are critical or meaningful for the children or adults in question. Determining appropriate visual cues to heighten or reduce in vision intervention programs, and possible sensory substitutions or modifications that may increase task efficiency, can be facilitated by an analysis of the visual demands of tasks (Lueck, 1997). For adults, critical tasks can be related to work, hobbies, recreational pursuits, and usual daily routines. For children and some adults, tasks also include specific activities related to educational pursuits. Providing assistance with these meaningful tasks will not only allow the individual to complete them successfully, but is also likely to foster a sense of personal adequacy and equality. This positive feedback is especially important for individuals who have recently lost their vision. Tasks that are meaningful, familiar, and concrete can be addressed in a positive manner while the individual faces the long-term impact of vision loss. An artist with retinitis pigmentosa who specializes in watercolors, for example, might be encouraged to work with black and white photographs (a visual environmental adaptation) and may later be

TABLE 7.1

Analysis of the Visual Demands of Tasks with Visual Environmental Adaptations and Sensory Substitutions: A Classroom Lecture

		VISUAL ENVIRONMENTAL ADAPTATIONS/SENSORY SUBSTITUTIONS*					
TASK AND VISUAL DEMANDS	SIZE OF MATERIAL	CONTRAST OF MATERIAL	LIGHTING CONDITIONS	COLOR OF MATERIAL	COMPLEXITY OF MATERIAL	POSITION OF MATERIAL	TASK DURATION
1. See chalkboard See 1-in. letters from 15 ft away written with colored chalk on blackboard in a room with overhead fluorescent lighting; assigned seat faces windows	Ask instructor to write letters about 2 in. high Change assigned seat to sit closer to instructor	Ask instructor to use white chalk on blackboard	Change assigned seats so that back is to windows to reduce glare				
2. See demonstrations Instructor is about 15 ft away; assigned seat faces windows	Change assigned seat to sit closer to instructor		Change assigned seat so that back is to windows to reduce glare				
3. See projected material Use of overhead projector with window blinds not drawn and room lights off; assigned seat faces window and is 10 ft away	Change assigned seat to sit closer to screen	Obtain print copy of over-head material prior to lecture Close window blinds					

4. Write notes Write notes in dimly lit room when viewing overhead projector	Use prescribed bifocal reading glasses on white paper	Use felt tip pen to write Use black ink Obtain lecture notes before class	Tape record lecture to supplement written notes Photocopy notes of a trusted friend if primarily needed to view projected material		Use reading stand to elevate writing paper
5. Read notes Read notes when writing in class; read notes for studying purposes after class	Use prescribed reading glasses	Write with felt tip pen Use black ink on white paper	Use task lighting on notes when studying	Use reading stand to elevate written material	Listen to tapes of lectures to reduce visual fatigue and studying time

* Most suggestions in this hypothetical example are visual environmental adaptations, but the use of a tape recorder is a sensory substitution.
Source: Adapted with permission of the publisher from A. H. Lueck, "Education and Rehabilitation Specialists in the Comprehensive Low Vision Care Process," *Journal of Visual Impairment & Blindness, 91* (1997), pp. 423–434.

encouraged to make a transition to sculpture (a visual environmental adaptation and sensory substitution).

Table 7.1 illustrates a systematic way to analyze the visual demands of critical tasks using attendance at a classroom lecture as the example. This analysis requires attention to the visual demands in terms of distance, size, color, lighting, position, duration, and complexity of that task. The task is analyzed into its various components so that the visual requirements of each component are identified. In the classroom lecture example, a student may need to watch demonstrations from a certain distance, read notes from a chalkboard at a certain distance, see projected slide material, write lecture notes, and read lecture handouts. Once the demands of the task are identified, appropriate compensatory methods can be suggested. Based on a person's visual abilities and available resources, a visual environmental adaptation or a sensory substitution or modification can be recommended for each component of the task to ensure that the task is completed successfully. In addition, instruction to improve the use of vision to complete task components may be recommended to reduce or alter the number, type, or intensity of the adaptations needed.

Visual environmental adaptations and sensory substitutions, discussed in more detail later in this chapter, are designed to encourage peak performance on a task, as in the following example:

> *A 55-year-old sales manager with age-related maculopathy reported difficulty reading the paperwork required for his job. He recently returned to his ophthalmologist, who found that he had 20/80 vision and small central scotomas in each eye. The eye care specialist explained this vision change and referred the manager to a low vision clinic, where new, higher power reading glasses and a closed-circuit television (CCTV) were prescribed for reading portions of his paperwork in 1.5 M print or smaller. It was found that directional lighting improved the manager's reading performance for print of larger sizes. He was evaluated to ensure he was using eccentric viewing (i.e., using an intact portion of the retina for viewing) and received instruction in visual skills related to reading. This was followed by training to use the new reading glasses and the CCTV as well as in the proper application of directional lighting. The manager found that he was better able to use the optical and electronic magnification devices for reading after the specialized vision instruction, and that directional lighting helped his reading. He also found that, for many tasks, he was able to read print larger than 1.5M without his new magnification devices when proper lighting was used.*
>
> *He could now use his vision to complete a critical vocational task with the appropriate assistive devices (i.e., new reading glasses, CCTV), visual environmental adaptations, (e.g., directional lighting), and vision instruction (in eccentric viewing and other visual skills for reading). Furthermore, as part of the low vision care process, the manager was referred to an agency providing a full array of rehabilitation services to evaluate other critical tasks*

in the home, workplace, or community where compensatory methods might be beneficial and to determine if additional services might be of assistance, such as attending a support group for people with low vision.

The following sections describe each of the main types of compensatory instruction for people with low vision and how they are used.

INSTRUCTION TO ENCOURAGE VISION SKILLS AND USE

To determine the most appropriate interventions to encourage visual skills and their use in functional tasks, it is important to identify and differentiate the types of visual skills and behaviors amenable to instruction as well as the ways in which they can be incorporated into intervention programs. Hall and Bailey (1989) indicate that there are three types of visual skills and behaviors:

➤ Visual attending behaviors have a major visual component and include such skills as fixating, following a moving object, shifting gaze, or scanning (see Sidebar 7.1).

➤ Visual examining behaviors have a major visual cognitive component and include such activities as inspecting, identifying, and matching visual material.

➤ Visually guided motor behaviors have a major visual-motor component and include such activities as reaching for, turning toward, and moving toward visual targets.

Visual skills and behaviors may be encouraged through instruction depending on the underlying visual capacities available to a given individual. One reason that comprehensive vision assessments are so important is that they provide critical information about a person's visual capacities, visual skills, and visual behaviors. This information can be used to determine if a visual skill or behavior may be responsive to intervention and the most appropriate interventions to use in specific instances, as in the following two examples:

Mrs. Grady, an elderly woman with age-related maculopathy and central scotomas is not aware that by tilting her head slightly to view eccentrically (thereby placing the visual image on an undamaged portion of the peripheral retina), she would be able to discriminate people's facial features. The underlying visual capacity to accomplish this task is there, and instruction in eccentric viewing techniques could help her improve her visual functioning.

By contrast, Tommy, a 10-year-old child with aniridia, cannot see objects smaller than 1 in. in height from 1 ft away based on his visual acuity test results and observational assessment. When preparing a visual environment for Tommy, high-contrast objects of regard must be at least 1 in. high at that

---

SIDEBAR 7.1

Visual Attending Behaviors

Visual attending behaviors include the following:

➤ **Fixating:** Pointing the eye so that the object of interest is imaged on the fovea or the preferred retinal locus (an alternative area of retina used for best vision when the fovea is damaged).

➤ **Shifting gaze:** Changing fixation to a new object of interest.

➤ **Scanning:** Making a series of fixations in order to inspect a large area visually.

➤ **Localizing:** Having an awareness of the location of an object of interest in the environment from visual, auditory, or kinesthetic cues so that one can fixate toward it.

➤ **Tracking or following:** Maintaining fixation on a moving object of interest using pursuit movements. Pursuit movements are smooth, involuntary eye movements that keep the object of attention imaged on the fovea as the object is moving or as the head is turning, or both. Pursuit movements occur when an object is moving, as in tracking or following, but also occur with head turns when one is looking at stationary objects.

➤ **Tracing:** Making a series of saccadic eye movements (rapid changes in fixation from one point to another) to shift fixation progressively along a line or a border.

Source: Adapted from D. Cline, H. W. Hofstetter, & J. R. Griffin, *Dictionary of Visual Science,* 4th ed. (Radnor, PA: Chilton Trade Book Publishing, 1980).

distance: his basic visual capacity to see details is not likely to change with instruction.

According to Hall and Bailey (1989), there are three basic types of instruction programs: visual environmental management instruction, visual skills instruction, and visually dependent task instruction (instruction in vision use in specific functional tasks). These are explained in the following sections.

Visual Environmental Management Instruction

Visual environmental management instruction involves the preparation of specially designed environments that promote the use of vision by fostering the development of visual attending, visual examining and visually guided motor behaviors. Visual cues are selected or controlled to encourage desired visual behaviors. There is little need for instructor intervention once the proper environment is established, since the carefully prepared environment itself motivates the person to use his or her vision. The identifying characteristics of visual environmental management instruction can be found in Table 7.2. This type of training is most relevant for young children with developing vision and for people who have recently lost their vision and are learning to use it efficiently.

A 2-year-old child with optic atrophy is playing in a room with colored bean bags on the floor that contrast vividly with the color of the carpet. A brightly colored laundry basket is next to the bean bags. The child is visually interested in these toys and independently decides to play with the bean bags by moving them into and out of the laundry basket. Since the bean bags are of contrasting color to the surroundings and are highly visible, the child looks at the toys, examines them, and makes direct reaches for them, thereby engaging in visual attending, visual examining, and visually guided motor behaviors. The child is motivated by the toys and does not need encouragement from an instructor to play with them.

Environmental modifications need to be gradually reduced (or faded) as much as possible as a person gains more effective vision skills and behaviors. For the child in the example, smaller bean bags will eventually be provided that have less contrast with the carpet. A smaller, less vividly colored container could be substituted for the laundry basket. The goal is to encourage the person to develop skills with the least intrusive environmental modifications.

Visual Skills Instruction

Visual skills instruction, according to Hall and Bailey (1989), involves instruction to promote the acquisition of visual attending behaviors (e.g., fixating on one object or glancing from one object to another) that have not developed or that have developed at a rudimentary level. Instruction in this area often focuses on fixation, scanning, and following skills for near and distance tasks (Berg, Jose, & Carter, 1983; Bureau of Education for Exceptional Students, 1992; Watson & Berg, 1983). The identifying characteristics of visual skills instruction are summarized in Table 7.2. It is important, whenever possible, to infuse instructional activities of this type into daily routines (e.g., a favored reading activity for an adult or playtime for a child) and to fade (reduce the level of) any specially designed visual cues so that the task becomes as normalized as possible, as illustrated in the following example:

A program is being designed to teach Jorge, a 7-year-old boy with visual and multiple impairments, to begin to use visual attending behaviors in

TABLE 7.2

Characteristics of Instructional Programs to Encourage Use of Vision

TYPE OF PROGRAM	DESCRIPTION	TARGET POPULATIONS	METHODS	EXAMPLES
Visual environmental management instruction	Person-directed learning of visual attending, visual examining, visually guided motor behaviors	People whose visual skills and behaviors are still developing	Select or control visual cues to encourage desired visual behaviors	Increase visibility of pictures in books used at free reading time to encourage visual attending
	Within functional tasks	People who have experienced recent vision loss who are learning to use their visual capabilities	Heighten or decrease cues in intensity, depending upon training goals	Reduce visibility of ball in rolling ball game to increase visual following to low contrast target and to promote use of nonadapted target for socialization
	In visually altered, naturally occurring environments		Fade heightened cues whenever possible	
			Provide a variety of environmental opportunities to learn skills	
Visual skills instruction	Instructor-directed training of visual attending behaviors: fixating shifting gaze scanning localizing tracking/following tracing	People who do not have or have rudimentary visual skill	Undertaken in isolated setting with the intention of fading the use of this setting and generalizing to usual settings where skills will be applied	Increase complexity of figure-ground in targeted tasks
		People recovering from neurological insult (Erin & Paul, 1996)	Undertaken in functional activities	Provide eccentric viewing training
		People who have experienced sensory deprivation (Erin & Paul, 1996)		Increase print reading efficiency

| Visually dependent task instruction | People who have developed visual skills | Instructor-directed training in functional tasks to encourage visual attending, visual examining, and visually guided motor behaviors.

Integration of vision into tasks using existing visual skills behaviors (visual cognitive or visual-motor tasks) | Identify key tasks where vision is efficient means for task completion

Heighten stimuli as necessary; fade stimuli gradually if possible

Encourage application of vision in specific task by direct teaching, pointing out methods and cues for efficient task completion

Plan for fading instructor-directed instruction

Generalize to other settings | Scan for recipes in cookbook

Find words in dictionary

Locate house numbers

Use vision to catch a ball |

Source: Adapted with permission of the publisher from A. H. Lueck, "Education and Rehabilitation Specialists in the Comprehensive Low Vision Care Process," *Journal of Visual Impairment & Blindness, 91* (1997), 423–434.

functional tasks. Repeated observations of Jorge in his home and school settings have indicated that he rarely attends to tasks using his vision, preferring to use touch for exploration instead. To locate specific food items on his wheelchair tray, he uses a raking hand motion and does not look down at the tray. Jorge has a visual acuity of at least 20/400, based on electrodiagnostic and acuity card assessment techniques, and his visual fields are normal. Jorge's teacher of children who are visually impaired believes that she will not be able to introduce instruction effectively to promote visual attending behaviors in the child's classroom since he is highly distracted by the noise and activity around him. She decides to introduce an intervention program in a quiet room where environmental variables can be controlled, and then move targeted instruction to the natural environment as soon as Jorge performs visual attending skills on a more regular basis. The teacher plans eventually to infuse instruction into his snack time and lunch lessons in his classroom, and decides to design a lesson using related items in the isolated setting. She plans to focus on promoting visual fixation and visual search behaviors.

To begin the instructional program, the teacher presents a favorite food at snack time (a peeled banana) that is high in visual contrast to the background color of the black wheelchair tray. She focuses a directional lamp on the tray to encourage Jorge's visual attention to the food item. The banana has an aroma, and this makes it easier for the child to know that the banana is present without using tactile cues. Jorge is encouraged to look for the item with his eyes before he reaches in his typical trial-and-error, raking motion without looking. He understands and responds to the verbal request readily. When he responds, he is given a small piece of banana to eat before he has the opportunity to engage in any nonvisual reaching behavior. Eating the banana provides positive reinforcement for the visual search and fixation behaviors and reduces the frequency of Jorge's usual nonvisual search movements. The peeled banana is then moved slightly to a different position on the tray to encourage Jorge to conduct a brief visual search to locate the banana again, and the process is repeated.

The teacher decides that Jorge must attend visually to the banana without a verbal prompt before moving on to the next phase of the lesson, in which the banana is broken into smaller pieces, and the child is encouraged to look for each of them. For this phase, when Jorge looks at each piece, he is handed the piece to eat and encouraged to follow the piece as it moves from the table to his hand. The goal of the lesson is first to encourage visual search and fixation (which has not been used by the child in this task with a large target and has only been seen fleetingly in other tasks) and then to encourage visual search and fixation with smaller items. The teacher plans to incorporate food items of less intense contrast into the lesson, and the directional lamp will eventually be eliminated to make the situation as similar to typical mealtimes as possible.

Once Jorge demonstrates regular visual attending behaviors with a predetermined frequency (e.g., three out of four trials), the child's instructional aide, classroom teacher, and caregiver are invited to observe the child in the isolated setting. The instructional team then comes up with and implements complementary activities to encourage the child to use these visual skills during snack time and lunch time in his classroom and at home. It is likely that once the child learns to locate the food item visually, he will then move on to even more purposeful visual behavior in which he reaches for the banana independently in order to eat it.

The critical distinction between visual skills instruction and the next type of instruction discussed—visually dependent task training—is that visual skills must first be acquired before they can be applied to more complex visual behaviors in a variety of specific tasks. The acquisition of visual skills may require instruction in an isolated setting using heightened stimuli to encourage acquisition of the visual skills. When basic visual skills have been acquired, there is usually less need to conduct instruction in these isolated settings and visual cues used to motivate visual behavior may not need to be so intense. Use of the acquired visual skills can then be encouraged in a variety of tasks in which vision is the most efficient means of task completion for a specific person (visually dependent task instruction or visual environmental management instruction).

Visually Dependent Task Instruction

Training of vision use in specific functional tasks, also called visually dependent task instruction (Hall & Bailey, 1989), is undertaken to increase and optimize efficient use of existing visual attending behaviors in tasks that can be completed more efficiently with the use of vision. It also promotes the development of visual examining and visually guided motor behaviors. In visual skills instruction, the person with low vision does not demonstrate facility with basic visual attending behaviors (e.g., fixating or following). In visually dependent task training, a person has demonstrated these skills but does not use them in certain tasks in which the use of vision would ensure their completion with greater efficiency (e.g., locating a part of a favorite toy or following an image moving across a computer screen).

Visually dependent task instruction includes encouraging visual attention to task components using systematic, contingent reinforcement techniques for some children (Goetz & Gee, 1987), the application of eccentric viewing techniques for functional near and distance tasks (Chapman, 1996; Goodrich & Quillman, 1977), and special visual perception training related to visual impairment (Barraga & Morris, 1980; Overbury & Quillman, 1996; Trudeau, Overbury, & Conrod, 1990). It promotes the increased application of visual attending behaviors to cognitive or motor tasks, expanding the opportunities to use and develop visual examining and visually guided motor behaviors. The identifying characteristics of visually dependent task instruction can be found in Table 7.2.

In the example of Jorge described previously, once he learned visual fixation and visual search skills related to food items on his tray, he moved to visually dependent task instruction which encouraged him apply those visual skills in tasks at snack time and lunch time to guide his reaching behavior more efficiently. The distinction between visual skills instruction and visually dependent task instruction can be subtle, but the differentiation is important. Placing Jorge into an instructional situation in which he was expected to execute a reach based on vision before he had acquired the abilities to search and attend would have been premature. Once he had acquired those visual skills, however, he could be encouraged to perform the reach based on visual information in functional tasks such as eating in his busy classroom.

Another example of visually dependent task instruction involved a young lawyer with Stargardt's disease who had experienced a recent major loss of vision. She was determined to use eccentric viewing when reading and was able to trace visually along a line of print, but was having difficulty applying these skills in sustained reading tasks required for her work. Her instructor decided to provide the lawyer with daily exercises, graduated in level of difficulty, to increase her reading speed and duration. The highly motivated client practiced at home and worked with longer reading tasks as well on her homework assignments. In three weeks, the instructor noted that his client's facility on sustained reading tasks had improved considerably. The application of acquired visual skills, eccentric viewing, and following (or tracing) along a line of print improved with practice and exemplifies visually dependent task instruction.

Within each of these three types of instruction programs—visual skills instruction, visually dependent task instruction, and visual environmental management—visual stimuli within the environment are regulated by instructors to stand out to greater or lesser degrees depending upon the goals of vision instruction exercises (Hall & Bailey, 1989). For example, a toddler may be encouraged to search for a favorite doll whose dress was changed from bright red to pale pink to encourage him or her to search for a stimulus that is less visible. Eccentric viewing training may begin with large, single letters presented on a chart before its introduction in a complex reading task with smaller print. Learning to trace (i.e., follow along) a line of print may begin with materials that use large letters or words and large spaces between lines.

VISUAL ENVIRONMENTAL ADAPTATIONS

Visual environmental adaptations—modifying elements in the environment to facilitate the use of vision—are needed by many people with low vision. This type of compensatory method differs from visual environmental management instruction in that these modifications will not be gradually reduced as part of a program to promote and fine-tune visual behaviors that are expected to improve over time. This method is used with adults and children who have experienced a vision impairment over a long time period of time and whose visual abilities are not likely to improve with instruction, and with people who have completed instruction to encourage vision skills and use. In essence, *visual environment adaptations* differ from *temporary modifications* to encourage vision use because the former are permanent changes in the way a task is performed by a particular individual in order to promote his or her participation in usual activities of daily life. An exception occurs when visual environmental adaptations are temporary solutions for task completion while a person is completing a vision instruction program or when less intense adaptations are able to replace the temporary solution, as in the following two examples:

> *A young child is presented with high-contrast, translucent pictures on a light box to encourage visual identification of two-dimensional objects. After several months, her teachers have decreased the amount of light emanating from the light box and introduced pictures printed on paper under normal illumination. The use of the light box and special pictures was a temporary adaptation to encourage vision use, since the child can now identify objects from pictures without the special modifications.*

> *Anna Cohen, an elderly woman who lives with her son and daughter-in-law, requires assistance each day to take her medicines. She is not able to read the labels on her medicine bottles, even with her handheld magnifier used under task lighting. After a visit from a rehabilitation teacher, she learns that, once her medicines are placed in a segmented pill container that separates medicines for each day, she can take her daily medicines without assistance despite not being able to read the bottles' labels. The pill container was a more appropriate method for Mrs. Cohen since visual environmental adaptations (handheld magnifier and task lighting) are not helpful to her in this task.*

Environmental adaptations for persons with progressive visual loss must be reevaluated periodically since they are likely to require more intense stimuli or other compensatory methods as their vision changes. A strong caution is appropriate here: it is often not possible to determine beforehand that instruction to improve vision functioning will have no results. It is best to attempt a program in visual skills and use, and use permanent visual environmental adaptations only after it has been systematically determined over time that the instruction program has had no effect on an individual's vision functioning. This is especially true for children with visual and multiple impairments.

Visual environmental adaptations are used in usual activities of daily life and may include changes in lighting, contrast, color, size, distance, position, and duration. Adults and children can be encouraged and trained to determine optimal adaptations independently based on a thorough and realistic understanding of their visual abilities. In some instances, particularly reading, a comprehensive assessment provides information to determine adaptations that encourage peak performance on critical tasks. An elderly person with cataracts, for example, might benefit from the use of a directional lamp for reading or from the use of colored electrical tape wound around the handle of a clear plastic hairbrush to make it easier to locate visually. A student in elementary school with albinism might benefit from facing away from the windows to view the blackboard and classroom demonstrations to minimize glare. Detailed information about environmental modifications for children and adults with low vision can be found in Chapters 8, 9, and 10.

SENSORY SUBSTITUTIONS

Sensory substitutions or modifications—using other senses in place of vision—can be provided directly, or individuals can be instructed in their use and availability so that they can choose an appropriate alternative as needed. Instruction in these modifications includes the use of special adaptive techniques and devices that compensate for impaired vision such as braille, sighted guide or long cane skills, speech output devices (e.g., talking clocks or computers with speech output), raised lines on checks, audiotapes, sighted readers, and adaptive needle threaders. Determining appropriate sensory substitutions or modifications can be accomplished by analyzing both the visual skills and behaviors required in a specific task and the person's visual capacities. The visual modality may not be the most efficient method for completing certain tasks, and visual environmental adaptations may not be sufficient.

Suggesting sensory substitutions requires careful, considered analysis, especially for adults with recent or progressive vision loss and for school age children who do not want to stand out from their peers by using adaptive equipment. Decisions about teaching alternative modes for reading and writing require careful analysis of comprehensive assessment data that goes beyond the assessment of functional vision detailed in this volume. When determining the most appropriate reading mode for adults, for example, Ponchilla and Ponchilla (1996) recommend that variables such as a person's age, learning ability, tactile ability, previous reading level, and reading goals be taken into consideration along with visual ability. Koenig and Holbrook (1995) have developed a process to determine appropriate learning and literacy media for students with visual impairments that considers sensory information including use of vision, touch, and hearing, as well as information on additional disabilities that can have an impact on learning. Since choosing the appropriate reading medium for a person with low vision needs to take into account a complex array of variables, the team approach is required in the educational decision-making process (Holbrook & Koenig, 2000). Information from various team members is also taken into account when establishing rehabilitation goals for reading media and determining services required to reach these goals with clients in rehabilitation settings (Wolffe, 1996).

ASSISTIVE DEVICES TO MAXIMIZE VISION USE

Instruction in the use of assistive devices that involve vision (e.g., optical devices, CCTVs, and computer-generated images) encourages their application in the context of usual activities of daily life. Instructional approaches with these devices are best arranged in consultation with ophthalmologists or optometrists and the person who will be using the device. Optometrists and ophthalmologists can provide critical input about the proper use of prescribed eyeglasses in conjunction with assistive devices, and information about the most appropriate image size, working distance, color, contrast, or polarity (whether the image is dark on a light background or vice versa), given the nature of the device, a person's visual condition, and other factors related to his or her learning profile. The person using the device can make personal decisions regarding preferences for such factors as color, contrast, polarity, as well as those related to cost, comfort, appearance, and effectiveness. A person's performance with specific devices should be compared to determine the most appropriate assistive devices, and may include the use of speech output and braille displays for computer users who have low vision (Whittaker, 1998.). See Chapters 8, 9, and 10 for more information about instruction in the use of assistive devices. Detailed guidelines for evaluating and recommending a range of assistive systems for individuals with low vision are beyond the scope of this book, but can be found elsewhere (Such & Whittaker, 1999).

INTEGRATING INFORMATION FROM ALL SENSORY MODALITIES

Guidance in coordinating the use of sensory input from all modalities during usual activities of daily living is especially important for infants and young children, (Lueck, Chen, & Kekelis, 1997) and for individuals who experience a sudden vision loss. Infants and young children need to maximize the use of their nonvisual senses to learn about their environment more fully. Persons who experience a sudden vision loss may require instruction in specific adaptive techniques (e.g., determining that water is boiling in a pot by the sound, that a transparent glass has been filled with water through tactile feedback, or that distant traffic is approaching using sound cues). For example, a middle-aged computer technician with reduced visual acuity and visual fields due to glaucoma could benefit from training from an orientation and mobility specialist to use object sounds, echoes, and smells in conjunction with visual cues to identify features in the environment and to establish his position in the environment.

CONCLUSION

A variety of methods must be considered to assist individuals with low vision in completing their usual tasks of daily life successfully, efficiently, and independently. Health care, education, and rehabilitation professionals need to work together and with consumers and their families to develop the most effective approaches for a given individual. Although the overriding principles of compensatory methods are the same regardless of a person's age, many issues specific to children and adults must be considered to create and deliver appropriate programs effectively. These specific issues will be presented in the three chapters that follow. Specific techniques used with young children and individuals with visual and additional disabilities who have developmental delays differ significantly from those used with students who have a more academic orientation. They are, therefore, reviewed separately in Chapters 8 and 9. Techniques used with working age adults and elderly people with low vision are reviewed in Chapter 10.

REFERENCES

Barraga, N., & Morris, J. (1980). *Program to develop efficiency in visual functioning.* Louisville, KY: American Printing House for the Blind.

Berg, R. V., Jose, R. T., & Carter, K. (1983). Distance training techniques. In R. T. Jose (Ed.), *Understanding low vision* (pp. 277–316). New York: American Foundation for the Blind.

Bureau of Education for Exceptional Students (1992). *A resource manual for the development and evaluation of special programs for exceptional students. Volume V–E. Project IVEY: Increasing visual efficiency.* Tallahassee: State of Florida Department of Education.

Chapman, B. G. (1996). Eccentric viewing methodology. *Journal of Vision Rehabilitation, 10,* 4–6.

Corn, A. L., DePriest, L. B., & Erin, J. (2000). Visual efficiency. In A. J. Koenig & M. C. Holbrook (Eds.), *Foundations of education* (2nd ed.): *Vol. II. Instructional strategies for teaching children and youths with visual impairments* (pp. 464–499). New York: AFB Press.

Erin, J. N., & Paul, B. P. (1996). Functional vision assessment and instruction of children and youths in academic programs. In A. L. Corn and A. J. Koenig (Eds.), *Foundations of low vision: Clinical and functional perspectives* (pp. 185–220). New York: AFB Press.

Goetz, L., & Gee. K. (1987). Teaching visual attention in functional contexts: Acquisition and generalization of complex motor skills. *Journal of Visual Impairment & Blindness, 81,* 115–117.

Goodrich, G. L. & Quillman, R. D (1977). Training eccentric viewing. *Journal of Visual Impairment & Blindness, 71,* 377–381

Hall, A., & Bailey, I. L. (1989). A model for training vision functioning. *Journal of Visual Impairment & Blindness, 83,* 390–396.

Koenig, A. J., & Holbrook, M. C. (1995). *Learning media assessment of students with visual impairments,* (2nd ed.). Austin: Texas School for the Blind and Visually Impaired.

Lueck, A. H. (1997). Education and rehabilitation specialists in the comprehensive low vision care process. *Journal of Visual Impairment & Blindness, 91,* 423–434.

Lueck, A. H., Chen, D., & Kekelis, L. S. (1997). *Developmental guidelines for infants with visual impairment: A manual for intervention.* Louisville, KY: American Printing House for the Blind.

Overbury, O., & Quillman, R. D. (1996). Perceptual learning in adventitious low vision: Task specificity and practice. *Journal of Vision Rehabilitation, 10,* 7–14.

Ponchilla, P. E., & Ponchilla, S. V. (1996). *Foundations of rehabilitation teaching with persons who are blind or visually impaired.* New York: AFB Press.

Salvia, J., & Yssledyke, J. E. (1991). *Assessment* (5th ed.). Boston: Houghton Mifflin.

Such, G. V., & Whittaker, S. G. (1999). Computer assistive technology for the low vision patient. In R. L. Brilliant (Ed.), *Essentials of low vision practice.* Boston: Butterworth-Heinemann Publishers.

Trudeau, M., Overbury, O., & Conrod, B (1990). Perceptual training and figure-ground performance in low vision. *Journal of Visual Impairment & Blindness. 84,* 204–206.

Watson, G., & Berg, R. V. (1983). Near training techniques. In R. T. Jose (Ed.), *Understanding low vision* (pp. 317–362). New York: American Foundation for the Blind.

Whittaker, S. G. (1998). *Choosing assistive devices when computer users have impaired vision.* Paper presented at the *Center on Disabilities' Technology and Persons with Disabilities Conference.* Available at www/csun.edu/conf/1998/proceedings/csun98_043.htm.

Wolffe, K. E. (1996). Adults with low vision: Personal, social, and independent living needs. In A. L. Corn and A. J. Koenig (Eds.), *Foundations of low vision: Clinical and functional perspectives* (pp. 322–339). New York: AFB Press.

Interventions for Young Children with Visual Impairments and Students with Visual and Multiple Disabilities

AMANDA HALL LUECK AND TONI HEINZE

Young children learn by being in the world and observing people, nature, activities, procedures, and cause-and-effect relationships. Much of this information is acquired through the visual channel. This visual information is a powerful motivator and stimulator for children to move out and explore, to search for more information, and to interact with their world. This interaction, in turn, is critical for their development of accurate and functional concepts about the world around them. It is also a powerful force for initiating actions, reacting appropriately, acquiring problem-solving abilities, experiencing the reinforcing effects of actions, and establishing a sense of curiosity and control over their environment. Figure 8.1 depicts this stimulating, reinforcing role of vision and interaction in learning.

As Figure 8.1 demonstrates, this learning cycle begins with early movement, even prenatally, as the developing infant moves and stretches without intention and then shifts position in preparation for birth. At birth, the natural urge for movement continues and builds, with the child moving arms and legs, hands and feet, as a natural part of his or her behavior. Soon, however, this movement becomes more and more intentional. From the beginning, vision provides a primary and powerful stimulator and motivator for the child to move, explore, and interact with the environment. Through vision, the environment entices the child, helping to promote his or her critical curiosity and the sense that the world is an extremely interesting place.

This developing curiosity about the world leads to increased movement, which becomes more and more intentional and deliberate. Early concepts begin to form as the child interacts more and more with the world through swiping, reaching, searching, handling, comparing, experimenting, and problem-solving behaviors. Increased movement and interaction lead to the development of more specific

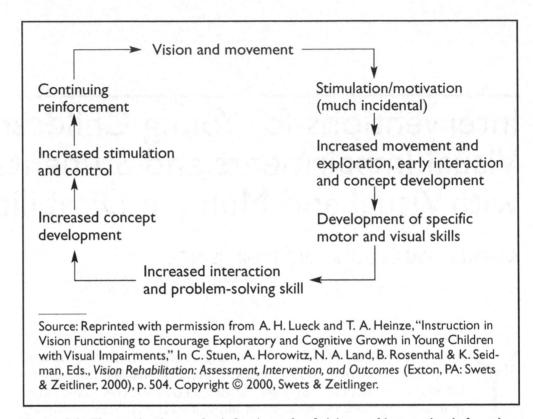

Figure 8.1. The motivating and reinforcing role of vision and interaction in learning.

and refined visual and motor skills. The child moves from fixating to following, shifting gaze, and scanning. In his or her gross and fine motor development, the child moves from supportive and righting behaviors to crawling, creeping, walking, and manipulating objects. The child also begins to integrate visual-motor skills and visual perceptual skills in functional contexts.

The child's increased experiences in interacting with the environment, with visual and motor abilities playing a critical role in this interaction, also result in more accurate, expanded, and varied concepts. These include an understanding of body image and spatial relationships, attributes and comparative concepts, cause-and-effect relationships, object permanence, part–whole relationships, conservation, and functionality (or the function and use of objects). This experience base was highlighted by Jan (2000) when he stated that "the development of the brain depends on the quality and quantity of interaction with the environment."

The child's success in using developing visual, motor, and thinking skills, and the environment's reinforcing role, continue to support the child's developing sense of control and motivation to initiate activities on his or her own. This in turn provides continuing reinforcement for the child to look, move, explore, interact, solve problems, and continuously refine concepts and skills.

In ideal circumstances, this cycle is a very positive one. A visual impairment alone or coupled with a motor impairment, however, can adversely affect this cycle. Many children with visual or motor impairments are at risk for missing significant critical visual information and stimulation due to their more limited opportunities for interacting with their environment. The implications of these reduced opportunities for exploration, interaction, concept building, problem-solving, and developing a sense of control are evident and far-reaching. Motivation to explore and develop both visual and motor skills may be reduced; attributes and functional characteristics of objects may be missed; object permanence, cause and effect, and spatial concepts may be delayed or only partially developed; and the ability to learn from imitation of models may be limited.

IMPORTANCE OF COMPENSATORY INSTRUCTION

Vision, therefore, plays a major role in overall development and learning. The ability to see is integrated with other functions to promote understanding and interaction with the environment, as well as appreciation of the things in it. Most important for children, vision guides cognitive and motor operations within purposeful behaviors so that children can comprehend, move, and maintain interest in their world. For children to develop in this fashion, they must be active participants in the learning process. In addition, vision affects social, emotional, cognitive, motor, and communication development and abilities, since information derived from visual input is processed and applied within these complex behavioral functions. As such, visual skills and behaviors must be taught within meaningful contexts and complex behaviors to provide adaptive significance and meaning for children who have visual impairments.

This chapter will emphasize ways to promote use of vision within critical and meaningful activities in typical environments, stemming from an early model proposed by Goetz and Gee (1987) and expanded upon by Hall and Bailey (1989). In addition, for infants who are just beginning to develop their visual skills, it is critical to incorporate strategies that promote vision use, encourage the application of vision within problem-solving tasks, and help infants verify and supplement their limited visual input through other sensory channels and through verbal feedback (Lueck, Chen, & Kekelis, 1997). Very young children with visual impairments need to be encouraged to apply their vision in usual daily activities in order to learn methods to compensate for their reduced visual functioning. This is also true for students with visual and multiple disabilities. Some children with visual impairments may not develop their full visual capabilities in naturally occurring environments and may require special methods to attract and maintain their attention in order to encourage development and use of their vision. These methods can sometimes be implemented through simple modifications in naturally occurring environments, depending on the skills and behaviors targeted for instruction. In some instances, it may be necessary to begin instruction in a specially designed environment, making the transition to more normalized settings and materials once the child has learned some basic skills.

Research is sparse on the efficacy of various methods of instruction to improve and encourage vision use in young children with visual impairments and children with visual and multiple disabilities. Available research indicates that instruction produces learning gains for children who have visual attending skills (e.g., fixating, following, shifting gaze) and must learn to apply these skills to other tasks (Goetz & Gee, 1987; Downing & Bailey, 1990). In addition, instruction in visual discrimination and recognition promotes performance gains on near tasks for children with low vision in the elementary grades (Barraga, 1964). Much emphasis has been placed in education programs on ways to maximize the development of visual attending skills for infants and toddlers. However, minimal research is available to show that these interventions result in increased visual skills and behaviors (Lueck, Dornbusch, & Hart, 1999). Until more research is available, we must rely heavily on limited findings about vision development and its use in young children with visual impairments and children with visual and multiple impairments combined with sound principles of teaching and learning in designing instructional approaches.

A great deal of material is covered in this chapter. This reflects the crucial need to optimize visual functioning so that young children with visual impairments and children with visual and multiple impairments can integrate their available visual information into more general skills and behaviors to reach their full potential. A discussion of general developmental and educational concerns for young children with visual impairments and for students with visual and multiple disabilities is outside the scope of this chapter. For more information regarding developmental concerns for young children with visual impairments see work by Lueck, Chen, & Kekelis (1997); Trief (1992, 1998); and Warren, (1994). For more information on educational issues for students with visual and multiple impairments see Chen (1999); Chen & Dote-Kwan (1995); Pogrund and Fazzi (2002); and Sacks and Silberman (1998).

INCORPORATING INSTRUCTION INTO DAILY ROUTINES

The goal of intervention with children who have low vision is not to develop visual skills and behaviors as ends in themselves; rather these visual skills and behaviors should be developed for functional purposes—that is, to accomplish tasks or carry out activities that have meaning to the individuals. The most efficient and meaningful way to accomplish this is to integrate and encourage the development of visual behaviors within daily activities.

Figures 8.2 and 8.3 provide examples of analyses of visual skills and behaviors within two typical activities, play and mealtime, and the corresponding exploratory and cognitive behaviors that can be promoted through the integration of those visual behaviors into that activity. (A blank copy of the form used to assist in the analysis of typical activities is provided in Appendix 8.1 to this chapter). By incorporating visual skills within routine activities such as play and feeding, instructors encourage the use of these skills to facilitate the child's exploratory, cognitive, motor and communication behaviors.

Play Activity

In the example detailed in Figure 8.2, the routine activity is play. Play can involve a wide range of visual skills, including the following:

➤ Basic visual control skills: fixation, tracking, shift of gaze, scanning

➤ Visual motor skills: reaching, visually guided crawling or walking

➤ Visual perceptual skills: discrimination of color, shape, size, position, figure-ground, visual closure, visual memory.

The use of these visual skills during play activities can facilitate the child's exploration and movement skills. For example, localizing a target requires shifting attention and scanning. Once localized, an interesting target can prompt visually guided reaching for that target, which, in turn, can encourage righting, creeping, crawling, or climbing to move toward the object. It can also lead to meaningful use of a child's hands to search, manipulate, and operate objects and surfaces involved in the play activity, thus promoting further cognitive growth.

The use of visual skills in play activities facilitates a child's cognitive development, including understanding of such concepts as attributes, body image, spatial/positional concepts, functionality of objects and body parts, cause and effect, problem solving, and object permanence in addition to a sense of curiosity and control over the environment and the making of choices.

In addition, communication abilities can be facilitated through the integration of such visual skills as fixating, shifting gaze, following, and discrimination through eye pointing or visual choice making during a play activity.

Mealtime Activity

Mealtime is a routine activity that lends itself well to the facilitation of visual skills and behaviors while promoting communication and conceptual understanding. For example, a child's plate and cup can be placed against a high-contrast mat, and food items can be placed on a high-contrast plate or napkin to make it easier for the child to localize them. He or she can be offered choices that facilitate fixating, discriminating, shifting gaze, as well as eye pointing to indicate choices. If the child has some self-feeding skills, this activity can reinforce many visual skills including: visual attending skills, such as shifting gaze and scanning to search for choices or visual following to observe the hand and food as they travel toward the mouth, and visually guided motor skills, such as reaching for a highly visible food item (or a spoon or fork, if used). For children who cannot feed themselves, visual attending skills can be facilitated by watching the caregiver's hand, pointing

Analysis of Daily Routines Form

DAILY SCHEDULE OF ROUTINES	CRITICAL ACTIVITIES WITH VISUAL COMPONENTS	VISUAL BEHAVIORS TO BE PROMOTED	EXPLORATORY BEHAVIORS FACILITATED	COGNITIVE BEHAVIORS FACILITATED
Play in living room after breakfast	Locating and investigating toys on carpet	Fixating on toys	Visual: scanning, searching, examining	Discriminating attributes (shape, color, size, position, etc.)
			Fine motor: swiping and reaching	Understanding of basic concepts (body image, spatial, object/ environmental), object permanence
		Scanning and searching for specific items	Visual: scanning, searching, examining	Developing a sense of control, discriminating attributes, understanding object permanence
			Fine motor: swiping and reaching	Understanding basic concepts (body image, spatial, object/ environmental), object permanence
		Shift of gaze	Visual: scanning, searching, examining	Understanding object permanence
			Gross motor: righting, creeping, crawling, walking	Understanding basic concepts (body image, spatial, object/

			environmental), object permanence
		Fine motor: handling and manipulating	Understanding the functionality of toy, making it work, cause and effect; problem solving
	Visual discrimination	Visual and motor exploration as above	Understanding the functionality of toys
Imitating an action performed by caregiver with toy	Shift of gaze	Visual and motor exploration as above	Comparing attributes and behaviors, imitating actions, curiosity
Indicating choices	Eye pointing	Visual exploration as above	Communication (language, eye pointing; gestures); social interaction; developing sense of control
	Visually guided reach	Fine motor: purposeful reaching	Understanding object permanence, attributes of objects
	Visually guided travel	Gross motor: crawling, walking to an intended goal	Understanding object permanence, attributes of objects, and travel path

Figure 8.2. Sample form for analyzing daily routines to promote visual behaviors and encourage exploration and cognitive growth: play activity.

Analysis of Daily Routines Form

DAILY SCHEDULE OF ROUTINES	CRITICAL ACTIVITIES WITH VISUAL COMPONENTS	VISUAL BEHAVIORS TO BE PROMOTED	EXPLORATORY BEHAVIORS FACILITATED	COGNITIVE BEHAVIORS FACILITATED
Breakfast	Locating food items on table	Fixating on cup, utensil, food	Visual: scanning, searching, examining	Discriminating attributes (shape, color, size, position, etc.)
			Fine motor: swiping and reaching	Understanding of basic concepts (body image, spatial, object/ environmental), object permanence
		Scanning and searching for specific items	Visual: scanning, searching, examining	Developing a sense of control, discriminating attributes, understanding object permanence
			Fine motor: swiping and reaching	Understanding basic concepts (body image, spatial, object/ environmental), object permanence
		Shifting of gaze among items on table	Visual: scanning, searching, examining	Understanding object permanence
			Gross motor: righting, creeping, crawling, walking	Understanding basic concepts (body image, spatial, object/

			environmental), object permanence
Caregiver pointing to food items	Visual following, visual discrimination	Fine motor: handling and manipulating	Understanding the functionality of utensils, making them work, cause and effect; problem solving, developing a sense of control
		Vision: following, examining	Discriminating attributes
Indicating choices	Eye pointing	Visual exploration as above	Communication (language, eye pointing; gestures); social interaction; developing a sense of control
	Visually guided reaching	Fine motor: purposeful reaching	Understanding object permanence, attributes of objects
	Visual discrimination	Vision: visual examining	Understanding functionality of utensils, imitation of use
		Visual-motor: eye-hand coordination	

Figure 8.3. Sample form for analyzing daily routines to promote visual behaviors and encourage exploration and cognitive growth: mealtime

to choices, and following the caregiver's hand as it brings food to the child's mouth. Figure 8.3 gives some examples of exploratory and cognitive behaviors facilitated through encouraging the use of vision during a breakfast activity.

INCORPORATING INSTRUCTION INTO INTERVENTION PROGRAMS

The importance of maximizing visual functioning to support the growth and development of children with visual impairments has been reflected in federal mandates requiring the provision of early intervention services in this country. Identification of children with visual impairments, assessment of their needs, and creation of instructional programs designed to meet these identified needs follows a formalized process structured around Individualized Family Service Plans (IFSPs) for children under age 3 and Individualized Education Programs (IEPs) for children 3 years and older. Such programs are put together based on team assessments and team decision-making processes.

The IFSP Process

For young children and their families, the major outcomes that are expected to be achieved through intervention are identified and set out in the IFSP through collaborative assessments and dialogues between children's caregivers and the team of service providers (McGonigel, Kaufmann, & Hurth, 1991). It is here that activities and behaviors that are important functionally within the family are determined. These outcomes are derived from identified family priorities and concerns as well as from an understanding of children's strengths and interests. Resulting programs must fit the learning needs of each youngster and involve the child and family as active participants in the teaching and learning process, with instructional goals infused into usual daily routines in natural settings (Dunst, Trivette, & Deal, 1988), as illustrated in the previous sections. As already noted, incorporating instruction into daily routines ensures that teaching will occur regularly and in meaningful contexts for young children and their families. It discourages instruction of isolated skills that are not integrated into relevant tasks and promotes activities pertinent to real-life issues for families and children. It is important to note that the IFSP process is a family-centered activity, focusing on family needs as well as those of the child, as shown in the following example:

> *A father states that he would really like his 2-year-old daughter to follow his movements visually. The IFSP team encourages this goal by suggesting that the father work on this daily when he changes his daughter's diaper after dinner every evening as usual, and when he plays with her in the living room before she goes to bed each night. He is encouraged to wear clothes that contrast highly with the wallpaper, remove distracting objects in the rooms so that his daughter can more easily follow his movements, move*

at a specified distance and pace from her to encourage visual following, and talk to his daughter as he moves around the rooms so that sound cues and descriptive language are coupled with visual cues.

In this example, the family's desired outcome is that the child be able to follow movements of a family member at home using her vision. This request involves the caregiver and the child in the teaching and learning process. Instruction is implemented daily by the family member during typical routines.

More complete descriptions of the IFSP process are provided elsewhere (Chen & Dote-Kwan, 1998; McGonigel et al., 1991). Sidebar 8.1 outlines the key features of the IFSP process.

The IEP Process

The IEP process serves students with visual impairments over the age of 3, including those with additional disabilities. For students with visual and multiple disabilities, family participation in all phases of assessment, instruction, and evaluation is necessary to identify students' learning styles, motivators, and behaviors in natural contexts. It is also the key to determining critical, age-appropriate activities in school, home, and community settings within which instruction will occur. For older students, activities are categorized into five broad domains: vocational, leisure and recreation, domestic, community, and functional academics. Instructional programs are designed to develop identified skills by engaging students in meaningful activities in typical environments alongside their nondisabled peers. Compensatory techniques to promote basic skills and to facilitate task completion through adapted materials or methods are incorporated into critical activities identified by the IEP team. The overall goal is to ensure a student's participation in school, home, and community environments at present and in the

---

SIDEBAR 8.1

Key Features of the IFSP Process

➤ Serves children below age 3

➤ Focuses on family and child's needs

➤ Includes ongoing collaborative assessments with family

➤ Determines child and family outcomes from family priorities and concerns as well as child's strengths and interests

➤ Involves family participation in teaching and learning process

➤ Incorporates instruction into daily routines

Key Features of the IEP Process for Students with Visual and Multiple Disabilities

➤ Serves students 3 years and older

➤ Involves family participation in all phases of assessment, instruction, and evaluation

➤ Identifies student's needs for instruction, learning styles, motivators, and behaviors in natural contexts

➤ Determines critical age-appropriate goals

➤ Instruction occurs in school, home, and community settings

➤ Involves vocational, leisure/recreation, domestic, community, and functional academic domains

➤ Instruction occurs in typical environments with nondisabled peers to the extent possible

future. More complete discussions of this type of assessment and instructional planning process are available elsewhere (Chen & Dote-Kwan, 1995; Erin, 2000; Falvey, 1989; Lueck, 1998; Silberman & Brown, 1998). See Sidebar 8.2 for key features of the IEP process.

Students with visual and multiple impairments may not grasp specific basic skills, including visual skills and behaviors, without purposeful and systematic instruction (Lueck, 1998). Basic skills include actions or behaviors that promote larger actions common to a variety of activities, such as walking (a motor skill), using touch cues (a communication skill), sorting (a cognitive skill), waiting in line (a social skill), completing a task (an activity performance skills), or visually searching for a dropped sound-making toy (an integrated sensory skill). Purposeful exposure to activities that include specific basic skills along with systematic instruction to learn the conceptual and the performance base underlying many of them may be required for students with visual and multiple disabilities. When additional basic skills can be acquired, the need for adaptations, including visual environmental adaptations, is decreased or the types of adaptations selected are likely to be less intrusive (Lueck, 1998), as demonstrated in the following example:

It has been determined from a comprehensive assessment process that Marisa, a 13-year-old girl with cognitive delay and severely reduced visual acuity, would benefit from choosing her own food in a fast food restaurant

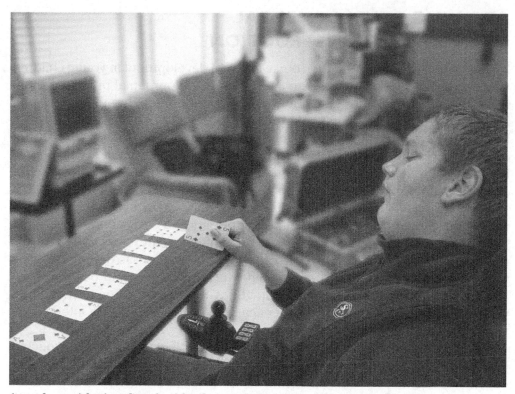

A student with visual and multiple impairments is engrossed in a simple card game that encourages him to apply visual and motor skills in a functional recreational activity that he enjoys. *(Robert Barkaloff)*

that her family visits often. To facilitate this process, she has been taught tactile signs that represent various food items served at the restaurant so that she can ask for them herself. In the past, she had been given photographs of food items but could not identify named items by pointing to them. Therefore, tactile signs were introduced as an adaptation. Recently, Marisa's teacher of students with visual impairments determined that she could indeed identify simple pictures if they were sufficiently large and of high contrast. After learning to identify five items visually, Marisa now uses a picture menu to choose her food when ordering at the restaurant from the server rather than having an intermediary translate the tactile signs. Some instruction to identify the pictures and use the menu took place in the classroom and some in the natural environment of the restaurant. This instruction was provided by both school staff and family members during outings to the restaurant. Although Marisa requires a visual environmental adaptation, the current adaptation is closer to a normalized experience, since she can choose from a variety of items presented on an adapted menu that is easy to transport, and she can order directly from the restaurant staff.

APPLYING DEVELOPMENTAL MILESTONES TO INSTRUCTION

It is important to understand the course of visual development in young children with unimpaired vision and how to apply these developmental principles to infants and toddlers with low vision (for more information, see Hyvarinen, in press). It is also important to understand how general developmental milestones can be affected by vision loss. A review of these many milestones and how they are affected in children with vision impairments is outside the scope of this book, but a number of authors have addressed these issues in detail (Blanksby, 1994; Eksted, Lastine, & Paul, 1996; Hyvarinen, 1988; Langley, 1998; Lueck et al., 1997).

When using any scales or checklists listing skills or behaviors in a developmental progression, it is crucial that instructors strive to devise ways to train targeted skills or behaviors within meaningful contexts, rather than to teach skills only in isolation. Instructors can examine usual daily routines to determine times when targeted skills are used and within which instruction can occur. For example, visual following can be encouraged with a bright spoon at mealtime; visually locating a sound-making object can be encouraged during interactions with a caregiver at bath time.

Very young children with severe visual impairments may not follow expected developmental progressions identified for children with unimpaired vision because they may not see well enough to accomplish certain tasks. Children with visual and multiple impairments may also have other health issues that preclude their performance of the cognitive, linguistic, or physical aspects of certain tasks. It is important to take this into consideration when designing instructional protocols for these youngsters. It is also important to be especially attuned to the communicative behaviors of these young clients, who, because of their age, developmental readiness, and other circumstances, may not express their needs and abilities in a straightforward manner. Instruction for children with visual and multiple disabilities is best implemented using ecological models of assessment and instruction developed for children with severe disabilities, as discussed in this chapter under Incorporating Instruction into Intervention Programs. Such ecological models make no assumptions about developmental progression. Instead they focus on identifying and training children in basic visual skills needed to complete a critical, functional, age-appropriate activity targeted for instruction, and on providing this assessment and training within the child's relevant environments and life tasks.

COMPONENTS OF AN INSTRUCTIONAL PROGRAM

Visual functioning must promote broader developmental activities or meaningful, functional skills. To accomplish this, an instructor must understand the general principles of vision instruction methods available so that he or she can choose appropriate methods and infuse into these the broader goals for young children with visual impairments and for students with visual and multiple im-

SIDEBAR 8.3

Planning a Functional Vision Instruction Program

➤ Determine the child's current visual skills and behaviors through assessment activities.

➤ Determine visual skills and behaviors to target for instruction based on the child's strengths and interests, input from caregivers or significant others, and assessment findings.

➤ Select one or more types of instruction programs to address targeted skills.

➤ Select appropriate stimuli, routines, and environments.

➤ Use diagnostic teaching when appropriate.

➤ Combine all components into ongoing activities implemented by professionals and family members in daily routines or functional activities in natural environments.

pairments. This section describes approaches to designing various aspects of functional vision instruction programs, which are summarized in Sidebar 8.3.

Determining Visual Skills and Behaviors to Target for Instruction

The visual skills and behaviors to be addressed in a functional vision instruction program are determined based on findings from the child's functional vision assessment and from input from caregivers and significant others as well as the child. The child's repertoire of visual behaviors needs to be determined along with information concerning when these behaviors are used and what motivates the child to use them. Visual behaviors can be categorized as visual attending behaviors (described in Chap. 7), visual examining behaviors, and visually guided motor behaviors. Figure 8.4 lists some visual behaviors within each category that are amenable to instruction and presents a form that can be used to record observations of these behaviors within specific tasks, using the example of a 12-month-old visually impaired infant with cerebral palsy. Instruction needs to focus on visual behaviors that are not present or are seen only fleetingly during specific tasks. They can be skills that the child is likely to acquire, ones that

Observations of Visual Behaviors

VISUAL BEHAVIOR TO CONSIDER FOR INSTRUCTION	SPECIFIC SKILL	WHEN OBSERVED	MOTIVATOR OR CONDITIONS USED
Visual Attending Behaviors			
Fixating	Regard of mother's face	When diaper changed by mother	Mother moved face close to talk to baby
Shifting gaze	Alternately looks from mother to father	In high chair at lunch time	Parents looked at and talked to baby from close distance
Scanning	Looked around and located favorite teddy bear	Playtime in playpen	Play in familiar environment
Localizing	Looks directly toward dog	Playtime on floor	Dog barked nearby
Tracking for following	Follows spoon to mouth	During snack time on mother's lap	Colored spoon, moved slowly towards mouth
Tracing	Behavior not observed	—	—

Comments:
Did not observe the above behaviors for objects farther than 3 ft away.

Visual Examining Behaviors

Behavior			
Looking attentively	Watched mother prepare mashed banana	On high chair tray at lunch time	Used red plate so that banana was highly visible
Identifying	Looked directly at spoon when asked "Where is the spoon?"	During snack time on mother's lap	Favorite pudding on spoon; enjoys interaction time with mother
Choosing visually	Behavior not observed	—	—

Comments:
Did not observe the above behaviors for objects farther than 3 ft away.

Visually Guided Motor Behaviors

Behavior			
Head turning toward visual goal	Looks directly toward dog	Play time on floor	Dog barked nearby
Imitating	Behavior not observed	—	—
Gross motor movement toward visual goal	Behavior not observed due to motor limitations	—	—
Reaching	Reached toward teddy bear	Play time in playpen	Play in familiar environment
Manipulating part of object	Grasped and pulled tail of teddy bear	Play time in playpen	Play in familiar environment
Other			

Comments:
Did not observe the above behaviors for objects farther than 3 ft away.

Figure 8.4. Determining a child's repertoire of visual behaviors. Examples are given for a 12-month-old infant who is visually impaired and who has cerebral palsy.

require refinement, or ones that the child has already acquired but must be applied to specific tasks or to a wider variety of tasks, as in the following example:

A 1-year-old child with optic nerve hypoplasia and high myopia may demonstrate visual attending behaviors (fixating, following, scanning, shifting gaze) and visual examining behaviors (looking attentively, identifying, choosing visually) but may not have demonstrated any sustained visually guided reaching behavior. The child does turn her head toward a visual goal. Her mother is concerned that the child is not reaching for objects using her vision. At the IFSP meeting, the team decides to address this concern and plans a program to facilitate reaching. It begins with a plan to encourage the child to reach for the mother's face in close proximity and, later, toward favored sound-making objects introduced in contact with the child's body and then moved slightly away at midline. This will be done during some diaper-changing times and after mealtime in the morning by the child's caregivers.

Instruction programs must take into account factors that can affect a child's ability to process visual information, such as movement (i.e., stationary or moving objects and the speed of movement), different light levels, familiarity with the surroundings, familiarity with objects or people involved with a task, presence or absence of competing sensory stimuli, and the effects of positioning effects (i.e., lying down, sitting, or standing). These effects are discussed in detail later in this chapter.

Selecting Instructional Programs

Once the targeted skills and behaviors are determined, the type of instruction program is selected. It may involve one or more approaches, should be flexible, and requires careful monitoring of outcomes so that task variables are adjusted for subtle changes in behavior. The three primary methods, visual environmental management, visual skills instruction, and visually dependent task instruction, were discussed in Chapter 7 and are summarized in Sidebar 8.4. They are also detailed in the case study at the end of this chapter. Their use with young children and students with multiple disabilities is described in the following sections.

VISUAL ENVIRONMENTAL MANAGEMENT INSTRUCTION

A visual environmental management program involves the creation and use of carefully determined surroundings that encourage a student to use his or her vision. A visual environment is created that is specially organized to select or control visual cues to encourage desired visual behaviors (attending, examining, visual-motor). This type of program encourages student-directed learning of visual attending, visual examining, and visually guided motor behaviors within functional tasks and in natural situations that have been modified to encourage

Designing Components of a Functional Vision Training Program

Visual Environmental Management*

1. Determine appropriate visual environmental and adaptations and sensory substitutions.

   ➤ Consider functional vision evaluation, observation, and input from caregivers and significant others.

   ➤ Consider functionality and age appropriateness.

   ➤ Consider motivational factors.

2. Place child in environment with time to explore and experience.

3. Monitor behavior and note any behavioral changes.

4. Adjust environment as needed.

   ➤ Heighten or fade visual or other sensory cues to promote visual behaviors.

5. If behavioral changes are not noted after a specified period of time:

   ➤ Consider alternative instructional strategies.

   ➤ Adaptations that heighten child's ability to notice materials may need to be continued indefinitely.

Visual Skills Instruction*

1. Select training context.

   ➤ Use in familiar routines if possible.

   ➤ Sometimes slightly altered familiar routines are more successful for teaching new skills, since some children may not be comfortable with changes in familiar routines.

   ➤ Sometimes a diagnostic teaching context must be established before skills can be infused into daily routines.

   ➤ Consider functionality and age appropriateness of tasks in which skills are taught.

   ➤ Consider motivational factors for the child.

2. Develop an instructional strategy to train new visual skill or to refine an inconsistent one.

   ➤ Make the environment visually comfortable for child.

Source: Reprinted with permission of the publisher from A. H. Lueck, H. Dornbusch, & J. Hart. "An Exploratory Study to Investigate the Effects of Training on the Vision Functioning of Young Children with Cortical Visual Impairment," *Journal of Visual Impairment & Blindness*, 93 (12) (1999), pp. 778–793.
*Adapted from A. Hall & I. L. Bailey, "A Model for Training Visual Functioning," *Journal of Visual Impairment & Blindness*, 83 (1989), pp. 390–396.

(continued on next page)

➤ Consider addition of other sensory cues to increase motivation.

➤ Consider decreasing extraneous visual cues.

➤ Consider providing initial tactile or auditory cues, if necessary, to initiate the use of vision by children who have CVI.

➤ Develop a plan to infuse into daily routines if skill first taught in diagnostic teaching setting.

3. Develop an instructional strategy for task performance of critical skills in which visual skill is infused.

➤ Develop a plan to fade from most to least prompting.

➤ Allow child time to respond.

4. Implement and monitor program.

Visually Dependent Task Instruction†

1. Select instructional context.

➤ Determine the necessity of vision for task completion.

➤ Consider functionality and age appropriateness of task.

➤ Consider motivational factors.

2. Develop an instructional strategy to promote use of established visual skill.

➤ Identify the critical visual moment (i.e., the precise portion of critical skill in which vision use increases task efficiency).

➤ Determine cues or prompts required to encourage vision use at the critical visual moment.

➤ Continuous looping teaching strategy (i.e., failure to use vision at the critical visual moment results in termination of trial and the initiation of the beginning of a new trial) should only be considered for older children with multiple disabilities.

➤ Methods of instruction for very young children will vary with each child, and the continuous looping strategy may not be appropriate for this population.

3. Develop an instructional strategy for task performance of critical skills in which visual skill is infused.

➤ Develop a plan to fade from most to least prompting.

➤ Consider time delay in prompting for older children with multiple disabilities.

➤ Methods of instruction for very young children will vary with each child.

4. Implement and monitor program.

†Adapted from L. Goetz and K. Gee, "Functional Vision Programming: A Model for Teaching Visual Behaviors in Natural Contexts," in L. Goetz, D. Guess, & K. Stremel-Campbell, Eds., *Innovative Program Design for Individuals with Dual Sensory Impairments* (Baltimore, MD: Paul Brookes, 1987), pp. 77–97.

specific visual behaviors and skills. The target population is children whose visual skills and behaviors are still developing or children who have recently lost or gained vision and are learning to integrate their remaining visual skills and behaviors. In this approach, methods are used to motivate a student to look and to apply vision independently within the specially modified environment. These methods may include the following:

➤ Selecting or controlling visual cues to encourage desired visual behaviors (e.g., providing a brightly colored doll on a beige carpet to encourage the child to look at it).

➤ Heightening or decreasing the intensity or visibility of cues, depending upon instruction goals (e.g., presenting a light-colored cereal snack on a dark-colored background to increase visibility and encourage eye-hand coordination. Later, the contrast of the background is decreased to encourage reaching to items of reduced contrast compared to their background.

➤ Fading heightened cues whenever possible as instruction outcomes progress to make the transition to a more normalized environment (e.g., placing colored electrical tape around a coat hook to increase its visibility, and removing the tape when the child is able to locate the coat hook without the cue).

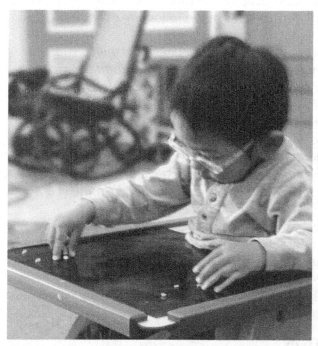 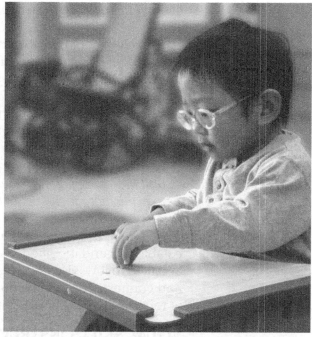

This child learns reaching and visual scanning with small objects when cereal is placed on a contrasting background during snack time (left). After the child's skills are developed through the use of high contrast in the task, his snack is placed on a low-contrast background (right) to promote the development of visual skills and behaviors in a more typical situation. *(Robert Barkaloff)*

➤ Providing a variety of opportunities in different settings to learn targeted visual skills and behaviors, (e.g., encouraging a child to learn cause and effect behaviors using vision by providing, in different locations at school and home, toys with highly visible buttons to press or highly visible switches that produce various effects when activated).

In the visual environmental management approach a student must be given time to explore and experience a naturally occurring environment that has been specially modified to encourage visual skills and behaviors initiated by the student. Behavior is not directed by a teacher, but it is carefully monitored, with behavioral changes noted. Visual cues are adjusted by the instructor to conform to the student's learning needs. Determining the appropriate environmental modifications must take into account a student's functional vision, caregiver preferences, functionality (meaningfulness and practicality) of the instruction task, age-appropriateness, and the student's motivation level. Cues may be faded if the student achieves a desired behavior or increased if the instructor determines that their intensity is insufficient to capture a student's attention. The goal of this approach is to reduce gradually the level of the cues needed by a student to encourage visual behaviors. When further fading of special cues no longer encourages visual behaviors on the part of the student, then the exceptional cues used to that point are identified as the student's usual visual requirements. If students do not respond to this approach, then a more systematic, method for altering the environment may be required, as in the following example:

> *A teacher would like to encourage Jasmine, a 6-year-old girl with visual impairment and cognitive delay, to participate in a rolling ball game at recess. In the beginning, the teacher provides a group of children with a highly visible beeper ball to attract Jasmine's attention and to encourage her and her peers to be interested in the task. As Jasmine becomes more accustomed to following the ball and playing with the other children, the teacher provides a less vivid ball without sound that more closely resembles balls regularly used on the playground. The teacher is finally able to introduce a ball that all children regularly use on the playground, and Jasmine is able to participate in the usual ball game with her peers.*

The child thus controls her interactions with the ball, but the environment is established and modified by her teacher. In the process, the child develops the ability to follow, visually, a fast-moving target that is gradually decreased in size and contrast. This is accomplished within a critical activity—playing with peers at recess—in the school environment.

VISUAL SKILLS INSTRUCTION

Visual skills instruction involves systematic instruction in basic visual skills. It promotes the acquisition of visual attending behaviors such as fixating, following, visual search, shifting attention, scanning, and localizing (see Chaps. 5 and 7 for descriptions of these terms). It is teacher-directed instruction that is usually implemented in special settings within a functional activity for that student. It often initially involves one-on-one instruction with the teacher and the student. Once a targeted visual skill is attained and demonstrated regularly in the special setting, the visual skill must be reinforced and generalized by infusing skill instruction into functional activities in natural settings. This type of instruction is appropriate for students who have not demonstrated a visual skill or who have used it at a rudimentary level in a particular activity. It is also appropriate for students recovering from neurological injury, students who have experienced sensory deprivation, and students who have never had the benefit of vision instruction (Erin & Paul, 1996).

Although visual skills instruction is best done within familiar routines or critical activities that are functional, age-appropriate, and motivating to the child, a teacher may first need to encourage certain skills in a less distracting, more controlled environment. The goal is to generalize and reinforce emerging skills learned in a controlled setting by eventually infusing them into activities in the student's usual daily routines or critical activities. This method often requires a diagnostic teaching context before skills can be taught within more complex settings to learn which methods are best to employ in natural contexts for a specific student. Diagnostic teaching combines assessment and instruction in such a way that assessment information is gathered continually. This information is used immediately to change instruction in order to make learning more efficient (Koenig & Holbrook, 1995). It involves the systematic trial and evaluation of a variety of instructional strategies (including materials, methods of presentation, and methods of feedback), and the modification of instruction to reflect the strategies that work for a particular student (Salvia & Ysseldyke, 1991). For purposes of visual skills instruction, diagnostic teaching involves continuous evaluation by the instructor of visual cues and prompting strategies used in isolated settings. (For a discussion of prompts, see the next section, Visually Dependent Task Instruction.)

Adjustments to instruction are gradually made that lead to the goal of permanently transferring instruction to more normalized environments. Thus, instruction in isolated settings is done with the intention of leaving those settings as quickly as possible. Special instruction techniques include the following:

➤ Making the environment visually interesting to a student

➤ Making the environment comfortable for the student

➤ Adding sensory input when appropriate to increase the student's interest and motivation

➤ Decreasing extraneous visual cues as appropriate

➤ Providing an initial auditory or tactile cue for students with cortical visual impairment, who often require alternative sensory input for the visual sense to "kick in" (Steendam, 1989; see the section on Cortical Visual Impairment later in this chapter)

➤ Preparing a plan to reduce levels of prompts and heightened sensory cues

➤ Developing a plan to infuse skills into daily routines or critical activities if a skill is first taught in a diagnostic setting.

Instruction should allow children with visual and multiple impairments sufficient time to respond, given their unique needs. Monitoring a student's progress is necessary to determine the visual cues to be used, how and when instruction should be moved to a more normalized setting, reduction of prompt levels, and decisions regarding continuation of instruction if gains are not made over a specified time period. The following is an example of visual skills instruction:

Joe is not shifting his gaze from one object to another at 10 months of age. His early intervention teacher is working with the family to encourage the child's visual behaviors. At playtime, Joe's mother is now encouraging him to look at an illuminated toy to his left, then sounding another illuminated toy to his right in a dimly lit room to encourage him to shift his gaze. Once the infant demonstrates shift of gaze in this context, the room lights will gradually be raised and the sensory cues changed until he performs the activity in natural room illumination with nonilluminated, silent toys. In addition, once Jeremy shows slightly more than rudimentary shift of gaze, his father will also start to encourage this behavior during the baby's daily morning bath routine using floating toys in the infant tub and at each mealtime with his bottle and finger foods.

VISUALLY DEPENDENT TASK INSTRUCTION

Visually dependent task instruction encourages a student's use of vision in a wider range of tasks. It involves systematic instruction to expand a student's use of available visual skills in critical tasks or daily routines. It is teacher-directed instruction that encourages the application of existing behaviors (visual examining or visually guided motor) to tasks that can be completed more efficiently using vision. This type of approach is most appropriate for students who have developed visual skills but do not apply them to specific tasks that could be performed more efficiently using these existing visual skills.

In visually dependent task instruction, first delineated by Goetz and Gee (1987) for students with significant cognitive delays as well as visual impairments, key functional tasks are identified within daily routines or critical activities in which vision would be an efficient method for task completion given a student's visual capabilities. Tasks are chosen that a student is motivated to complete. The point at which vision use would enhance task performance (called the critical visual moment) is identified. Cues or prompts to encourage vision use at a critical visual moment are then identified, depending on the student's visual, cognitive, and motor capacities. Visual cues within identified tasks may need to be heightened in the beginning of the instructional process, but should be faded gradually to more normalized cues whenever possible.

During instruction, if a student with visual and multiple impairments who has cognitive delay does not use vision at the critical visual moment in a given trial, the trial should be terminated and a new trial initiated by the teacher; this is called a continuous looping strategy. For example, in teaching a student to hang a jacket on a coat hook, the student may not consistently use vision to locate the hook (the critical visual moment). The student may search for it tactilely, even though the teacher has determined that the student can readily see the hook and that a visual search is more efficient than a tactile search for that student with that activity. In the lesson sequence, when the student uses vision to locate the hook, he or she then holds the hook with one hand and places his or her jacket on the hook with the other. If the student does not reach for the hook using vision, the teacher asks him or her to repeat the task of looking visually for the hook before he or she is allowed to finish the task sequence.

This continuous looping technique should be considered for older children with visual and multiple disabilities who experience cognitive delay. Methods of instruction for very young children and for children with no cognitive delay will vary with each child. The continuous looping strategy may discourage learning for these groups of children since they may benefit from self-initiated experiential learning, as in environmental management instruction (described previously). For these children, artificially ending an activity that may have a meaningful exploratory component for them could discourage experiential learning and might reduce future exploration.

In visually dependent task instruction, as in visual skills instruction, a plan to fade the teacher's prompts from most intrusive to least intrusive prompts should be in place as the student gains mastery of the task using vision at specified points. The skills used in the task can be applied to other tasks in other settings as appropriate to further reinforce and generalize the use of available visual skills. The instruction program should be monitored to determine how and when prompts can be gradually decreased and visual or other sensory cues can be normalized. For many children, visual cues may need to remain at a heightened level of intensity, depending on their visual capacities related to specific cues, as in the example at the end of this section.

A detailed discussion of the use of prompts for young children with visual and multiple impairments is provided elsewhere (Chen & Dote-Kwan, 1995). Lueck et al. (1997, p. 21) provide a list of prompts from least to most intrusive that apply to students with visual impairments:

➤ *Natural cue:* Offering an object for the child to see or feel elicits the desired action.

➤ *Gestural cue:* Movement or gesture indicates the desired action to the child and elicits the desired response.

➤ *Direct verbal cue:* Verbal request for the action elicits desired response by the child.

➤ *Modeling:* Demonstration of the action to the child elicits the desired response. Students who are blind should be encouraged to place both hands on the modeler's hands to feel the movement.

➤ *Physical prompt:* Physical contact is provided, which can range from touching the student's hand to guiding the child through part of the action to elicit the desired response.

➤ *Physical guidance:* The instructor's hand is placed over the student's hand in full physical contact to complete the desired action. This is sometimes described as hand-over-hand assistance.

In an example of visually dependent task instruction, Samantha, a 7-year-old girl with visual, cognitive, and physical impairments is learning about cause and effect by pushing a button that initiates a short verbal request on a simple communication device in her classroom. Samantha does not use vision to locate the button; instead she uses a raking motion with her right hand to find the button prior to pushing it. She is able to push the switch when it is located on a table or tray in any position in front of her: to the left, right, or center. The verbal request programmed into the device is for a favorite toy she can have before free play time in her classroom.

A functional vision assessment indicates that Samantha is able to see the button but that she rarely uses her vision to scan and locate objects during her school day. Her teacher of students who are visually impaired has therefore devised a systematic instruction program to encourage the student to look prior to reaching for the button on her communication device. Samantha is encouraged to use her eyes to locate the device, which is moved from center, left, and right on her wheelchair tray. To obtain a toy, she is required to push the button on the device, which then relays a verbal request. When she locates the button visually, and makes a relatively direct reach to push it, she is given the toy. If she made a raking motion without looking for the device, the teacher asks her to start again, and the position of the device is altered. To encourage Samantha to look at the button at the critical visual moment, the teacher taps on it while verbally requesting that her student "look at the button with her eyes." In addition, the teacher has made the button more visible by painting it a bold, primary color (red) against a high-contrast background (white). It previously was a light tan button on a white background.

SELECTING APPROPRIATE STIMULI, ROUTINES, AND ENVIRONMENTS

Attributes of visual stimuli can be adjusted during instruction so that their visibility is increased or decreased, depending on the instructional goal. These attributes include the following:

➤ Size

➤ Contrast

➤ Complexity

➤ Illumination

➤ Duration

➤ Color

➤ Position

➤ Distance

When first working with children with visual impairments, the instructor needs to assess the environment to be certain that visual stimuli are presented optimally to promote the student's full use of available functional vision. Sidebar 8.5 presents examples of adjustments to the attributes to consider when arranging the visual environment of children with visual impairments. In instruction

---

SIDEBAR 8.5

Attributes of Visual Stimuli to Be Considered in Arranging the Visual Environment of Young Children with Visual Impairments

The following adjustments in various attributes of visual stimuli can be made to promote the full use of students' functional vision:

Size

➤ Make objects larger.

➤ Move child closer.

➤ Use optical devices for magnification.

Contrast

➤ Increase contrast.

➤ Objects and details of low contrast may be difficult for some children to see (e.g., facial features, stairs, drop-offs).

Complexity

➤ Reduce "visual clutter" on tabletops, desks.

➤ Present objects against a plain background in the classroom (e.g., a solid-color wall).

➤ Present simple pictures without fine lines.

(continued on next page)

Color

➤ Use bold, primary colors (red, orange, yellow, green, blue, violet) or black and white to capture children's attention.

➤ Present a range of colors, including pastels, to those with less impaired vision.

Illumination

➤ Avoid light shining directly into a child's eyes from directional lights or when lying on back on the floor looking at overhead lights, or looking at windows.

➤ To increase lighting, move light source closer or child closer to light source (do not shine light source directly into child's eyes).

➤ Allow children time to adapt from light to dark and from dark to light.

➤ Sunglasses may help some children who squint in bright light; check with eye care specialist.

Position

➤ Find the position in which a child is most visually alert when encouraging visual skills.

➤ Provide instruction in visual tasks in a child's most visually alert position; usually this is a position that the child can maintain with little difficulty and promotes head, neck, arm, and hand movements.

➤ Allow children to bring materials unusually close to the eyes to see them or to move up close to see things better.

➤ Some children with visual impairments see best when they tilt their heads; do not discourage this behavior.

➤ For children with visual field loss, maximize ability to use intact field in the classroom (e.g., for children with left field loss, place them on the left side of the classroom or workgroup to maximize right field use; for children with lower field loss and little head control, bring instructional materials up to intact visual field area).

Duration

➤ Allow children more time to complete visually demanding tasks or tasks that require viewing visual details.

➤ Be aware that some children tire more quickly than others on visual tasks; be sure to give them breaks with less visually demanding tasks.

programs, many of these conditions may be modified to encourage vision use with less conspicuous stimuli so that children learn to function in more normalized environments (see the discussion later in this chapter, From Heightened to Normalized Visual Stimuli). The determination of appropriate visual stimuli depends on the student's visual profile, the instructional situation, and the specific instruction goal. This information should be obtained from comprehensive vision assessments and from an understanding of the cues that motivate a child to explore, move, and learn.

A variety of methods to optimize stimuli in beginning instructional programs are summarized in Sidebar 8.6 and are discussed in the following sections. These methods are recommended for initial instruction programs. Other variations may be applied once instruction has commenced and the instructor has a clearer understanding of the child's visual capabilities.

Small Worlds

The environment can do much to motivate and reinforce the child's looking, moving, and exploring behaviors. One such method to facilitate curiosity in the environment for young children with visual impairments using visual environmental management involves the setting up of so-called small worlds—delimited areas within a child's reach that contain objects and surfaces with enhanced visual, tactile, or auditory cues within the child's sensory capacities (Heinze, 1980, 1985). These can encourage reaching and exploring and facilitate the development of curiosity, basic concepts, as well as spatial and causal relationships. These small worlds can be varied as the child's skill levels increase. Use of small worlds integrates visual environmental management instruction into broader developmental learning goals. Small worlds should be made up of items naturally found in the various environments in which the child lives and plays, but the items may be arranged in closer proximity, with enhanced backgrounds, or with greater variety than would naturally occur, depending on the child's current level of visual, cognitive, and motor functioning. Some considerations in setting up small worlds are summarized in Sidebar 8.7.

When setting up a small world for a child with low vision, information from the child's comprehensive vision assessments will provide valuable information about the types of items he or she finds especially interesting, how close items must be to be visible, what degree and type of contrast and lighting are necessary, and the size and color of items to include. In addition to these visual characteristics, items that move and have tactile and auditory interest should be included, at least initially. The child's motor abilities must also be taken into consideration. These small worlds must not be so filled with stimuli that they are overwhelming. Small worlds can be built around naturally occurring situations, such as the following:

➤ An area on the floor bordered by a couch, large pillow, or the side of a toy chest; with a blanket or rug with interesting textual, visual, and auditory elements

Methods to Optimize Stimuli During Instruction in Initial Training Programs

The following methods may be useful to optimize visual stimuli during initial instructional programs:

Familiarity

➤ Begin with familiar objects and move to less familiar ones.

➤ Introduce *familiarity training* (discussed later in this chapter) to teach students about stimulus attributes when appropriate.

Visibility

➤ Present heightened stimuli when a child is learning a new skill or concept. Later reduce the intensity of the stimuli, being sure that the stimuli are still visible to the child.

➤ Introduce *light structuring* (discussed later in this chapter) for students with minimal visual interest in their surroundings when appropriate.

Figure/Ground

➤ Isolate specific visual variables at first and, later, infuse with other variables.

➤ Provide more space between objects and later move them gradually closer together.

➤ Provide less compelling stimuli around the target variable and move to more compelling stimuli.

Concept or Skill Acquisition

➤ Heighten visual cues to facilitate acquisition of conceptual and performance skills.

Use of Other Senses

➤ Confirm visual input through other sensory modalities.

➤ Adjust for the impact of competing sensory stimuli.

➤ Optimize the use of other sensory modalities as well as vision. Some children, particularly those with cortical visual impairment, may require auditory or tactile input to "trigger" awareness to use of visual input (e.g., touching an object first to induce active visual examination of it.)

SIDEBAR 8.7

Small Worlds for Young Children with Visual Impairments

The goal of creating small worlds is to facilitate the development of children's curiosity, basic concepts, and spatial relationships through active exploration and reaching in naturally occurring or specially prepared environments that encourage the use and integration of vision and other sensory input. The following are some key considerations in setting up such an environment:

➤ Start within the child's visual and motor levels.

➤ Use items naturally found in typical settings that will entice, encourage, reward, and reinforce any attempts to look, move, follow, reach, and explore.

➤ Choose materials that provide visual, tactile, and auditory motivation and that do things when activated to encourage initiating and developing a sense of control.

➤ Broaden the "worlds" as the child grows and develops increased mobility, visual skills, and curiosity.

➤ For larger spaces (areas within the home and preschool), several small worlds can make up the overall space.

and objects that can be activated placed on the floor; and created walls. A family member may participate.

➤ Pots, pans, and utensils in a low kitchen cabinet to which the child has easy access.

➤ A toy box in the living room for exploration during family time after dinner.

➤ Toys, containers, and other items set up for exploration during bath time.

➤ A safe exploration area in a classroom that is slightly partitioned off and used during free play time.

➤ A sand box (or cornmeal box) with toys and objects for exploration in a covered outdoor play area.

Positioning of items is important. For example, if a 1-year-old child is only able to sit with support, the proximity and positioning of items and surfaces must be considered. They must be close enough so that he or she can initially feel them with little effort or as a result of accidental swiping. If the child is able to reach or creep, then items must be positioned to be accessible but also must provide continuing variety to encourage him or her to keep moving and exploring. Such selection and arrangement will facilitate not only the child's visual and exploratory behaviors but also his or her sense of planes, basic spatial relationships, and object permanence. Items that will entice, encourage, reward, and reinforce any attempts to look, move, follow, reach, and explore are critical. Items that can be activated should also be included to encourage the child to initiate his or her own activity and develop a sense of control.

As a child's visual and motor skills develop and he or she is able to scan and search, crawl, or even walk, these small worlds can be broadened to require increased effort and use of his or her growing skills. They should continue to provide a rich variety of visual, tactile, and motor activities that will reinforce his or her efforts and encourage her continued exploration. Once his or her increased visual and movement skills allow greater freedom, items can occur more naturally, and familiarity with the environment should be emphasized. If the child is able to move about larger spaces, such as within the home or preschool, several small worlds can make up the overall space and the child can be familiarized to each of the smaller units and then make a transition from one to another.

Familiarity Training

Most babies, young children, and students with visual and multiple disabilities are more disposed to learning when they are comfortable and content, in familiar environments with familiar people, and using familiar objects in familiar routines. Some youngsters will be less affected by environmental changes than others due to individual differences in temperament and their previous exposure to diverse settings and people. A child's performance and abilities can change dramatically when a familiar person, place, or thing is altered in his or her established routine. It is best to begin with familiar people or objects, and slowly introduce objects with different visual attributes to a child's instructional repertoire. The instructor needs to remember, however, that children must be actively engaged with their environment to learn from it. If children become habituated to an object or person to the extent that they are no longer interested in looking at or interacting with it, a novel stimulus that generates increased interest needs to be introduced to promote learning.

Familiarity training is one technique to facilitate a youngster's ability to discriminate, recognize, and select desired items more accurately and quickly from a field of possible choices. It involves knowing *what* to look for. This technique is based on the premise that the more familiar a child becomes with a particular object, picture, or symbol (and still maintain an interest in it), the more quickly and accurately the child can identify that target. Even with limited cues available, the child will become more able to make accurate judgments (i.e., use the process of visual closure, or mentally filling in partial cues) based on repeated experience. This type of training is especially beneficial for very young children and students with cognitive delays who may not pick up this information incidentally because it provides structured development of such discrimination and

SIDEBAR 8.8

Familiarity Training

The goal of familiarity training is to assist children in recognizing critical elements of objects and environments in order to facilitate visual identification. It consists of the following elements:

➤ Provide experiences with objects, pictures, or symbols under ideal environmental conditions and at the individual's present level of functioning.

➤ Call attention to critical features of the object: use both visual and tactile exploration along with verbal description.

➤ Work toward accuracy and consistency in recognition and discrimination, starting with a few choices that are very different from each other.

➤ Gradually vary the distance, position, location, background, contrast, figure-ground, lighting, or illumination. Work toward continued accuracy and consistency in recognition and discrimination at each level of change, increasing choices and decreasing differences.

➤ Continue variations until the object, picture, or symbol is recognized under realistic or natural conditions.

➤ Take advantage of logical environmental context clues involved in knowing where to look for something (e.g., paper towels are more likely to be found near the sink than near the seating area of the kitchen).

recognition skills. It is also appropriate for children mainstreamed into a general education classroom or adults learning about a new skill or environment. This familiarity can be developed through several sequential steps that are described here and summarized in Sidebar 8.8.

First the item (e.g. object, picture, or symbol) is presented alone to the child under ideal environmental conditions. These conditions would include ideal lighting and glare control for the student's ocular condition, a background with high contrast and no distractors (low figure/ground), and ideal positioning and proximity to the student (enabling the child to explore the item both visually and tactilely). For example, at the initial stage, a child's red nylon jacket with brightly patterned knit trim around the bottom, down the sleeves, and around the hood would be placed in front of the student against a high-contrast and low figure–ground background. Lighting and glare control would be adjusted to suit the child's ocular condition. The youngster would be encouraged to explore the jacket both visually and tactilely, getting as close to it as he or she wanted. While the child is exploring, the teacher would call attention to the critical features of the jacket (i.e., characteristics that would be especially noticeable by the student and would serve as discriminators when comparing this jacket with those of other family members or classmates). These might include the red color, the bright pattern in various locations on the jacket, the silky feel and sheen of the nylon. The child should be encouraged to explore these features both visually and tactilely.

Next, the child would be presented with the opportunity to select the object from among several others, still under ideal conditions. At this stage only a few alternatives, each very different from the child's own jacket, would be presented, and several selection opportunities should be provided. The goal is to work toward accuracy and consistency of the child's selections.

Gradually, the teacher can vary the proximity, position, location, background contrast, degree of distraction by figure-ground elements, and the lighting variables. The jacket could be placed at a slight angle or with a sleeve folded underneath. It could be placed at a slightly greater distance from the child necessitating that his or her selection depend on visual cues alone. A slightly distracting background or less highly contrasted background could be used, or the lighting could be less than ideal. At this stage, changes in the variables should be gradual and involve only one or two of them at a time. The accuracy and consistency of the child's selections should be confirmed at each level of change before any additional variations are made. As the child progresses, the selection alternatives can be increased in both similarity and number.

As the child progresses, the teacher can continue to introduce variations until the object, picture, or symbol can be selected by the child under realistic or natural conditions. The child's jacket could be presented hanging over the back of a chair, hanging on a hook in the classroom or by the door, and with variations in lighting provided. Initially, when the item is placed in more naturally occurring settings, it might be beneficial to start again with less similar alternatives and limited background confusion, and then gradually build up to more similar alternatives placed more closely together and even overlapping (e.g., on coat hooks).

In addition to increasing the recognizability of objects through familiarity training, students can become more efficient in locating desired items by using context clues (knowing *where* to look for the item) with this method. For example, by familiarizing students with relevant environments, their attention can be called to the logical or frequent location of specific items in certain locations. The teacher or parent can work with the child in making experienced logical "guesses" about where he or she might find a particular item. Making such guesses and checking to see if they are correct can facilitate more efficient searching by decreasing the areas that require searching. For example, a youngster can learn that paper towels are kept near the sink (which is a larger and more visible target); therefore, she can go to the sink and systematically search for the paper towels in that area, rather than searching the entire kitchen.

From Heightened to Normalized Visual Stimuli

At the beginning of instruction programs, visual stimuli should generally be much more intense than the student's basic visual capacities would require to motivate the child to look at them and to complete the instruction tasks. If the cues are not sufficiently bold and easy to discriminate, the child must work harder to see in order to complete a task. Once a child understands the concept behind a task and actively participates in it with these high-intensity cues, the cues can gradually be made less conspicuous to encourage finer and finer visual discriminations by the child. The instructor needs to be certain that the child can still discriminate the less conspicuous stimuli. For some visual functions, stimuli must always be some degree above basic visual capacities for the student to feel comfortable using his or her vision to complete the task. For very young children learning to use their vision, their basic visual capabilities (e.g., visual attending, visual examining, and visual-motor behaviors) may change as they become more efficient in the use of their vision.

For example, it was determined that 2.5-year-old Ahmed could discriminate objects that were at least 1-in. high from 6 in. away. The IFSP team worked with the child's mother to encourage him to attend to near vision tasks such as looking at picture books. Initially the picture books selected for reading during a daily midmorning quiet time had bold, simple images that were at least 2 in. high. The mother held the books about 6 in. from the child. As Ahmed gained interest and proficiency with the pictures, books with pictures at least 1-in. high held 6 in. away were incorporated into his reading program. Because Ahmed was doing so well in learning to use his vision, it was next decided to introduce more complex pictures with more details that were at least 1-in. high, as well as simpler pictures that were 1/2 in. high from 6 in. away. Ahmed participated with interest in these tasks, enjoying the pictures, his successes, and his interactions with his mother.

Six months later, a functional vision assessment shows that Ahmed can now discriminate objects at least 1/2 in. in height from 6 in. away. It is not likely that Ahmed's visual acuity increased, but his ability to attend to the more difficult visual task may have increased with instruction and with his overall developmental maturation.

An important point to remember in vision instruction is that heightened cues must be faded whenever possible. The goal is to have a student interact with cues as close as possible to cues used in his or her typical environments: at home, school, or in the community. Since it is highly likely that myriad visual cues will not be visible to many children with low vision due to their organic limitations, heightened cues for a specific child should be faded until they reach his or her comfort level, which is often still more intense than required by his or her basic visual capacities. That precise comfort level can be determined as instruction progresses. If a child requires highly conspicuous cues to encourage engagement in a task due to cognitive or behavioral issues, such high-intensity cues may need to be maintained. If these high-intensity cues are unrealistic in naturally occurring environments, then alternative sensory approaches may be more useful and should also be encouraged.

Structuring Light Levels

Light structuring is a method that uses gradual changes in illumination to promote visual awareness and attention for students with minimal visual interest in their surroundings. It is among the many ways to enhance the visibility of elements in the environment to give children useful information. (Check with a student's eye care practitioner before using these methods for students who are very sensitive to light or who have seizure disorders that may be triggered by bright light.)

The light-structuring process involves sequential and individualized adjustments to the lighting in the environment to enhance visibility and increase the child's chances for visual awareness and attention to tasks within it. This process may require modifications for students who are light sensitive or very sensitive to glare, which can be determined based on results of the low vision evaluation and the functional vision evaluation. If the child is sensitive to bright light, then care must be taken to avoid glare. Lighting should not be made so bright that the child's visual system becomes overwhelmed and his or her vision is reduced. An approach to light structuring is described in the following sections and summarized in Sidebar 8.9.

Instructors need to work within the natural environment on functional tasks or in daily routines whenever possible. If the child's ocular condition necessitates special modification that cannot be attained in that environment, one can either determine another activity with the same visual goals that is amenable to environmental modification in the natural setting, or begin instruction in a temporary diagnostic teaching situation in which the environmental modifications are introduced and gradually faded as the child's skill levels increase.

If the child has difficulty attending or concentrating on specific visual items or tasks, be certain that figure-ground problems have been eliminated. Background stimuli may be stronger than the stimulus that the child is targeted to observe, and the child may be overwhelmed. One way to increase visibility is to increase the lighting difference between the background and the foreground by increasing illumination on the task and/or decreasing the light in the background. This should be done gradually, increasing the lighting difference only as much as is necessary to enable the child to attend and develop basic looking skills. Providing more lighting difference than necessary will require a more extended transition back to more naturalistic conditions later. High-contrast background colors along with high-intensity table lamps and dimmer switches on lamps and overhead lighting allow for flexibility in contrasted lighting levels.

Once the child shows some visual awareness in a task, the instructor can work on basic skills such as fixating, focusing, following, shifting gaze, reaching, exploring, visual matching, and selecting. When the instructor notices consistently accurate behaviors, more natural lighting conditions can be introduced, depending upon the individual child's visual capacities. The child needs to be encouraged to practice targeted visual skills at each lighting level. If this process has been occurring in a temporary diagnostic environment, the visual skills, once

Light Structuring

The goal of light structuring is to make sequential and individualized adjustments to lighting in the environment to enhance the visibility of visual stimuli and to increase a child's chances for visual awareness and attention to tasks within it. It consists of the following elements:

➤ Work within the normal environment on functional activities or within daily routines whenever possible.

➤ Be certain that modified lighting conditions used in light structuring do not create glare or overwhelm the child's visual system with too much light for those sensitive to bright light.

➤ If the child has difficulty focusing on a desired task, increase the lighting difference by using extra illumination on the object and decreasing background light.

➤ Increase lighting difference only as much as necessary to promote effective looking behaviors.

➤ Work on basic skills within the task: looking, tracking, shifting gaze, handling, reaching, matching, selecting.

➤ Gradually return to more natural lighting conditions (as much as possible given the individual child's visual capacities) so that skills and behaviors can be readily transferred to everyday situations. As with familiarity training, provide opportunities for the child to demonstrate accurate and consistent behaviors at each change of the lighting level.

➤ Remember that some children will always require additional lighting on tasks (or reduced background lighting), depending upon their visual conditions.

established, can be encouraged in natural environments so that they become generalized and reinforced. Additional lighting on tasks and glare control may always be required, depending upon a particular child's visual needs.

One sequence of lighting alternatives could progress as follows:

➤ A light box with a dimmer switch in a dimly lit room

➤ A directional lamp with a dimmer switch in a dimly lit room

➤ A light box with a dimmer switch in a normally illuminated room

➤ A directional lamp with a dimmer switch in a normally illuminated room

➤ Normal room illumination only

Isolating Visual Elements in the Environment

It is sometimes necessary to isolate visual elements in the environment to encourage a child to attend to them. As always, any modification of a child's usual environment should be gradually faded as much as possible, depending on his or her visual capacities. Some ways to isolate visual variables include the following:

➤ Present objects singly.

➤ For tasks requiring a choice, present two objects some distance apart on a contrasting background.

➤ Present objects against a contrasting background of a single color. Remember that the background behind objects should be simplified as well as the background underneath them.

➤ Choose pictures with a minimum of detail.

➤ Present pictures of single objects rather than as part of a complex scene.

➤ Outline a picture or symbol in red or embed the picture in a boldly outlined box.

➤ Shine a directional light onto an object in a dimly lit room.

➤ Present a self-illuminated object such as a lighted toy.

➤ Present transparent pictures or partially opaque objects on a light box, and gradually dim the level of background lighting.

Heightening Visual Cues

Sometimes students with visual impairments and additional disabilities may not understand the conceptual and performance skills that underlie a basic activity. It may be helpful, in some cases, to heighten visual cues while teaching conceptual or performance skills, and then fade the heightened cues once the child has mastered the skills, as is done in the following example:

Raul, a 10-year-old boy with visual and multiple impairments is asked to open a door in an unfamiliar classroom where his class has gone for a special activity. He does not respond to a teacher's verbal request to open the door. The doorknob appears and operates differently from the one in his regular classroom that he opens every day, and this silver doorknob does not contrast strongly with the silver-gray door. The teacher in the unfamiliar classroom makes the erroneous assumption that the boy does not know how to open doors. Raul's vision teacher realizes that the boy has not been exposed to this type of doorknob and that he has difficulty seeing it. She affixes a piece of paper of contrasting color to the door behind the doorknob. Then she shows him the doorknob, explains and shows how the doorknob works, and encourages him to try opening the door. Once Raul learns to open the door, his vision teacher can remove the high-contrast background color. She finds that the child still uses his vision to complete the task. In this instance, the environment required modification to encourage the boy's vision use for instruction only: to allow Raul to conceptualize how the unfamiliar doorknob worked. He understood the concept of opening doors, but did not have the concept of how to operate this particular doorknob. Now he is able to operate this type of doorknob without any modifications.

Interrelationships of Visually Related Variables in the Environment

Visual variables are defined here as attributes of visual cues or visual tasks that can be modified, such as size, contrast, illumination, and visual complexity. These variables affect a child's efficient use of his or her vision, and there is an interrelationship among them, particularly lighting, contrast, size, and (a nonvisual variable) level of task difficulty. If one of these attributes, or variables, is less than optimal for a particular child, it becomes more important that other variables be at optimal levels.

Some examples include the following:

➤ When lighting is less than optimal for a particular child, he or she has greater need for optimal size, contrast, and task familiarity.

➤ When lighting is optimal, a child may function efficiently even though one of the other variables may be less than optimal (e.g., less contrast, smaller object size, or less familiarity with the task).

➤ If the size of an item or task is smaller than optimal, it will be more critical that the lighting and contrast are optimal and that the task be familiar or of limited difficulty.

➤ If a task is new or relatively difficult, it will be more critical that the lighting, contrast, and size are optimal.

➤ If the task is familiar or relatively simple, the child has a greater chance of being successful even though the lighting, contrast, or size may be less than optimal.

Although optimal levels for all these visual variables would be best, this is not always possible, and what is optimal for one child may be different from what is optimal for another. Teachers and parents must be attentive to situations in which any one of these visual variables may be less than optimal and consider how manipulating the other variables might impact the child's efficiency.

Light Pairing

When a child does not react visually to objects, or even to light, on a consistent basis, but there is still some question as to whether vision may play a useful role in his or her learning, light pairing may be useful diagnostically (Smith & Cote, 1982). It is used as a form of diagnostic teaching (see the earlier section on Visual Skills Instruction) to determine if concentrated vision instruction may lead to increased vision use and if vision is a potential learning channel. Light pairing involves assisting the child's transition from attending to input experienced through other senses to that experienced visually and is summarized in Sidebar 8.10. (Check with a child's eye care practitioner before using this method with students who are very sensitive to light or who have seizure disorders that may be triggered by light.)

The teacher first identifies a nonvisual object that the child responds to (e.g., a noise, toy, or other tactile item). When that item is presented to the child, the instructor also shines light onto the object. At first, light is presented each time the interesting item is presented. Then the light is presented first, followed by the interesting item. Next, the light is presented first, followed only intermittently by the interesting item. Then, if necessary, the light is presented alone, and the child is encouraged to attend to it briefly, follow it, and reach for it. This light only phase should be very brief but should involve different kinds of lights presented from different positions in the child's field of vision. This may not be necessary for some children. Very soon after this, the light is presented with a variety of other objects related to motivating and functional tasks, and again the child is encouraged to attend, follow, shift gaze, and reach for these objects, or otherwise engage in the meaningful tasks. Finally, objects and tasks are presented without the light, and the same behaviors are encouraged. These behaviors should be conducted in natural environments as early as possible in the instructional process. If the child is able to successfully progress through the stages presented, he or she has made a transition from attending only to nonvisual stimuli or situations to those which are visual; he or she has also developed basic visual skills, demonstrating potential for using vision as a contributing learning channel.

Optimizing the Instructional Setting

Sometimes a natural setting is not the most effective way to introduce instruction that will target specific visual skills. There may be too many distractions from competing sensory stimuli, the child may be uncomfortable in new surroundings or with unfamiliar people, or it may not be possible to isolate targeted visual skills sufficiently to encourage learning. If initial instruction is done apart from normalized settings, it needs to be transferred to usual settings as soon as possible to reinforce and generalize learning and to encourage children to practice skills as the need naturally arises. Guidelines for selecting appropriate instructional settings are presented in Sidebar 8.11.

In some situations teaching visual skills within routines that are slightly altered may be more successful for children who require activities that do not deviate

Light Pairing

The goals of light pairing are to encourage children who do not appear to use their vision consistently to do so, and to determine whether vision is a potential learning channel for a specific child. It involves a transition from nonvisual to visual awareness, attention, and exploration using a light source as an intermediary step. It consists of the following elements:

➤ Identify a nonvisual (auditory or tactile) object or activity that engages a child's interest (e.g., noisemaking toy or chenille stuffed animal).

➤ Initially, always shine a light source on this object or activity to attract the child's visual attention.

➤ Change to presenting the light source first, and then the favored object or activity.

➤ Then shine the light source first and only intermittently pair this with the favored object or activity.

➤ Present the light only and work with basic attention, following, and reaching skills. This training phase should be very brief and may not be necessary for some children. Experiment with different kinds of light and from different positions.

➤ As soon as possible, pair new, functional objects and meaningful tasks with the light to capture the child's interest.

➤ Gradually fade the use of the light source by presenting it intermittently with the new objects, and then not at all.

➤ Work on the following skills within this activity: awareness, looking, following, reaching, manipulating consistency.

➤ If necessary, physically move in synchrony with, and then guide, the child's body or hands (so-called coactive movements) in the beginning, to demonstrate behaviors.

➤ Move activities to natural environments as early as possible in the instruction process.

Source: Adapted from A. J. Smith and K. S. Cote. *A Resource Manual for the Development of Residual Vision in Multiply Impaired Children* (Philadelphia: Pennsylvania College of Optometry, 1982).

> **SIDEBAR 8.11**
>
> # Guidelines for Selecting Appropriate Instructional Settings
>
> Sometimes natural settings are too distracting to encourage learning. The following principles apply to the selection of appropriate instructional settings:
>
> ➤ Familiar settings may be more conducive for learning.
>
> ➤ Natural settings enable children to participate in usual activities with peers.
>
> ➤ Instruction within daily routines for infants and toddlers promotes consistency, regularity, and normalization.
>
> ➤ Instruction within critical and meaningful activities in usual environments for students with visual and multiple disabilities promotes motivation to learn, consistency, and normalization.
>
> ➤ Diagnostic teaching can assist in determining appropriate methods, materials, prompts, and cues for instruction.
>
> ➤ Slight alteration of a usual routine may motivate a child to modify an established behavior pattern targeted for change.
>
> ➤ Keep as a goal the infusion of an instructional program into typical settings in home, school, or community, to promote learning and inclusion.

from habitual patterns. A slight change may encourage children to alter their usual behavior patterns slightly so that learning takes place. It is important that the change not be so great that the student becomes frustrated or confused.

For example, 9-year-old Ayisha, who has visual and multiple impairments, regularly removes her milk carton from a tray and places it next to her snack on a classroom table at snack time. She reaches toward the tray of milk cartons as her teacher brings it around the classroom table and grasps any milk carton without looking. In fact, she rarely looks at most things she wants to obtain before reaching for them. Ayisha's teacher wants to encourage her to reach directly for the milk carton using her vision to guide her reach. The teacher has determined that the milk carton is large enough for Ayisha to see, and she knows that she is motivated to obtain it. When encouraged to do this in her usual routine, Ayisha is resistant to change. She is quite comfortable with the familiar snack time scenario. Her teacher decides to alter the routine slightly so that the child is more willing to adjust her behavior. The teacher places all the milk cartons on a revolving tray in the center of the snack table. Ayisha likes to turn the rotating tray, but because it is so large she can only reach across a small segment of it from a seated position. When all the other children have taken their milk cartons, Ayisha is encouraged to turn the tray until her carton is within reach. She is encouraged to watch the tray until the carton is close. She can then reach directly for her milk and place it next to her plate as she usually does. The instructor systematically teaches the child to complete this task until she is familiar with it. Once this is accomplished, Ayisha can attempt to reach for her milk while several other cartons are still on the tray.

Confirming and Augmenting Visual Input Through Other Senses

Children with low vision confirm and augment input from their vision with information from other sensory systems. It is important not to overlook the use of other sensory systems when designing instruction programs for students with low vision. It is critical to present situations that not only enhance visual skills and behaviors but also help the child learn how to coordinate visual information with information from his or her other sensory modalities. Implementation will depend on a child's specific visual and other abilities, and should be done within the context of age-appropriate, functional activities. Within these rich sensory experiences, the child can be encouraged to pay attention to and usefully correlate the wealth of sensory information available. Care must be taken not to overwhelm children with too many stimuli at one time, especially children with cortical visual impairment. Ways to foster multisensory learning include the following:

➤ Establishing learning environments that promote the association of real objects with their pictorial representations or with three-dimensional models.

➤ Encouraging children to associate food items with their aromas.

➤ Encouraging children to identify rooms in the home and school or stores in the community by their aromas or typical sounds associated with them.

➤ Providing art activities that supply auditory and/or tactile feedback in addition to visual feedback, such as finger painting with colored gelatin mixed with the paint.

➤ Encouraging multisensory experiences within daily living activities such as cooking (rolling cookie dough by hand on a high-contrast surface), cleaning, or washing clothes.

➤ Identifying objects by their sound or touch, and then confirming guesses with visual input, This can be done, by having the child reach into a "guessing box" to identify an object by feel or sound and then pull out the object to confirm its identity using his or her vision.

➤ Making photo albums of a child's activities at home, school, and in the community for periodic review.

➤ Presenting and reviewing a videotape of a real experience that has a rich multi-sensory component, such as a visit to the beach, a zoo, or a pizza parlor.

➤ Encouraging children to associate people with their voices.

➤ Promoting gross motor play in rich sensory environments such as sand boxes, water, and grassy areas.

➤ Taking trips to the fruit and vegetable sections of grocery stores and exploring the food items there.

Use of Other Senses

Since many children with low vision rely heavily on nonvisual input, it is important to consider the role this sensory information can play in a specific learning situation and to encourage the meaningful interplay of tactile, visual, auditory, and olfactory feedback. The specific goal of a compensatory program will determine how other sensory modalities will be used to promote learning. Cues from other modalities may serve various functions in a program to promote vision functioning in a variety of ways:

➤ Additional sensory cues may be added to a task to increase a child's motivation to participate.

➤ Additional sensory cues may be added to a task for children with cortical visual impairment, since they may require a sound, touch, or olfactory stimulus to initiate the use of vision. Once the child is using his or her vision, these additional sensory cues may need to be reduced so that the child focuses primarily on visual processes.

➤ Additional sensory cues may need to be reduced so that a child can focus primarily on available visual cues, without being distracted by additional sensory input.

➤ Additional sensory cues may be added to a simplified task to make it more typical once the child is applying a visual skill or behavior learned in isolation.

Minimizing Sensory Distraction

When presenting multisensory experiences, it is important that the wealth of sensory information not overwhelm students and reduce their focused interaction on objects and events around them. For example, an extremely noisy environment is not conducive to learning for some students and can be extremely disorienting for them. A noisy environment can also be counterproductive for students who are highly distractible. They will shift brief moments of attention from one competing auditory stimulus to another, never really engaging in higher order thinking skills since they do not focus long enough to extract and process information. In such an environment, the motivation to look, examine, and act upon visual stimuli can be minimal.

A visually busy environment can also be highly distracting to many children, especially when they are learning new skills. The background against which a visual task is presented should encourage children to focus on the task. For example, teachers or caregivers who are presenting lessons in sign language should wear solid-color clothing that contrasts highly with their hands. Some people wear gloves in a color that contrasts with their clothing. A classroom demonstration should be made against a solid color background so that a child can focus on the teacher and not be distracted by nonessential stimuli on the wall behind the teacher. Near vision materials should be presented on a high-contrast background of a single, solid color to encourage the child to look at them.

Tactile distractions can also divert a child's attention from learning opportunities. The instructor or caregiver may need to regulate carefully what is available for the student to touch, pull, push, hold, scratch, or rotate so that he or she performs these operations as part of the instruction program and not instead of it.

OTHER FACTORS THAT AFFECT INSTRUCTION

In addition to the methods of instruction that are selected to improve a child's visual functioning, an instructor needs to be aware of other factors that may affect the course of instruction. These may include stereotypical or other maladaptive behaviors, the child's physical position, and his or her physical or biological state.

Neurobehavioral Adaptations

Neurobehavioral adaptations are unusual visual behaviors that may compensate for a visual disability (Good & Hoyt, 1989). Some behaviors, begun when a child is very young, such as unusual head tilts and unusually close viewing distances (Lueck et al., 1997), may continue to have adaptive value whereas others, such as eye poking, prolonged light gazing, and flicking a hand in front of the eyes, should eventually be discouraged. The IEP or IFSP team needs to work in conjunction with the student's eye care specialist to learn the adaptive function of any unusual visual behaviors and to determine whether they should be encouraged or discouraged.

When working with children to discourage maladaptive behaviors, it is essential that other activities that have adaptive value be introduced to replace maladaptive ones. For example, if a child stares at the windows and shakes his or her head side to side when left alone, it is important to substitute an activity that has meaning to the child in place of the perseverative light-gazing behavior. The child might be positioned to face away from the windows and given some functional activity with visual and tactile feedback that attracts his or her attention.

Even with such interventions, it may be difficult to redirect children from engaging in maladaptive behaviors once they become habitual (Brambring & Troster, 1992). It is especially important, therefore, to work with caregivers and service providers to promote meaningful use of available vision in early infancy, thereby reducing the development and persistence of maladaptive behaviors.

Positioning

Depending upon their physical conditions, children may be more alert and ready to learn in some positions than in others. For children with physical impairments in addition to visual impairment, it is best to conduct instruction to promote visual functioning when they are not also putting energy into maintaining their posture or position. For example, a child may be in a prescribed stander for 30 min daily to promote his or her leg strength. During this time, the child is concentrating on maintaining the standing position, and it may be difficult for him or her to focus on additional sensory tasks. Later, when the child is rested and sitting in his or her wheelchair for group story time, vision instruction tasks can be introduced. He or she is comfortable, alert, and ready to engage in interesting and enjoyable activities. Determining the best positions or postures for vision instruction can be determined during a functional vision assessment with input from physical or occupational therapists. As long as children can focus on visual tasks in the positions selected, visual activities should be encouraged when children are in a variety of positions (Rainforth & York-Barr, 1996).

Biobehavioral States

Learning patterns of young children and children with visual and multiple disabilities may alter dramatically when they are tired, hungry, upset, ill, uncomfortable, have taken certain medications, or have experienced seizure activity. Instruction to promote vision functioning is most effective when children are alert, comfortable, and well. Smith and Levack (1996) present a method to assess biobehavioral states, ranging in their classification from sleep/inactive to awake/alert to awake/agitated, to assist in determining the most effective learning situations for particular children. Activities that encourage alerting or quieting may be introduced to alter biobehavioral states in preparation for instruction (Smith & Cote, 1984). For many children it is best to alternate activities that are quite active and energetic with ones that are more quiet and calming to give children time to reenergize and integrate what they have learned. Some children, especially those with cortical visual impairment (see the following section), require a complete break between activities. Others may require high-energy physical activity to reach an alert state before instruction can be valuable to them. Instructors need to be sensitive to the unique needs of individual children and modify instructional activities accordingly.

SPECIAL STRATEGIES FOR CHILDREN WITH CVI

Cortical visual impairment (CVI), also called cerebral visual impairment, caused by disturbance of the posterior visual pathways and/or the occipital lobes of the brain (Blind Babies Foundation, 1998) is the leading cause of visual impairment in young children in industrialized countries. It can affect vision in different ways depending upon the location, extent, and onset of the damage to the brain (Hoyt, 2002). Children with CVI may manifest one or more of a variety of behaviors related to this condition that are not seen in children with ocular visual impairment. Although many intervention techniques for children with CVI may overlap with those appropriate for children with ocular visual impairments, in children with CVI these techniques may address different underlying causes. It is important for caregivers and practitioners to understand these differences in order to create and administer effective intervention programs.

The visual behaviors of children with CVI have been reviewed by a number of authors (Blind Babies Foundation, 1998; Groenveld, Jan, & Leader, 1990; Jan & Groenveld, 1993; Jan, Groenveld, Sykanda, & Hoyt, 1987; Steendam, 1989). Children with CVI may see differently than they usually do when they are tired, sick, taking medications, or under stress. They may look directly at an object and not know that it is there. They may reach directly for an object, although they may not be looking directly at it. They may move about without bumping into objects that one would not expect them to see. Children with CVI may be highly distracted by competing sensory stimuli, and may not be able to separate out which to attend to. They may therefore function more effectively in environments with fewer distractions. They may need to experience an object through other senses than their vision first (e.g., touch or smell an object first) to initiate the use of their vision (Steendam, 1989). It may also be easier for them to notice a moving than a stationary object. They may locate objects visually but look away before reaching for them, possibly due to difficulty they experience in processing visual and motor tasks simultaneously. They may have difficulty separating figures from their background in both two and three dimensions. As such, they may be attracted to explore a nonfunctional part of an object, and not notice the object as a whole. They may be sensitive to light or, conversely, stare at light sources. They may have better color vision than form vision since mechanisms in the brain that detect color are often still intact (Blind Babies Foundation, 1998). Children with CVI may "shut down" when they become overloaded by sensory stimuli, and this point of saturation may come more readily for them than for children without CVI. Children with CVI often do not look directly at faces, which can be a serious impediment in the process of bonding with their caregivers.

Some investigators prefer the term cerebral visual impairment since some children have visual impairment due to subcortical white matter insults (e.g., periventricular leukomalacia) (Hoyt, 2002). In addition, researchers and ophthalmologists are only beginning to understand the complex visual processing issues associated with brain dysfunction that affect vision in children, as well as their educational implications (e.g., Dutton, Day, & McCulloch, 1999; Hoyt, 2002; Hyvarinen, 1999, n.d.).

Brain damage early in life can affect a number of cognitive visual functions distinct from those related to visual field, visual acuity, contrast sensitivity, and color perception. Dutton and his colleagues (Dutton et al., 1996; Dutton, 1999) report that the following cognitive visual functions are affected:

➤ Recognition of people, shapes, or objects

➤ Orientation in physical space

➤ Depth perception (e.g., difficulty differentiating low-lying surfaces, estimating accuracy of visually guided movements, and with accommodation and convergence used for tracking in the third dimension)

➤ Perception of movement due to impaired tracking (e.g., difficulty seeing fast-moving objects)

➤ Simultaneous perception (e.g., figure-ground difficulties, difficulty in differentiating crowded images)

➤ Visual memory (e.g., difficulty with copying tasks)

➤ Visual imagination (e.g., difficulty with visual concepts as applied in art and design)

➤ Visual attention (e.g., looking away from material or tiring rapidly of visual tasks)

➤ Processing time (e.g., longer time is required).

Until more research-based information is available, general guidelines for working with children with CVI can be offered, with an understanding that each student must be evaluated for his or her unique needs and behavior patterns. A multidisciplinary team approach is best when working with children with vision loss due to brain damage because of the multiplicity of areas which may be affected (e.g., neurological, physical, cognitive). Sidebar 8.12 presents suggested instructional practices to use with children who have cortical visual impairment. As mentioned earlier, many of these approaches are also useful with children with ocular visual impairments, but these approaches specifically address the visual cognitive processing issues experienced by children with CVI.

ASSISTIVE DEVICES

In addition to instruction to make maximum use of their vision, some young children with visual impairments can benefit from the use of assistive devices. These can include optical devices and electronic magnification as well as augmentative and assistive communication devices for children who also have speech limitations.

Instructional Strategies for Students with Cortical Visual Impairment

PATRICIA MORGAN

Overall Strategy

➤ Schedule visual experiences for the time of day when the student demonstrates optimal visual functioning.

➤ Slow down.

➤ Simplify the task.

➤ Space visual information so that it is viewed in manageable units.

➤ Be specific about what you want the student to see and to do.

➤ Sequence the task.

➤ Provide structure and sameness in each presentation.

Adapting the Environment
Goal: To provide an environment that allows the student with CVI to respond to the visual information presented.

Provide an environment that is free from visual clutter
➤ Work surface: be sure that the work surface does not have a pattern.

➤ Background surfaces and spaces: be sure that the learning environment has only essential visual information; decorative items hanging from the ceiling, "busy" bulletin boards or walls, spaces filled with objects, or carpets with visual patterns will make it difficult for the student with CVI to select visually the desired visual target and attend to it.

➤ Clothing of the person(s) presenting the visual target(s): wear solid, dark colored clothing or a smock, if you are in the child's visual field when the visual target is presented.

Provide an environment with proper lighting
➤ Watch for glare on all surfaces, and eliminate it as much as possible.

➤ Maximize indirect lighting sources.

➤ Minimize the use of fluorescent lighting.

➤ Position the student with his or her back to the windows.

➤ Dim the lights if the student experiences photophobia (light sensitivity).

(continued on next page)

Reduce the amount of competing sensory information

➤ Provide a quiet environment; constant background noise tends to lull many children, whereas intermittent noises are unexpected and seem to startle them or reduce their ability to stay visually focused.

➤ Eliminate any unnecessary odors (perfumes, food odors, etc.).

➤ Maintain a comfortable room temperature; if the room is too warm, children may be lethargic; if it is too cold, muscle tone will be increased.

➤ Reduce unexpected movement in the visual field.

Adapting the Presentation of Materials

Goal: To adapt the presentation of material so that children can use their visual abilities to learn new concepts.

Enhance the visual targets

➤ Keep visual information simple, constant, and predictable.

➤ Use real objects in natural sequences to aid in the understanding of the real visual environment; limit the use of toys that provide a degree of abstraction that is too difficult for the child to interpret and are made of plastic. (These items have the same taste, smell, temperature, and tactile information.)

  ● Provide high contrast between the object to be viewed and the background.

  ● Light-colored foods on dark cutting boards or plates.

  ● Eating utensils of contrasting colors.

  ● Shoelaces in two bright colors, so that the left is different in appearance from the right.

  ● Pastel pictures, colored over with fluorescent or primary colors.

➤ Use color.

  ● When teaching the identification of objects, keep the color of common objects constant until the concept has been established to some degree; later, other colors can be added.

  ● Letters and numbers that have color shading around them (such as red or yellow) may attract the visual interest of some children and may provide more visual stimulation than black letters on a white field.

➤ Eliminate unnecessary visual details or information.

  ● Use correctional fluid to mask any details that are not necessary on worksheets, symbols for communication boards, etc.

  ● Cut or fold the paper so that the visual information is presented in smaller units.

  ● Use markers to mask part of the information.

➤ Widely separate objects or units of visual information, so that each item can be viewed individually.

  ● Use picture books with simple, single pictures on a page.

  ● Leave spaces between visual targets on visual displays when introducing alternative and augmentative communication devices (see Appendix 8.2 for more information).

  ● Hand letter beginning reading words, so that there is more space between the letters than in typed printing.

  ● Use a computer to create and print reading materials with expanded spacing.

When possible, present visual material in the student's best visual field
➤ Allow the child to position the materials herself or himself for optimal use of the available visual field.

➤ Observe the student and determine whether she or he views two-dimensional material better in the horizontal or vertical plane.

Provide verbal, auditory, visual, or tactile clues to the location of the visual target or task so that the student will know where to look
➤ Verbally describe the location of the target, known as "verbal cueing" (e.g., "Your doll is by your foot").

➤ If the student is fascinated with light, dim the environment and aim a penlight onto the visual target. This helps to reduce the background "clutter" and provides an emphasized visual target.

➤ Position visual targets on a light box.

➤ Add a sound to the visual target (this can be as easy as tapping on the item).

➤ Create boundaries to the location of a stationary target, by using a tray, a piece of contrasting background paper, etc.

➤ Mark a desired place in the environment: bold symbol might indicate your classroom door; a strip of reflective tape might identify the location of the soap dish in the bathtub.

➤ Run your hand down the child's arm to his or her hand to direct his or her visual attention to an object or fine motor task

➤ When presenting a moving visual target, tap the side of the student's body, then bring the object in from that side.

➤ Teach the student to slide (without lifting) a finger across units of visual information, such as pictures, shapes, numbers, letters, and words.

Clearly identify the visual task for the student
➤ Verbally indicate the beginning and the end of each task.

(continued on next page)

SIDEBAR 8.12 CONTINUED

➤ Mark the physical placement of tasks and objectives:

- Top or beginning of a page.

- Bottom or end of an assignment.

- Left side of the line of symbols, if the student is expected to move visually from left to right. If the student is to view a series of symbols on an augmentative communication device, mark the left side of the device with a red line, while having the child wear a red band on his or her left hand.

- Location for his or her answer. A bright pink line might be used to indicate where the child is to write.

Ritualize the presentation of the tasks
➤ Use the same materials consistently.

➤ Repeat known sequences. Have the child help set the table in the same sequence for a regular meal time lesson; have the child do reading workbook exercises in the same sequence.

Pace the presentation of material, so that it is neither too slow nor too fast

Use a tone of voice that is interesting and calming, but not boring or startling

Watch the facial expression of the child when you are presenting new visual information
➤ At times, students with CVI fade out on overload; do not make changes in presentation during these moments.

Accommodate other disabilities as much as possible, to allow all available energy to be concentrated on the visual tasks
➤ Position children with physical impairments so that their head is not hanging forward, if necessary and, if appropriate, provide head support to avoid involuntary shifting of the visual field.

Provide consistency between home and school
➤ Communication with family members or other caregivers will help to provide similarity in the style of approach.

➤ Use of the same materials, in the different environments, is often beneficial.

Low Vision Optical and Electronic Devices

There has been little research on the introduction of low vision optical devices to young children with low vision. Ritchie, Sonksen, & Gould (1989), conducted a study in which stand magnifiers were introduced to children with low vision aged 18 months to 6 years. They found that children with better visual acuity (i.e., ability to discriminate a 12M Snellen letter at 10 cm) and who had the developmental skills necessary to make use of their stand magnifiers (including the ability to attend to instructional materials as well as sufficient language and cognitive skills) benefited most from the devices. In a study of a group of children aged 3 to 6 years who were prescribed a variety of near and distance optical devices, most children were more enthusiastic about the use of distance devices (monocular or binocular telescopes) than near devices (Nott, 1994). Nott indicated that distance devices may offer more significant enhancement of viewing than near devices for children at this age. She reasoned that children of this age need not rely solely on optical magnification to see near material since they can bring the material quite close to the eye for magnification, using their available accommodative abilities. To view material at a distance, however, they may need optical magnification. Nott emphasized the importance of team work among eye care specialists who work with children with low vision, parents, and teachers of students who are visually impaired to maximize successful prescription and use of optical devices. Ritchie et al. (1989) emphasized other factors that contribute to the successful introduction of low vision devices to young children:

➤ The experience of professionals in working with young children with visual impairments

➤ The approach taken to explain information and encourage the child's use of devices

➤ The use of a wide range of materials suitable for preschool children to determine which device might work best for which children

➤ An initial trial period of 6 to 8 weeks to work with the device at home

Although research on the use of closed-circuit television systems (CCTVs) for young children is not available, these electronic devices are being used in practice in direct instruction programs with a caregiver or teacher for highlighting detail and to promote matching, selecting, and tracking skills with preschool and older children. These devices are also being incorporated into play and exploration activities for young children to promote conceptual development in conjunction with vision skills use. Systematic instruction in their use needs to take into account children's physical, visual, and developmental levels. (See Chap. 9 for sequential instruction methods in the use of optical and electronic devices that can be modified to fit the unique needs of young children and children with visual and multiple disabilities.)

For children who may benefit from the early use of optical and electronic magnification devices, several suggestions are presented in modified form from Project VIISA (1999), a teaching resource developed by teachers, parents, and administrators for those working with very young children with visual impairments:

➤ Have the child complete a low vision evaluation first and receive directions for use of the device recommended.

➤ Ask the prescribing ophthalmologist or optometrist if it is possible to start with optical devices of lower power; they are easier for young children to use, and lower power telescopes require less adjustment.

➤ Ask the prescribing ophthalmologist or optometrist to suggest the lowest power that can be used with an electronic magnification device. This will enable children to see more material on the screen at one time. Some children (e.g., those with CVI) may benefit from having less information on the screen to reduce visual clutter. In such cases, a higher amount of magnification may be advisable. This needs to be determined for each child individually.

➤ Emphasize the device's functional use and application across tasks and environments (playing games, looking at nature, eating in a restaurant, etc.).

➤ Start with highly stimulating activity sessions and match the length of each session to the attention span of the child (Cowan & Shepler; 1990). These sessions could include finding "secret" details on two similar objects or pictures; identifying distant objects (such as signs for ice cream or toy stores); then traveling to the locations and playing hide and seek).

➤ Encourage the child to use the device independently in functional activities whenever possible.

For the young child's use of low vision optical and electronic devices to be most effective, it is helpful for families to have an understanding of basic optical principles and environmental factors that affect vision use, including the following:

➤ Basic concepts of light and optics

➤ Basic principles of corrective lenses

➤ Types of magnification, different devices, and their use with different tasks

➤ How a prescribed device works and its particular uses

➤ Concepts of color, contrast, lighting, functional acuity, and fields

➤ Methods to reduce glare

➤ Use of nonoptical devices alone and in combination with optical devices (Project VIISA, 1999)

➤ Effects of reduced visual fields created by magnification devices (e.g., discriminating part-whole relationships and determining a whole object from its parts)

As mentioned earlier, Ritchie et al. (1989), indicate that children need to understand the use of optical magnification devices to benefit the most from them. This principle likely applies to electronic magnification devices as well. Children need to understand the following in order to use these devices most advantageously:

➤ Positioning the device and material to be viewed for optimal performance, and maintaining those best positions

➤ Manipulating illumination for specific tasks to eliminate any shadows created in using the device

➤ Focusing a telescope or electronic magnification device for the clearest image

➤ Localizing the target

➤ Scanning, tracking, and systematic search techniques

➤ Tying the parts of an image together to understand the whole when using magnification devices

Children using these devices need to master the skills of localizing, fixating, scanning, tracking, and discriminating visual characteristics with unaided vision, and then with the use of the chosen device (Watson, 1989). For children who can benefit from the use of low vision optical and electronic devices at an early age, their use can facilitate the development of concepts, increase independence, promote self-esteem and curiosity, and encourage basic skills for using low vision devices that can be expanded upon as they grow older. Teachers must be careful, however, to base their use on individual assessment, linking device use to the relevant and specific goals for each child. It should also be noted that many activities critical to the development of concepts, curiosity, motor skills, and environmental interaction in very young children may be inhibited by the use of devices that can restrict children's visual fields as well as their physical manipulation of and interaction with objects.

Communication Devices

Many children with visual and multiple impairments require special devices to assist with communication when their speech is limited. These devices vary in complexity from a simple, switch-operated device that outputs a single spoken word or phrase to more complex devices that allow students access to various sets of pictures or symbols associated with many spoken words, phrases, or sentences (Taylor & Murphy-Herd, 1998). It is important that vision specialists provide input regarding the size, complexity, distance, contrast, and positioning of visual symbols on these devices as part of the collaborative IFSP or IEP team. The necessary information is determined from results of the eye examination, low vision evaluation, the functional vision evaluation, and the learning media assessment. The size of the symbols can be determined based on the individual child's visual acuity and the distance the assistive device will be from the student (see Table 5.3 in Chap. 5).

Photographs, pictures, or line drawings are often used in conjunction with communication devices. Some students can see photographs while others cannot. Color photographs are generally easier to decipher than black and white ones since the former have greater contrast. The eye care specialist can help to determine whether photographs can be used or whether other alternatives such as noncomplex pictures or outline drawings would be easier for a student to discriminate, and can also determine the optimal size of these images.

The eye care specialist can also help to determine if tactile symbols may be beneficial to the student. The positioning of the device will depend upon the way in which the student is expected to interact with the device as well as any visual field or oculomotor limitations the student may have. For example, if a student has limited use of the left hand only, the device should be positioned so that the child makes maximum use of that hand. If the child also has a left visual field loss, the symbols must be placed so that they are visually accessible. This may mean that the device should be positioned slightly left of center rather than to the far right side in order to promote both left hand use and visual functioning. The child will have to turn his or her head slightly to the left in order to use his or her intact right visual field. The exact area to locate the device in relation to the student must be determined by observing the student with the device. Guidelines on the use of visual displays for augmentative and alternative communication devices can be found in Appendix 8.2.

CASE STUDY: Justin

A case study of a young child with visual and multiple disabilities serves to clarify and illustrate the process of pulling together all the factors considered in this chapter into a functional vision intervention program. Training such as this in turn facilitates cognitive growth and exploration. Sidebar 8.13 describes the process in general.

Background

Justin is 3 years, 1 month of age and was diagnosed with cortical visual impairment by his ophthalmologist. He has hydrocephalus and has just recuperated from surgery to repair the bones in his skull that had fused together, causing pressure on his growing brain. It was reported by his mother and home counselor that Justin's vision had regressed following this latest surgery. Justin is nonambulatory, can sit with slight assistance, can reach and grasp with his left hand, and has only limited use of his right hand. He communicates by making two or three specific facial expressions that his parents acknowledge and reinforce. He also repeats some sounds (e.g., ah, boo, baa) as well as cries and fusses to indicate his needs and wants. Justin lives with his mother, father, and teenage brother in an urban area where he receives services from a home counselor with training in visual impairment education as well as physical therapy and occupational therapy. Justin does not attend a school program, primarily because his parents were concerned about his exposure to illnesses since he is medically fragile.

Factors to Consider for Instruction in Visual Functioning

➤ Determine current level of visual functioning from results of ophthalmological, optometric, low vision, and functional vision evaluations.

➤ Use a transdisciplinary model for assessment and intervention.

➤ Involve parents in assessments, the determination of instructional goals, and implementation of programs.

➤ Determine systematically the repertoire of children's visual attending behaviors, visual examining behaviors, and visually guided motor behaviors.

➤ Determine as a team a functional vision instruction program that considers visual environmental management, visual skills instruction, and visually dependent task instruction.

➤ Use appropriate visual cues and appropriate sensory environment to encourage visual behaviors.

➤ Incorporate instructional programs in young children's daily routines or critical activities for students with visual and multiple disabilities implemented by caregivers or other significant persons in the children's lives.

➤ Incorporate visual functioning goals into routines that the students, caregivers, and professionals enjoy.

➤ Incorporate visual functioning goals into functional, age-appropriate activities.

➤ Consider students' positioning, response time, and level of alertness in designing instructional protocols.

➤ Reinforce visual behaviors targeted for systematic instruction by focusing on them as they occur naturally in additional activities throughout the day.

➤ Adjust the instructional program (visual cues, frequency and level of prompts, and reinforcement procedures) as behavioral changes occur to promote independent functioning in naturally occurring visual environments.

➤ Continue instructional programs over an extended period of time.

➤ Monitor students' progress regularly and systematically.

➤ Revise instructional protocols when methods are not successful.

Source: Adapted with permission of the publisher from A. H. Lueck, H. Dornbusch & J. Hart, "An Exploratory Study to Investigate the Effects of Training on the Vision Functioning of Young Children with Cortical Visual Impairment," *Journal of Visual Impairment & Blindness, 93*(12), (1999), pp. 778–793.

Visual Assessment

Reports by his ophthalmologist indicated that Justin had cortical visual impairment with no refractive error and pupils that were briskly responsive to light. The last report, prior to Justin's major surgery, indicated improved visual fixation with no nystagmus or strabismus.

A functional vision assessment was conducted with a teacher of visually impaired students, a home counselor, an orientation and mobility specialist, and Justin's mother present. It indicated that Justin was able to fixate on objects, but his fixations were fleeting and he did not appear to use his vision to examine objects. Justin did not appear to shift gaze between two objects on repeated trials in various locations. He did, however, appear very briefly to follow objects that were presented at midline then moved slowly just to the left or right of midline.

When presented with silent objects at eye level, Justin reached directly for them when they were slightly to the left and right of midline as well as centrally. He crossed midline to reach for objects with his left hand. Objects had to be of high tactile, auditory, and visual interest for Justin to respond to them visually, and he often lost interest in them after one or two presentations. When he reached, Justin appeared to look at objects eccentrically, making it very difficult at times to determine whether or not he was looking at the objects. It appeared that Justin was more likely to look at objects after he had touched them, a common characteristic of children with cortical visual impairment. It also appeared that Justin was more likely to fixate briefly on objects that were moved into his field of view and was not likely to fixate on stationary objects, which is another common characteristic of children with cortical visual impairment.

Justin only occasionally initiated a visual search for objects he heard that were extremely compelling for him (e.g., a flashlight covered with a favorite noisy, soft tissue paper). Justin's preferred mode of exploration was tactile, searching on his tray for objects, picking them up with his left hand, sometimes putting them in his mouth, then throwing them on the floor for an adult to retrieve. One of his trays had a bowl-like depression built into it that Justin explored constantly. He would search the bowl tactilely with his left hand, pick up an object, and throw it down as part of his favorite retrieval game with his parents. Justin was not noted to search tactilely for objects other than those located on his tray. Justin's mother reported that he was most alert in his stander, which he used for 1 hour at a time.

Determining Skills for Intervention

Justin's mother, home counselor, and the orientation and mobility specialist considered that encouraging Justin to extend his area of exploration from the tabletop to an area slightly above the tabletop would increase the repertoire of skills he needs to interact meaningfully with his surroundings. The group also believed that encouraging more independent play was an area of need for Justin. Justin showed the ability to search visually for objects that he heard when he reached directly for the flashlight covered with tissue paper. These needs and abilities were incorporated into a functional goal related to vision for Justin: to increase the frequency of his visually guided search and reach for objects presented just below eye level but slightly above the tabletop. Figure 8.5 presents a form that facilitates the consideration of individual elements in establishing an intervention program, using the intervention designed for Justin as an example. (A blank copy of this form appears in Appendix 8.3 to this chapter.)

Intervention Design

This intervention was completed at home and integrated into Justin's playtime in his stander. An addition to Justin's play station was a tabletop enclosure made from a piece of heavy, white poster board folded into three sections. The poster board was positioned so that it remained upright on the flat surface of the stander tray in order to block out visual input from the surrounding environment. The standing position was selected for Justin since he was reported to be most alert when standing. The enclosure was introduced to reduce competing visual cues so that Justin would be more inclined to focus on new playthings placed inside it. Children with cortical visual impairment are often confused by a plethora of visual stimuli, often focusing on noncritical visual cues that distract them from those needed to complete activities successfully. A metal stand was placed inside the enclosure, with a wire running across the top, and from that wire was hung a smooth stick with colored feathers attached at the bottom. The toy was jiggled and spun, since moving objects are more readily seen by children with cortical visual impairment, and a small bell was also attached to attract Justin's attention further. These cues were added since sound and movement were noted to encourage Justin's visual behaviors. The toy could be moved along the wire to Justin's left and right or center. Attached to the wire with elastic, the toy would spring back slowly when pulled. Justin was not able to throw the toy down for retrieval by an adult, but he received kinesthetic feedback from it when it was pulled, and he could retrieve the toy independently. Justin's mother implemented the instruction and record-keeping activities with some help from Justin's father.

The visual goal of this activity was for Justin to make direct visually guided reaches for the hanging feather toy when the enclosure was removed for independent play. The developmental goal was for Justin to interact meaningfully with objects in his environment without assistance.

The intervention of the enclosure used visual environmental management to provide an environment that facilitates viewing of critical visual stimuli. For Justin, however, this was preceded by visually dependent task instruction to encourage use of skills (visual search and visually guided reaching) that Justin had but did not apply to tasks that could be completed more efficiently using vision.

Form for Designing an Intervention

Goal	*To interact meaningfully with objects in the environment during play time without assistance*
Activity components	*Free play with toys within reach on stander* *Direct reaching for motivating toys* *Sustained, independent play with meaningful exploration of objects and their relationships*
Visual behaviors involved	*Scanning, fixating, visually guided reach, following, visual investigation*
Modifications to the environment	*White enclosure to reduce visual distraction from toys* *Toys of high contrast against white background* *Toys attached with rubber band to wire strung across top of enclosure to provide kinesthetic feedback and visual feedback* *Toys interesting to tactile, auditory, and visual senses*
Nonoptical devices	*White enclosure*
Optical devices	*None*
Probable best sensory approach for accomplishing task	*Combined visual, tactile, auditory* *Reduction of distracting stimuli*
Specific skills to teach	*Manual exploration and manipulation* *Understanding of cause and effect (when toy is pulled it bounces back)*
Probable best vision instruction components to use	*Visual skills instruction* *Visually dependent task instruction* *Visual environmental management*

Figure 8.5. Sample form for designing an approach to activities with visual components: Justin's intervention program.

Outcomes

Justin had a highly ritualized play routine that was familiar and rewarding to him. When a new toy, object location, and type of feedback were introduced, Justin did not appear interested in interacting. In fact, he protested by crying and fussing when the activity was first introduced. During the initial environmental management instruction sessions without direct adult intervention, Justin was learning about a completely new visual and tactile environment. He did interact with it, but his interactions were minimal. He did, however, demonstrate the ability to interact with his surroundings in a new way when visually dependent task instruction was introduced using adult reinforcement of his reaching responses. Justin did not appear motivated to reach for the feather toy until his mother introduced verbal and physical reinforcement techniques. It is likely that this visually dependent task instruction increased Justin's visual reaching behavior for this activity. Later, Justin's mother reported that she often let him play independently with toys hanging from the wire using the enclosure. She indicated that he enjoyed his independent play and that she could leave him alone in play for the first time. She also introduced new toys: a soft clown doll with shiny metallic clothes, which Justin pulls, as well as an orange ball that he hits. After initial instruction, Justin was able to benefit from visual environmental management instruction. He was curious about new toys and independently initiated interactions with them.

CONCLUSION

This chapter emphasizes that functional vision is not a detached set of skills and behaviors that operate in isolation and focus solely upon the discrimination of elements in the environment. Functional vision in fact operates in conjunction with other sensory, motor, and cognitive systems, and these coordinated functions enable children to master ways to explore and understand their world. The successful design of intervention programs must not only take into account the way these systems operate within each child but must also consider factors associated with the child's family and environment so that goals, objectives, and strategies are tailored to the unique capacities, needs, and circumstances of individual students. The following chapter reviews compensatory instructional techniques for academically oriented school age students with low vision to apply the principles described here in support of school and other activities.

REFERENCES

Barraga, N. C. (1964). *Increased visual behavior in low vision children.* New York: American Foundation for the Blind.

Blanksby, D. C. (1994). *Visual assessment and programming: The VAP-CAP handbook.* Victoria, Australia: Royal Victorian Institute for the Blind.

Blind Babies Foundation (1998). *Pediatric diagnosis facts sheets: Cortical visual impairment.* San Francisco, CA: Author.

Brambring, M., & Troster, H. (1992). On the stability of stereotyped behaviors in blind infants and preschoolers. *Journal of Visual Impairment & Blindness, 86,* 105–110.

Chen, D. (Ed.). (1999). *Essential elements in early intervention: Visual impairment and multiple disabilities.* New York: AFB Press.

Chen. D., & Dote-Kwan, J. (1995). *Starting points: Instructional practices for children whose multiple disabilities include visual impairment.* Los Angeles, CA: Blind Children's Center.

Chen, D., & Dote-Kwan, J. (1998). Early intervention services for young children who have visual impairments with other disabilities and their families. In S.Z. Sacks & R. K. Silberman (Eds.), *Educating students who have visual impairments with other disabilities.* (pp. 303–338). Baltimore, MD: Paul Brookes.

Cowan, C., & Shepler, R. (1990). Techniques for teaching young children to use low vision devices. *Journal of Visual Impairment & Blindness, 84,* 419–21.

Downing, J., & Bailey, B. (1990). Developing vision use within functional daily activities for students with multiple disabilities. *RE:view, 21,* 209–220.

Dunst, C. J., Trivette, C. M., & Deal, A. G. (1988). *Enabling and empowering families: Principles and guidelines for practice.* Cambridge, MA: Brookline.

Dutton, G., Ballantyne, J., Boyd, G., Bradnam, M., Day, R., McCulloch, D., Mackie, R., Phillips, S., & Saunders, K. (1996). Cortical visual dysfunction in children. A clinical study. *Eye, 10,* 302–309.

Dutton, D. N., Day, R. E., & McCulloch, D. L. (1999). Who is a visually impaired child? A model is needed to address this question for children with cerebral visual impairment. *Developmental Medicine and Child Neurology, 41,* 211–213.

Eksted, R., Lastine, D., & Paul, B. (1996*). Individualized, comprehensive, evaluation of functional use of vision in early childhood (I-CEE).* Roseville, Minnesota: Minnesota Department of Children, Families, and Learning.

Erin, J. (2000). Students with visual impairments and additional disabilities. In A. J. Koenig & M. C. Holbrook (Eds.), *Foundations of education:* Vol. II. *Instructional strategies for teaching children and youths with visual impairments.* (pp. 720–752). New York: AFB Press.

Erin, J., & Paul, B. (1996). Functional vision assessment and instruction of children and youths in academic programs. In A. L. Corn & A. J. Koenig (Eds.), *Foundations of low vision: Clinical and functional perspectives* (pp. 105–220). New York: AFB Press.

Falvey, M. A. (1989). *Community-based curriculum; Instructional strategies for students with severe handicaps.* (2nd ed.). Baltimore, MD: Paul Brookes.

Goetz, L., & Gee, K. (1987). Functional vision programming: A model for teaching visual behaviors in natural contexts. In L. Goetz, D. Guess, & K. Stremel-Campbell (Eds.), *Innovative program design for individuals with dual sensory impairments* (pp. 77–97). Baltimore, MD: Paul Brookes.

Groenveld, M., Jan, J. E., & Leader, P. (1990). Observations on the habilitation of children with cortical visual impairment. *Journal of Visual Impairment & Blindness, 84,* 11–15.

Good, W. V., & Hoyt, C. S. (1989). Behavioral correlates of poor vision in children. *International Ophthalmology Clinics, 29*(1), 57–60.

Hall, A., & Bailey, I. L. (1989). A model for training visual functioning. *Journal of Visual Impairment & Blindness, 83,* 390–396.

Heinze, T. (1980). Increasing the visually handicapped child's interaction with the environment. Paper presented at the National First Step 1980 Conference for Preschool Handicapped Children. Myrtle Beach, South Carolina.

Heinze, T. (1985). Helping preschoolers to reach out and get to know their world. Paper presented at the Southwest Conference for Association for Education and Rehabilitation of the Blind and Visually Impaired. San Diego, CA.

Hoyt, C. S. (2002, July 9). Visual function in the brain-damaged child. *The Doyne Lecture.* Oxford, UK.

Hyvarinen, L. (1988). *Vision in children: Normal and abnormal.* Meadford, ON, Canada: Canadian Deaf-Blind and Rubella Association.

Hyvarinen, L. (1999). Visual perception in "low vision." *Perception, 28,* 1533–1537.

Hyvarinen, L. (n.d.). *Assessment of low vision for educational purposes.* Lake City, FL: Vision Associates.

Hyvarinen, L. (in press). Rehabilitation of visually impaired infants and children. In M. E. Marnett, M. Trese, M. A. Capone, S. M. Steidl, B. Keats (Eds.) *Pediatric retinal diseases: Medical and surgical approaches.* Philadelphia, PA: Lippincott, Williams & Wilkins.

Jan, J. (2000, June 7). *Medical considerations in serving young children who are visually impaired.* Paper presented at the Hilton Perkins Preschool Conference, Vancouver, B.C.

Jan, J. E., & Groenveld, M. (1993). Visual behaviors and adaptations associated with cortical and ocular impairment in children. *Journal of Visual Impairment & Blindness, 87,* 101–105.

Jan, J. E., Groenveld, M., Sykanda, A. M., & Hoyt, C. S. (1987). Behavioral characteristics of children with permanent cortical visual impairment. *Developmental Medicine and Child Neurology, 29,* 571–576.

Koenig, A. J., & Holbrook, M. C. (1995). *Learning media assessment of students with visual impairments: A resource guide for teachers* (2nd ed.). Austin: Texas School for the Blind & Visually Impaired.

Langley, M. B. (1998). *ISAVE Individualized systematic assessment of visual efficiency.* Louisville, KY: American Printing House for the Blind.

Lueck, A. H. (1998). Incorporating unique learning requirements into the design of instructional strategies for students with visual and multiple impairments—the basis for an expanded core curriculum. *Re:view, 30,* 101–116.

Lueck, A. H., Chen, D., & Kekelis, L. (1997). *Developmental guidelines for infants with visual impairment: A manual for infants birth to 2.* Louisville, KY: American Printing House for the Blind.

Lueck, A. H., Dornbusch, H., & Hart, J. (1999). An exploratory study to investigate the effects of training on the vision functioning of young children with cortical visual impairment. *Journal of Visual Impairment & Blindness, 93,* 778–793.

Lueck, A. H., & Heinze, T. A. (2000). Instruction in vision functioning to encourage exploratory and cognitive growth in young children with visual impairments. In C. Stuen, A. Arditi, A. Horowitz, M. A. Lang, B. Rosenthal, & K. Seidman (Eds.), *Vision rehabilitation: assessment, intervention, and outcomes* (pp. 504–507). Exton, PA: Swets & Zeitlinger.

McGonigel, M. J., Kaufmann, P. K., & Hurth, J. L. (1991). The IFSP sequence. In McGonigel, Kaufmann, & B. H. Johnson (Eds.), *Guidelines and recommended practices for the Individualized Family Service Plan* (pp 15–24). Bethesda, MD: Association for the Care of Children's Health.

Nott, J. (1994). The use of low vision aids by children under the age of seven. *British Journal of Visual Impairment, 12,* 57–59.

Pogrund, R. L. & Fazzi, D. L. (Eds.). (2002). *Early focus: Working with young children who are blind or visually impaired and their families.* New York: AFB Press.

Project VIISA (Vision Impaired In-Service in America) (1999). *Topic 13: Use of low vision aids with preschoolers. Training manual.* Logan, UT: SKI-HI Institute, Utah State University.

Rainforth, B., & York-Barr, J. (1996). Handling and positioning. In F. P. Orelove & D. Sobsey (Eds.), *Educating children with multiple disabilities. A transdisciplinary approach* (3rd ed., pp. 79–118). Baltimore, MD: Paul H. Brookes.

Ritchie, J. P., Sonksen, P. M., & Gould, E. (1989). Low vision aids for preschool children. *Developmental medicine and child neurology, 31,*509–519.

Sacks, S. Z., & Silberman, R. K. (Eds.). (1998). *Educating students who have visual impairments with other disabilities.* Baltimore, MD: Paul Brookes.

Salvia, J., & Ysseldyke, J. E. (1991). *Assessment* (5th ed.). Boston: Houghton Mifflin.

Silberman, R. K., & Brown, F. (1998). Alternative approaches to assessing students who have visual impairments with other disabilities in classroom and community environments. In S. Z. Sacks & Silberman (Eds.), *Educating students who have visual impairments with other disabilities* (pp. 73–99). Baltimore, MD: Paul Brookes.

Smith, A. J., & Cote, K. S. (1984). *Look at me: A resource manual for the development of residual vision in multiply impaired children.* Philadelphia: Pennsylvania College of Optometry.

Smith, M., & Levack, N. (1996). *Teaching students with visual and multiple impairments: A resource guide.* Austin: Texas School for the Blind & Visually Impaired.

Steendam, M. (1989). *Cortical visual impairment in children.* New South Wales, Australia: Royal Society for the Blind.

Taylor, R. G., & Murphy-Herd, M. (1998). Access technology with computers for students who have visual impairments with other disabilities. In S. Z. Sacks & R. K. Silberman (Eds.), *Educating students who have visual impairments with other disabilities* (pp. 469–504). Baltimore, MD: Paul Brookes.

Trief, E. (1992). *Working with visually impaired young students: A curriculum guide for birth–3 year olds.* Springfield, IL: Charles C. Thomas.

Trief, E. (1998). *Working with visually impaired young students: A curriculum guide for 3 to 5 year olds.* Springfield, IL: Charles C. Thomas.

Warren, D. H. (1994). *Blindness and children: An individual differences approach.* New York: Cambridge University Press.

Watson, G. (1989). Competencies and a bibliography addressing student's use of low vision devices. *Journal of Visual Impairment & Blindness, 83,* 160–63.

Analysis of Daily Routines

DAILY SCHEDULE OF ROUTINES	CRITICAL ACTIVITIES WITH VISUAL COMPONENTS	VISUAL BEHAVIORS TO BE PROMOTED	EXPLORATORY BEHAVIORS FACILITATED	COGNITIVE BEHAVIORS FACILITATED

Guidelines for Customizing Visual Displays for Students with Visual Impairments Who Have Severe Speech and Physical Impairments

DEBORAH TIERNEY KREUZER AND JILLIAN KING

Students with severe speech and physical impairments are increasingly using augmentative and alternative communication (AAC) to develop their communication skills. The educational team, consisting of the student, parents, vision specialists, teachers, speech-language pathologists, and motor specialists (along with others) determine when the use of visual materials facilitates communication. Visual displays refer to one way in which information is presented for AAC. Visual displays can be used as a teaching strategy when the method of response from the student is affected because of a reduction in fine motor skills. For example, after reading a selection, the student uses the visual display to select items, to indicate sequencing, to pick out the main idea, or to answer yes and no questions. The student demonstrates his or her knowledge by indicating choices of one or more visual items through an individualized method of selection such as touching a symbol, eye-gazing to a symbol, or pointing to a symbol.

Visual displays are also a way to represent thoughts and ideas when communicating with others: to indicate, for example, preference, request more information, and/or ask questions. Visual displays can use color, color cues, shapes, icons, and print in picture symbols, photographs, alphabet or number symbols placed on a board or an eye-gaze transparency (E-tran). Figure 1 shows a selection of four symbols representing "snack choices" in four quadrants of an eye-gaze transparency board used as a visual display. Visual displays can also be incorporated into more complex electronic voice output communication aids (VOCA) with visual symbols that can be customized.

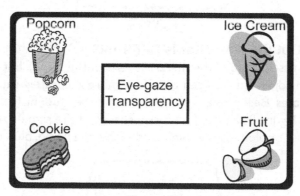

Figure 1

Source: Adapted with permission from the Bridge School, from Deborah Tierney Krueger & Jillian King, "Classroom Strategies: Solutions to Supporting Participation for Children with Augmentative and Alternative Communication and Assistive Technology (AAC/AT) Needs," *Vision & AAC*, No. 2 (Hillsborough, CA: The Bridge School, Winter 2000).

(continued on next page)

Maximizing the Use of Color Cues

Color can be used to enhance visual displays. Some students might not "know" the name of a color or see a color in the same way as a person who is not visually impaired, but they may still respond visually to color. Color-coding of displays (e.g., all nouns are red) and using color to encode messages (e.g., choosing "red" for the column and "2" for the row to bring up a message stored in a quadrant or section of the AAC device) are strategies used when designing more sophisticated visual displays.

Instructors can explore how best to incorporate color into a student's visual display by setting up a variety of tasks to answer the specific questions detailed in the following sections.

Does the Student Respond to Particular Colors?

Present several circles of the same color, along with one that is different, and watch to see if the child's eyes are drawn to the one that is different. Doing this activity with a light projection box can be helpful. (However, use of a light box for students who are very sensitive to light or who have seizure disorders that may be triggered by bright light is not recommended.) Note which colors the student is particularly regarding or noticing. Does he or she regard that color when it is presented against a variety of colored backgrounds or one or two in particular? Is the student responding to colors or to differences in shading? Ask the student to look at the color or colors that he or she likes best. Figure 2 depicts four circle shapes of the same size with three of the same color and one different (for example, red circle, yellow circle, red circle, red circle).

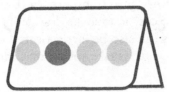

Figure 2

Can the Student Pick Out the One That Is Different?

This task is similar to the first one (and the materials remain the same), but you are cueing the student to find the one that is different. You can therefore more accurately gauge which colors the student actually discriminates. Begin here if you believe that the student has a good understanding of "same" and "different." Figure 3 depicts four circle shapes of the same size, with three of the same color and one different color (for example, red circle, red circle, blue circle, red circle).

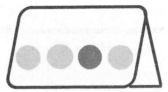

Figure 3

Can the Student Identify Specific Colors by Name?

Using the same materials, ask the student to find the "red" one or the "blue" one. Knowing this information is particularly important if you will be asking the student to use color to code displays.

Other suggestions for optimizing the use of color in visual displays are provided in the following sections.

In all activities, start with the primary colors and move toward pastels. Pastels may be difficult to discriminate for students with conditions including optic nerve atrophy and optic nerve hypoplasia.

Pay attention to the positioning of colors next to each other. Can the student consistently respond to, discriminate, or identify the color red if given a choice between red and yellow, but not if given a choice between red and orange? Shades of blues and purples may be difficult to discriminate, but the student may be able to identify purple if given a choice between yellow and purple. The student may not be able to differentiate between two dark colors when they are presented side by side as in Figure 4.

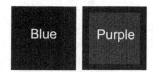

Figure 4

Vary the positions of the items that are "different," and present the number of choices that the student can handle at one point in time. For example, position and color can work together to facilitate access to the visual display by positioning a dark-colored square next to a light-colored square (see Fig. 5). An example of a visual display with four varied color choices could be: blue square, yellow square, green square, red square.

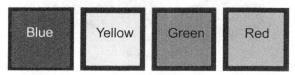

Figure 5

Maximizing the Use of Shapes

As with color, shapes can be used to enhance visual displays. Associating concepts or ideas (e.g., news from home is in the circle, news from school is in the square) and even grammatical/semantic categories with a particular shape can assist in associations and recall.

You can explore how best to incorporate shape into a student's visual display by setting up a variety of tasks to answer specific questions such as those reviewed below.

Does the Student Respond to Particular Shapes?
Present several red circles (keep color consistent) along with one shape that is different (e.g., red square). Watch to see if the student's eyes are drawn to or focus upon the one that is different. Note which shapes the student is particularly regarding or noticing (see Fig. 6).

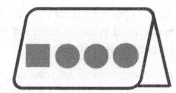

Figure 6

(continued on next page)

Can the Student Pick Out the One that is Different?

This task is similar to the first one (and the materials remain the same), but you are cueing the student to find the one that is "different" and can therefore more accurately gauge which shapes the student actually discriminates (see Fig. 7).

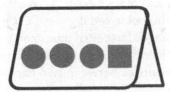

Figure 7

Can the Student Identify Specific Shapes by Name?

Using the same materials, ask the student to find, for example, the circle or the triangle. Knowing this information is particularly important if you will be asking the student to cue into particular shapes for meaning—for example, programming an arrow (see Fig. 8) that is contained in a rectangular shape as a "hot spot" that will facilitate the return to a main page on a dynamic screen display.

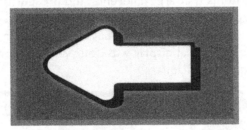

Figure 8

A simple progression for evaluating shapes is: circle, square, triangle, rectangle, star. Contrast is important for enhancing shapes on a visual display (e.g., a yellow square on a blue or black background will be highly visible). It is also useful to use thick black lines to outline and define a shape.

Selecting Icons

Iconicity refers to the visual relationship of a symbol to its referent (Lloyd & Blischak, 1992). A symbol is something that stands for or represents something else (Vanderheiden & Yoder, 1986). Icons (in the form of graphic or visual symbols) are commonly used in visual displays.

Using Meaningful Graphic Symbols

Among the many factors that need to be considered when the team is making decisions about which symbol system or combination of symbols to use is the ease with which a symbol can be associated with its referent. Beukelman and Miranda (1998) consider three levels in the symbol-referent relationship:

➤ *Transparent:* The meaning of the symbol is easily guessed in the absence of the referent (e.g., a photo or picture of a dog).

➤ *Translucent:* The meaning of the referent may or may not be obvious, but a relationship can be perceived between the symbol and the referent once the meaning is provided (e.g., the gesture or picture of a hand with the "thumbs up" position to depict "great").

➤ *Opaque:* No symbol-referent relationship is perceived even when the meaning of the symbol is known (e.g., the written word "dog").

It is important to start with the level of representation the student is able to understand. This level depends upon several key factors, of which cognition is one component. The understanding of complex or more abstract symbols may also be affected by the student's level of experience. Training opportunities that incorporate the use of symbols in natural settings are important for success.

Using Symbols at the Appropriate Representational Level

The representational level of a symbol refers to the level at which the student is able to understand the symbol and use it for communication. Symbols can exist at the following four levels:

➤ *Tangible:* The use of real, miniature, or partial objects.

➤ *Representational:* The use of photographs and line-drawing symbols.

➤ *Abstract:* The use of forms that do not have any suggestion for meaning, as in geometric forms or lines that do not have pictographic symbolism. (A square with a triangle on top could represent a house, however, and would not be considered abstract.)

➤ *Orthographic:* The use of letters, words, phrases, and sentences; this also includes braille.

Making Symbols Visually Distinctive

The use of "dissimilar" or "similar" icons is also a consideration in the design of visual displays for students who are visually impaired. Dissimilar icons can easily be discriminated because of the differences in numerous features or characteristics of the icon (see Fig. 9). Similar icons share more features and characteristics and may therefore be harder to discriminate for the student who is visually impaired (see Fig. 10).

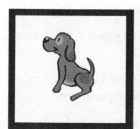 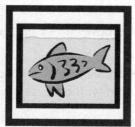   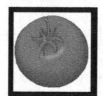

Figure 10

Figure 9

Even if the student is able to see the difference between more similar icons, it may take longer for him or her to complete this task than a task with dissimilar icons. In communication, every

(continued on next page)

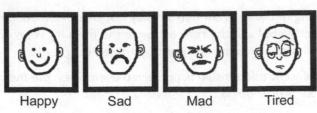

| Happy | Sad | Mad | Tired |

Figure 11

second counts; using more distinctive icons may facilitate quicker visual recognition and communication. For example, consider the typical visual display depicting feelings. A child is asked to describe his or her feelings by looking at an array in which each symbol has a similar face shape and only subtle features are changed to indicate mood (see Fig. 11).

By isolating or enhancing key features, symbols can be more visually distinctive. In Figure 12, "happy" is represented by a big smile and "tired" by the partial view of a woman sleeping with her head on a pillow.

Icons can also be made more distinct by incorporating color. In Figure 13, the icon for "mad" has been colored red to depict "I see red!" and the icon for "sad" has been colored blue to represent "I feel blue."

Figure 12   **Figure 13**

Spacing, Position, and Number of Symbols

It is important to pay attention to the spacing, position, and number of graphic symbols (including words). The following questions should be answered in determining the best use of visual displays for an individual student:

➤ Is the student able to track visually from left to right if three or more objects or symbols are placed together?

➤ Is it easier for the student to look at items if he or she moves his or her eyes down a column of icons and/or words?

➤ Is it helpful to place items 2 inches apart or more, or if icons and/or words have larger spaces between them? (Crowding can be a problem for children with cortical visual impairment.)

Visual Displays that Incorporate Print

Some students may benefit from the use of single word presentations in visual displays rather than running text; others may be able to complete more complex reading tasks that incorporate alphabetical spelling of words or the use of word prediction features in the AAC device.

When incorporating words into visual displays, teach students that words have shapes, particularly when they are spelled with lowercase letters. Students may learn to look at the ways in which letters are put together to form words. The ups and downs in the configuration of lowercase letters could contribute to the visual recognition of words. For example:

Looking   eyes

has a more distinctive shape than

LOOKING   EYES

In order to maximize reading skills, consider the use of a low vision reading program with optical character recognition (OCR) software that enables the reader to customize the size and presentation of print that is scanned into a computer. There are several modes of computer text presentation. Two methods for low vision reading are rapid serial visual presentation (RSVP) and elicited sequential presentation (ESP).

The RSVP method enables the reader to view one word at a time at the same location on a computer screen. The rate of presentation of print may be adjusted on the computer and each word is read at a uniform rate. RSVP has been helpful to students whose eyes cannot easily follow a line of print or return to text and find their place (Bliss & Young, 1998).

The ESP method is a variation of RSVP in which the reader controls the presentation rate on a word-by-word basis by means of a button press, rather than being presented with each word automatically (Arditi, 1999). Putting the pace of the presentation of each word into the hands of the reader allows him or her to allocate the amount of time spent on each word as needed, based on word length and difficulty (Arditi, 1999). This style of text presentation may be useful for a student who has sufficient motor skills to press a button.

Scanning Using Complex Visual Displays

Input from all team members working with a student is particularly important for students with severe motor impairments who access communication through scanning, since this technique involves the coordination of motor, visual, cognitive, language, and other skills. Scanning is a complex process involving a facilitator (i.e., a trained communication partner) or a complex electronic device. It can involve the presentation of material in visual, auditory, or a combination of visual and auditory modes. Scanning involves a facilitator or electronic system presenting (or scanning through) single items in a predetermined, systematic manner while the student waits until the item of choice has been reached. The student then indicates this choice by pushing a button or using eye movements, speech, or gesture (Beukelman & Miranda, 1998). This method is primarily for individuals who cannot choose from an array of several items (i.e., a selection set) due to lack of motor control.

When looking at the viability of complex displays for students with visual impairments, one must consider the issues of fatigue, combined auditory/visual processing, and motor response.

Fatigue
Using vision can be very fatiguing for a student with a visual impairment, particularly following periods where high demands have been placed on his or her vision. The instructor will need to answer the following questions: Is the student able to maintain focus on the AAC device, follow the scan

(continued on next page)

pattern, locate the desired item, and shift eye gaze between the switch site and the visual display for a reasonable period of time? In addition, the student may be looking to the facilitator or communication partner for confirmation or additional information, which places further demands on the communication exchange.

Combined Auditory and Visual Processing

It is important to assess the student's ability to process auditory information while visually focusing on the device, following the scan, and finally locating the desired item. The student needs to be able to perform these activities in order to utilize successfully a visual display that involves scanning.

Motor Response

The student's ability to execute a motor response needs to be considered. For example, is the student able to activate a switch to select an item while the choices are presented to him or her in an auditory, visual, or combined auditory/visual mode? Enhancing the features of the visual display to decrease the demands posed by visual materials may not be enough. At times, decreasing the visual demands and using auditory cueing (or auditory scanning) features found on most devices can result in an increase in operational use of a system. Carefully evaluating the student's success under conditions of auditory/visual scanning in combination, auditory scanning alone, and visual scanning alone will yield useful information.

Whether or not visual symbols are used to make selections, using the visual modality to reinforce selections will aid in the development of conceptual understanding that in turn contributes to the development of meaningful language. The use of concrete materials and/or visual representations (if the student demonstrates adequate cognitive understanding) may facilitate the communication process by motivating the student to initiate more requests and make more independent choices. In addition, the use of visual symbols combined with auditory information could aid in directing attention to the communication task by keeping the learner engaged instead of being distracted by other stimulating activities in the environment.

References

Arditi, A. (1999). Elicited sequential presentation for low vision reading. *Vision Research, 39,* 4412–4418.

Beukelman, D. R., & Miranda, P. (1998). *Augmentative and alternative communication: Management of severe communication disorders in children and adults.* Baltimore, MD: Paul Brookes.

Bliss, J. C., & Young, P. (1998). *Optimizing reading for visually impaired people.* Retrieved from http://www.csun.edu/cod/conf/1998/proceedings/csun98_110.htm.

Lloyd, L., & Blischak, D. (1992). AAC terminology policy and issues update. *Augmentative and Alternative Communication, 8,* 104–109.

Vanderheiden, G. C., & Yoder, D. (1986). Overview. In S. Blackstone (Ed.), *Augmentative communication: An introduction* (pp. 1–28). Rockville, MD: American Speech-Language-Hearing Association.

Designing an Intervention

Goal	
Activity components	
Visual behaviors involved	
Modifications to the environment	
Nonoptical devices	
Optical devices	
Probable best sensory approach for accomplishing task (visual, tactile, combined, other)	
Specific skills to teach (visual, exploratory, cognitive, communicative, other)	
Probable best vision instruction components to use (environmental management, visual skills, visually dependent task instruction)	

9

Compensatory Instruction for Academically Oriented Students with Visual Impairments

IRENE TOPOR, AMANDA HALL LUECK, AND JANICE SMITH

Low vision intervention focuses on maximizing the individual's ability to perform a variety of visual tasks identified as important and desirable. When a youngster is attending school and undertaking academic work, the focus differs, sometimes dramatically, from that of efforts designed for very young children and children with multiple disabilities.

Chapter 8 has reviewed intervention strategies related to vision use for school age students with low vision who have additional disabilities and whose programs focus primarily on functional and meaningful skills that promote participation in school, home, community, and vocational settings. This chapter describes the teaching of compensatory methods to academically oriented school age students with low vision, preschool through 22 years, who can benefit from one or more forms of such intervention.

The application of these methods is discussed within the context of the educational setting, where an interdisciplinary team works to provide a cohesive, integrated, and collaborative program for each student. Such teams can include the student, the student's parents, a teacher of students with visual impairments, an orientation and mobility (O&M) specialist, the general education teacher, and other professionals, including team members working outside the school district such as the ophthalmologist or optometrist.

A team process is vital in implementing the specialized program across various school, home, prevocational/vocational, and community settings. Team members contribute to the assessment process, jointly determine areas to target for instruction, and jointly develop individualized education programs (IEPs) that guide the instructional process. This chapter emphasizes the importance of a range of compensatory methods for students with visual impairments, delineates methods for the design of vision instruction programs, and provides guidance for instructional approaches in a major curricular area: literacy. The focus on the functional ability to read and write at a level commensurate with one's cognitive abilities is highlighted here because literacy skills provide the foundation for basic life skills in educational, occupational, daily living, recreation and leisure, and social-emotional activities (Lueck, Dote-Kwan, Senge, & Clarke, 2001).

WORKING WITH SCHOOL AGE STUDENTS

Changing Task Demands

One role of teachers of students with visual impairments, O&M specialists, and other professionals is to facilitate the instruction of school age students with low vision using methods that optimize their visual functioning to promote the successful performance of tasks of different lengths, complexities, and demands in many different environments. The demands of various tasks for students with visual impairments in school, at home, and in the community and workplace (for older students) change over time. Reading and writing tasks, for example, are usually shorter and less demanding in early elementary school. When students enter fourth grade, the print size of their texts decreases, reading passages and assignments become longer, and they receive writing assignments more frequently. In grades 5 through 12, students increasingly utilize reference materials, write term papers, and learn to read and interpret maps, graphs, charts, and tables. Students' interests in reading and writing tasks outside school may change from playing with toys that have simple labels to reading a book for pleasure to doing research on the Internet to find out where to purchase a favorite compact disc.

These changing task demands can lead to a decrease in visual performance for the following reasons:

➤ Students may lack an understanding of ways to manage their increasingly complex visual environments.

➤ Students may fail to apply their available visual abilities to critical tasks.

➤ Students may not have developed latent visual skills that can be applied to critical tasks.

Students' level of visual functioning and performance on critical tasks is documented and recorded in their functional visual assessment (see Topor & Erin, 2000; Erin & Paul, 1996; and Chap. 4). A functional visual assessment is conducted when the student changes school or class placement, if the student's vision status changes, or when his or her tasks or activities change. The interdisciplinary team helps students to utilize techniques and strategies that address these changing and multifaceted task demands.

The Expanded Core Curriculum

Teaching visual efficiency skills is not a new area of instruction. It is one of nine areas in the expanded core curriculum (Hatlen, 1996), and informs all areas of instruction. The expanded core curriculum for students who are visually impaired includes and goes beyond the core curriculum, which is most often limited to reading, math, science, and other academic subjects. It provides direct instruction in such areas as leisure and recreational skills, career and work skills, daily living skills, O&M skills, as well as functional vision skills. Such instruction enables students with visual impairments to gain the necessary additional skills needed to access information and their environments to promote full and independent lives. Instruction to improve visual functioning should be taught systematically in conjunction with other expanded core curriculum areas targeted for instruction, for children from preschool through high school years. Incorporating a program to promote visual functioning will have a significant impact on the ultimate goal for students with visual impairments: to be well prepared academically, socially, and emotionally to negotiate personal and career paths successfully, leading to fuller participation in society once they leave high school.

The Educational Team

The Individuals with Disabilities Education Act and the regulations governing its implementation dictate the development of an IEP for every student, based on the regular assessment of his or her needs and involving the appropriate members of an educational team, including the student and family. Through discussion, the interdisciplinary team reports and reviews assessment data to gain a shared understanding of a student's present levels of performance and educational needs as they relate to the expanded core curriculum for students with visual impairments. The team uses a group decision-making process to select those methods appropriate to the needs and abilities of the student, to establish instructional goals and objectives from selected core curriculum areas (including those that require the use of vision), and to identify related services and materials necessary for the student to benefit from the regular education program (Lewis & Allman, 2000). Appendix 9.1 to this chapter summarizes the contributions of various members of the interdisciplinary team.

DESIGNING AN INDIVIDUALIZED FUNCTIONAL VISION INSTRUCTION PROGRAM

One way in which teachers of students with visual impairments, O&M specialists, and other professionals can infuse effective functional vision instruction programs into the goals and objectives of the IEP is by applying the backward design approach proposed by Wiggins and McTighe (1998). This approach consists of three steps: (1) identify the desired results, (2) determine acceptable evidence of mastery, and (3) plan learning experiences and instruction. The following guide to designing and evaluating a vision training program reflects many of the critical elements of performance-based teaching, learning, and assessment identified by McBiles (1998).

Step 1: Identify the Desired Results

The first step in the process of designing a vision instruction program answers the following basic questions: What are the visual skills, behaviors, and attitudes required for the student to complete efficiently the critical tasks encountered today, in the near future, and on graduation within meaningful environments (home, community, school, and workplace)?

Critical tasks are those that are important to the individual to accomplish his or her goals in everyday, meaningful environments. For a school age student in an educational setting, these will include the tasks required to achieve the goals and objectives selected for a student's IEP as determined by the interdisciplinary team. Students with visual impairments may lack or need refinement of the skills, behaviors, or attitudes necessary to complete these critical tasks efficiently using their vision. Teachers of students with visual impairments and O&M specialists must work together with the student and the interdisciplinary team in identifying critical tasks, the student's abilities in relationship to those tasks, and the compensatory methods, if any, needed to complete the tasks.

First the team needs to identify and set priorities for critical tasks related to targeted instructional goals. These are the tasks encountered by the student in meaningful environments in the home, community, school, and workplace. For example, an instructional goal for a high school student with low vision is to pass a high school science class. Critical tasks targeted for instruction in this area that have a visual component would include (1) getting access to textbook material to complete assignments, (2) using word-processing programs to complete class assignments, and (3) completing laboratory exercises independently.

Next, the team evaluates the student's sensory abilities in relation to the sensory demands of each task. (See Chap. 7 for information on analyzing the visual demands of critical tasks.) For a student who has low vision to benefit optimally from an educational program, the student, parents, teachers, and other professionals must understand the following:

➤ The student's current visual skills, behaviors, and attitudes

➤ The student's capacity for visual intervention

➤ The means by which the student can learn visual skills

➤ The sensory requirements of the student's identified critical tasks

The educational team then determines if compensatory methods are required for the student to meet the visual demands of each critical task. If so, the team needs to identify the specific compensatory method or methods to be used by that student to meet the visual demands of each task. As discussed in Chapter 7 and later in this chapter, compensatory methods include the following:

➤ Visual skills instruction

➤ Visual environmental adaptations

➤ Sensory substitutions

➤ Integration of sensory experiences

➤ Assistive devices

For the high school student with low vision in our example, the following compensatory methods were recommended:

➤ Instruction in the use of books on tape and in the use of a prescribed low vision magnifier to access textbook material in order to complete her school science assignments.

➤ Instruction in the use of a special print-enlarging computer software program to use word processing programs to complete class assignments in academic subjects.

➤ Instruction in the use of a video magnifier and prescribed optical devices to complete laboratory assignments independently.

Step 2: Determine Acceptable Evidence of Mastery

In this step the team determines what mastery of these visual skills, behaviors, and attitudes will look like within meaningful environments (home, community, school, and workplace). The teacher of students with visual impairments and O&M specialist work with the student and the interdisciplinary team to develop written objectives for each compensatory method selected in Step 1 that addresses the goal in the IEP. Each objective should have the following characteristics:

➤ Specify the compensatory methods used to accomplish each critical task; the same compensatory methods may be applicable to more than one critical task.

➤ Be observable and measurable.

➤ Identify the specific performance criteria used by the teacher, the student, or others in evaluating performance.

➤ Build on what the student already knows and is able to do.

➤ Ensure that the student, family, and team members providing instruction have a shared understanding of the objectives and performance indicators.

➤ Determine what data will be collected, how often, and by whom.

➤ Determine how performance data will be communicated to members of the team including the student.

➤ Determine how performance data will be used to guide future learning opportunities.

Detailed information on the creation of measurable goals and objectives for IEPs for students with visual impairments is available elsewhere (Koenig & Holbrook, 2000).

Step 3: Plan Learning Experiences and Instruction

In this step the team determines what learning experiences will engage the student in developing the visual skills, behaviors, and attitudes identified in Step 1. The teacher of students with visual impairments and the O&M specialist work collaboratively with other team members to accomplish the following:

➤ Design instruction in the use of compensatory methods that will lead to successful completion of the critical tasks encountered by the student.

➤ Provide sufficient opportunities to practice and apply visual skills, behaviors, and attitudes within targeted activities in the IEP.

➤ Link learning experiences to the student's prior knowledge and experiences.

➤ Include the teaching of new concepts required for the successful completion of the task.

➤ Select learning experiences representative of different learning styles and types of intelligence (Lazear, 1991).

➤ Provide choices to students.

In *The Seven Habits of Highly Effective People,* Covey (1989) stated, "To begin with the end in mind means to start with a clear understanding of your destination. It means to know where you're going so that you better understand where you are now so that the steps you take are always in the right direction (p. 98)." By starting with the end in mind, the interdisciplinary team members will design learning opportunities that involve students with low vision in the direct application of visual skills, behaviors, and attitudes to critical tasks related to instructional goals that have an impact on their home, community, school, and workplace activities and promote optimal vision functioning as students grow and their needs and skills change.

Sidebar 9.1 lists some curricular areas that have visual components within which compensatory instruction can be infused to promote visual functioning

Sample Curricular Areas in Which Compensatory Instruction to Promote Visual Functioning Can Be Infused

Social/Emotional Needs
Socialization
Acceptable and unacceptable private and public
    behaviors
Appropriate nonverbal communication techniques
Appropriate body posture and movement awareness
Proper manners in eating and social situations

Recreation
Familiarity with a variety of social and recreational
    activities
Participating in a variety of social and recreational
    activities
Choosing leisure time activities

Sex Education
Grooming and hygiene skills and concepts
Understanding gender
Identification of male and female body parts
Child care procedures
Understanding verbal and nonverbal communication
    of sexual messages

Orientation & Mobility Needs and Concepts
Body image concepts for mobility
Environmental concepts
Spatial concepts

Travel Skills
Independent travel in simple and complex settings
Object location techniques
Use of vision for travel
Use of optical devices for travel
Use of public transit
Orientation skills for independent travel
Use of alternative routes for travel

Travel-Related Skills
Skills for pay phone use and location
Understanding functions of stores, businesses
Communication skills, verbal or nonverbal, for travel

Communication Needs
Reading
Writing
Typing and keyboarding

Devices for Reading and Writing
Optical devices
Closed-circuit television systems
Electronic notetakers
Computers with special adaptations
Other technology

Concept Development and Academic Needs
Body image
Understanding of basic concepts
Reference material use
Notetaking skills
Writing and recording skills

Sensory/Motor Needs
Purposeful exploration skills
Movement skills
Balance
Coordination of body parts in different positions
Fine motor skills

Daily Living Needs
Personal hygiene skills
Dressing skills
Clothing care skills
Housekeeping skills
Cooking skills
Money management
Social communication skills
Telecommunications skills
Written communication skills
Time skills

Career/Vocational Needs
Concept of work
Pride in one's work
Responsibility and commitment in the workplace
Job application skills
Resume skills
Proficiency in adaptive devices for work
Career awareness
Work experiences and job skill training
Obtaining material in specialized media

Source: Adapted with permission of the publisher from *Program Guidelines for Students Who Are Visually Impaired,* copyright © 1997, California Department of Education, P.O. Box 271, Sacramento, CA, 95812.

(Lueck, 1999). Examples of ways to infuse instruction related to visual functioning into critical tasks can be found in the case studies at the end of this chapter.

MOTIVATION OF SCHOOL AGE STUDENTS

When working with school age students, it is important to keep in mind that they may be sensitive to peer pressure and seek peer approval. They may choose not to use adaptive devices or techniques since the use of such materials may make them feel different from their classmates. When implementing educational plans for students, it is important to be sympathetic to students' need to fit in and, whenever possible, provide instruction in ways that encourage student cooperation and acceptance. Some possible methods for accomplishing this are detailed in the following sections.

Allow Students to Choose Critical Tasks

Students are often more interested and motivated to complete tasks that they feel are important to them. Encourage students to select *one* critical task as a starting point for instruction. This will often result in a successful outcome. The following story illustrates this point.

> *Jim, a high school junior, was reluctant to use low vision optical devices. His group of friends wanted to send e-mail messages to each other, and one member of the group prepared a list of everyone's e-mail addresses to share. Jim could not read the list, since the print was too small for him to decipher. He had been prescribed an illuminated handheld magnifier after a recent low vision evaluation but left it unused in his backpack most of the time. Jim mentioned his plan to send e-mails to his friends to his teacher of students with visual impairments and provided the teacher with a list of e-mail addresses. Jim asked that his teacher enlarge the list on a photocopier for him. The teacher asked Jim if he might want to try using his magnifier to read the list of addresses instead. His teacher told Jim that he could access the information much more quickly this way, especially when other friends wrote down their addresses for him. Jim told his teacher that he thought it would be too hard, but he was willing to try. Jim was able to read the list easily with the magnifier, and he went home that evening eager to begin his e-mail conversations with his friends from his home computer. His teacher will now encourage Jim to use his magnifier in other critical tasks related to goals and objectives in his IEP.*

Work With Families to Identify Critical Tasks

When working with students with low vision, it is important to remember that students, their parents, and their teachers may not be aware that students are not participating as fully or efficiently as possible in everyday activities or that there are other options for completing tasks than those currently used. Teachers and parents may not understand how much to expect from a student. They may be not be aware of the array of low vision devices or other compensatory methods that can promote a student's fuller independence and inclusion. For example, when a parent was asked if there were any family activities she wished her child could participate in, she commented that her son and his dad enjoyed going to the archery range together, but the son was unable to see the target while his father was shooting. A monocular telescope, prescribed by the student's low vision eye care practitioner, readily solved this problem.

Wait Until the Student Is Ready to Learn

Sometimes students are more focused on activities related to medical, family, and social issues; learning compensatory methods may not be a priority for them. Every instructor has had experiences with students who show little interest in completing lessons, using instructional materials, or focusing on instructional presentations. Determining the underlying reasons for this lack of interest is important and requires the cooperation of everyone on the interdisciplinary team. Sometimes the underlying factors affecting the situation can be readily addressed and sometimes they cannot. Sometimes moving ahead with lessons is appropriate; at other times, waiting until students have worked through issues that are more meaningful to them is wiser. The interdisciplinary team provides a supportive vehicle for guiding the educational plans of such students and for determining when instruction in compensatory methods should begin or resume.

Involve Classroom Peers

For younger children, working with a teacher of students with visual impairments or O&M instructor may be viewed as a special, favored experience. Involving classroom peers (i.e., one particular child, a small group, or the whole class) in some of these lessons as an occasional treat can assist in putting the compensatory instruction in a positive light for the student.

Encourage Experiences with Adult Role Models

Some preteenagers and teenagers will benefit from meeting successful adult role models who use the compensatory skills they are now in the process of learning or are about to learn. The adults may enlighten students about what possibilities are available to them, how to set goals for the future, and how learning certain compensatory methods may help them to realize their goals.

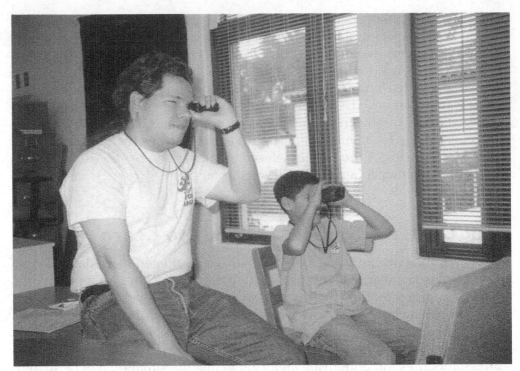

Exposure to adult role models can motivate students with low vision. A teacher who has a visual impairment instructs his student with low vision to use 6× binoculars to find a target. *(Irene Topor)*

Encourage Experiences with Peer Role Models

Since many students with low vision are enrolled in local school programs, they may not have met other students with visual impairments in social or academic situations. It may be helpful to arrange meetings that promote social interchanges among peers with low vision. This can be accomplished through weekend workshops, summer camps or programs, or other specially designed activities.

TEACHING COMPENSATORY METHODS TO OPTIMIZE VISUAL FUNCTIONING

Compensatory methods include instruction in visual skills and vision use, visual environmental adaptations, sensory substitutions, integration of sensory experiences, and assistive devices (see Chap. 7). For successful intervention, the methods selected must be infused within the critical tasks identified by the interdisciplinary team so that instruction takes place in functional and meaningful contexts. As compensatory methods are discussed in the following sections, existing programs and materials that contain instructional ideas, sequences, and procedures related to each method will be mentioned. However, the instructor must select and adapt pertinent elements of these curricula in order to infuse these instructional components effectively into targeted critical tasks determined for individual students.

Types of Programs

There are three basic types of visual functioning training programs: visual skills instruction, visual environmental management instruction, and visually dependent task instruction (see Chap. 7). Most academically oriented students who have had low vision from birth or early infancy have acquired basic visual skills by the time they enter elementary school. To be certain that these skills are applied efficiently, it is critical to introduce instruction in basic visual skills in preschool and kindergarten programs. Information about instruction in tracing, tracking, and scanning when visual impairment occurs later in life can be found in Chapter 10. Visual skills that promote effective travel include fixating, scanning, localizing, and following distant targets. Instructional protocols to promote these skills can be found in the program developed by Smith and O'Donnell (1992): *Beyond Arm's Reach: Enhancing Distance Vision*. Instructors are encouraged to infuse basic skills training into functional activities as soon as possible to increase motivation, practice opportunities, and to apply the skills directly into activities that are meaningful for students.

Some skills, such as eccentric viewing, finding the null point for students with nystagmus, or maximizing field losses, are discovered naturally by most children who have experienced low vision from birth or shortly thereafter. Some of these skills, such as eccentric viewing, must be reinforced through direct instructional methods when working with optical devices. Students with acquired vision loss may benefit from this type of instruction as well, based on assessment findings. (For methods to teach these skills to persons with low vision acquired later in life, see Chap. 10). Sidebar 9.2 presents some additional techniques for eccentric viewing instruction for school age students.

Optimizing Stimuli During Instruction

Heightened or reduced visual stimuli can be presented in instructional programs depending on the learning goal. Some principles for stimulus presentation are briefly reviewed here as they apply to school age students and will be discussed in more detail as they apply to literacy instruction for students with low vision later in this chapter. Additional information can be found in Chapters 8 and 10.

Attributes of visual stimuli that can be adjusted during instruction include size, contrast, complexity, illumination, duration, color, position, and distance.

Although more research is needed in this area, it is likely that students with low vision may benefit from learning new or difficult tasks using heightened visual cues (Lueck, 2001). These heightened cues need to be faded whenever possible, however, so that the student can operate effectively in normalized environments

SIDEBAR 9.2

Teaching Eccentric Viewing to School Age Students

Some students with central scotomas may require instruction to promote eccentric viewing (i.e., using a nonfoveal area of the retina to see details). This instruction should be completed prior to having the student use a telescope. Refer to Chapter 10 for detailed instructions on teaching eccentric viewing. The following are some special considerations for teaching this specialized technique to school-age students.

For students who are unfamiliar with the position of numerals on the clock traditionally used for eccentric viewing instruction, substitute lines running from the center of a circle to a shape at the edge (each direction can be a different color) and place a target in the center of the circle. Ask the student to move his or her eye slowly along each of the colored lines toward the shape at the edge and report if the target in the center of the circle becomes clearer or pops into view.

If procedures using the clock face or the modified chart above are unsuccessful, try placing a 2 cm hole in a patch in the area that will provide the student with the best eccentric viewing position. Consult with the low vision practitioner to determine this position. The student will see black unless the eye is moved into this position (see Berg, Jose, & Carter, 1983, p. 289).

The student can practice until the position can be maintained by:

➤ Viewing an object in a poster

➤ Watching television

➤ Using the eccentric viewing position while doing daily tasks (e.g., putting toothpaste on toothbrush or picking up utensils while eating).

in which high-intensity substitutions may not be possible. The degree of normalization depends on a student's vision, the difficulty and dimensions of the task, and the student's individual abilities (Corn, 1989). For example, a student in a school play may benefit from high-contrast props placed in strategic places on the stage to help her know where to stand during various portions of a complex scene as she is learning her part. When she has become familiar with the scene, any unneeded props can be removed and replaced by large X's on the stage floor made with masking tape of a high-contrast color.

Isolating visual variables encourages attention to them and may promote learning. To prepare the student for more normalized situations, gradual introduction of more complex formats or materials is recommended whenever possible. The

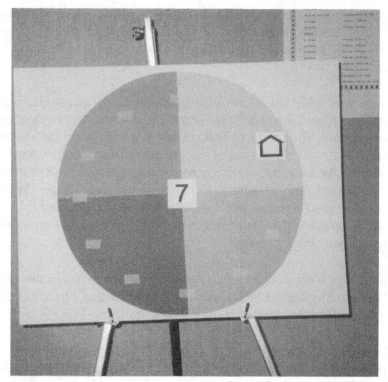

A modified eccentric viewing clock can be prepared for children by adding colors and using shapes instead of numbers. The student first finds a familiar shape in the center of a circle, and moves his or her eyes toward a shape in the periphery, reporting when the central shape becomes clearer or pops into view. Color quadrants are used as cues to help the student find the target symbol along the rim of the circle. *(Irene Topor)*

amount of normalization will depend on factors affecting the vision of individual students, as in the following example:

> *A workbook for Paul, a kindergarten student who is learning to read letters, includes complex pictures into which letters are embedded, making the letters harder to locate and decipher visually. Paul's teacher of students with visual impairments has remade these pages in the workbook, simplifying the illustrations while still retaining the letter identification task. Paul is, therefore, able to keep up with his classmates independently in group lessons. In addition, the teacher decides to use the original workbook pages for lessons designed to promote this student's visual perceptual skills. With time, Paul is able to work with more complex illustrations similar to those in the workbook.*

Competing sensory stimuli can reduce a student's focused attention on a specified task. Visual, auditory, and kinesthetic distractions may make it more difficult for students with low vision to process pertinent visual information, especially when learning new skills. Reducing the impact of competing sensory stimuli, especially in instructional situations, may facilitate learning for some students with low vision:

Anya, a student with low vision in a high school cooking class carefully measures her ingredients while listening to the cooking teacher's directions at the same time. The teenager is focusing so carefully on her measuring activity that she misses portions of the teacher's instructions about a special procedure for the next step in the recipe. Her teacher notices that Anya has stopped working and comes over to help her individually. When the teacher discovers what happened in talking with Anya, she decides to make it a practice to have all the students in the class pause to listen whenever she introduces a new procedure.

It is critical to present situations that not only enhance visual skills and behaviors but also help the student learn how to coordinate input from other sensory modalities to confirm and augment their visual input:

A third grader wants to learn how to make a diorama as part of a book report project. He asks his teacher how to construct some clay figures for his project. The teacher allows the student to see and feel a model containing similar figures so that the student can understand how the figures are constructed through the coordination of both visual and tactile input.

The goal of a compensatory program determines how other sensory modalities will be used to optimize learning outcomes. In some instances, additional input from other sensory modalities can be useful, at other times input from other sensory modalities may serve as a distraction for students. An example of the latter is that looking at the computer keyboard when learning keyboarding skills by touch may lead to less efficient keyboard techniques.

Interdisciplinary team members must be especially attentive to situations in which a specific visual variable may be less than optimal (e.g., insufficient lighting) in natural environments. They must consider how visual variables (e.g., contrast, size, color) can be adjusted to facilitate the student's visual efficiency. (See Sidebar 9.3 for some examples.) Additional information about visual environmental adaptations can be found in Chapter 10, which also provides, in Appendix 10.1, a list of specific household adaptations that may be appropriate for students with low vision and their families.

COORDINATING INPUT FROM ALL THE SENSES

Students with low vision have limited opportunities to observe others complete critical tasks. Although their visual system is impaired, students with low vision

Optimizing the Visual Environment

Students with low vision can benefit from environmental modifications illustrated in these examples:

Color

➤ Use objects with bold, primary colors (red, orange, yellow, green, blue, or violet) or black and white to capture attention.

➤ Avoid using colors that the student has difficulty seeing.

➤ Present a range of colors, including pastels, to students with less impaired vision.

➤ Use black or blue inks (avoid reds, greens, etc.).

Contrast

➤ Increase contrast by increasing the dark/light difference between an object and its background, or print and its background (e.g., use black ink, soft pencils, or fiber-tip pens on white paper; choose colored toothbrush that contrasts with toothpaste; provide soap and towels that contrast with bathroom walls and countertop).

➤ Use a variety of plain colored mats that can be placed on the student's work area and interchanged to contrast with materials.

➤ Add contrasting features to help identify critical environmental features (e.g., paint doorway trim a contrasting color, mark each stair with a strip of contrasting color).

Duration

➤ Allow students more time to complete visually demanding tasks or tasks that require viewing visual details.

➤ Break up standardized tests into smaller time intervals and administer over several days.

➤ Give breaks to students who tire on visual tasks more quickly than other students by interspersing visually demanding tasks with less visually demanding tasks.

➤ Teach students to rest their eyes while reading by glancing off into the distance for a few seconds every 10 to 15 mins. If they are wearing single-vision reading glasses, they need to look over the glasses when looking into the distance.

Figure-Ground

➤ Reduce visual clutter on table tops and desks; teach organizational skills (for example, placing different types of objects into bins and organizing them on shelves).

➤ Present objects or print against a plain background (e.g., a solid color wall; clean whiteboard or blackboard; plain colored paper products).

Illumination

➤ Use task lighting or directional lights to avoid light shining directly into student's eyes (do not position student looking directly into light source or shine light directly into student's eyes).

(continued on next page)

➤ Position student with back to windows or control lighting by adjusting window shades.

➤ Place source of illumination to side of student's eye with better vision.

➤ Move student closer to light source to increase illumination.

➤ Allow student time to adapt from light to dark and from dark to light.

➤ Before turning off the lights for movies or videos, announce to class so students have opportunity to find their seats.

➤ Use sunglasses, hat, or cap outdoors to control for glare. Check with low vision practitioner for shade and tint of glasses recommended.

➤ If student squints indoors, check with low vision practitioner for glare protection.

Position

➤ Allow students to bring materials unusually close to the eyes to see them or to move up close to see things better (e.g. books, computer monitor, or television).

➤ Use computer monitor stand with moveable arm to adjust distance.

➤ Choose a position that can be maintained with little difficulty and promotes the use of vision (e.g., foot rests, correct table height and monitor height).

➤ Some students with visual impairments see best when they tilt their heads; do not discourage this behavior.

➤ For students with nystagmus, place materials where null point can be used; if a student's null point is in down gaze, place materials on the desk rather than on a bookstand.

➤ For students with visual field loss, maximize ability to use intact field (e.g., for students with left field loss, place them on the left side of the classroom or workgroup; for students with lower field loss and little head control, bring instructional materials up to intact visual field area).

Size

➤ Make objects larger for students with reduced visual acuity (e.g., large-print calculators and date books, large-button remote controls for television and stereo).

➤ Make objects smaller for students with good acuity but severely constricted fields (e.g., use standard print textbooks instead of large print textbooks).

➤ Allow the student to sit closer to activities and objects and provide reference copies of posted information that is too small to be seen (e.g., menu at the student's favorite fast food restaurant).

➤ Provide computer enlargement software and instruction.

➤ Use large-print sheet music.

➤ Use large-print playing cards and game boards.

➤ Use optical and electronic magnification devices.

tend to rely heavily on the use of vision and are often unaware of the interplay of all their sensory modalities in the efficient completion of a task. Students with low vision may not realize that students who are fully sighted may appear to have better hearing when, in fact, they are integrating information about the speaker's lip movements provided by visual input. Students with low vision may also lack information about the limits in the use of vision in individuals who are not visually impaired. They may not be aware that their peers with unimpaired vision are also unable to read print at a certain distance away. They may not realize that peers have difficulty seeing in dimly lit environments and will use their sense of touch to complete efficiently tasks such as finding their house keys and opening a door in the dark.

Sensory systems include auditory (hearing), gustatory (smelling and tasting), kinesthetic or proprioceptive (moving in space), tactile (touching), vestibular (balancing), and visual (seeing). The central nervous system integrates information from all sensory systems and provides the foundation for sensory motor development, perceptual motor development, and cognition (Williams & Shellenberger, 1996). Instructional approaches are dependent on the student's capacity for accessing information through each sense, his or her capacity to learn to use one or more senses efficiently in the completion of the task, and his or her motivation. Teaching strategies need to take into account the potential contributions of all of the modalities involved in the completion of a task and their integration.

Although verbal guidance and feedback can be important features of instructional programs, it is important to give students with low vision time to examine things visually prior to providing verbal guidance. The verbal dimension may actually distract students from processing visual input effectively on some tasks (Corley & Pring, 1993a).

Tactile-kinesthetic feedback may be provided in instructional tasks such as writing, painting, woodworking, cooking, shuffling cards, playing board games, winding up and setting a clock, aligning and focusing a telescope, and tracing along a line of print while using a stand magnifier. For example, paper with raised lines can serve as a line guide, providing tactile-kinesthetic feedback for students learning to write.

During intervention, the instructor may need to help the student to attend selectively to a task through a sense other than vision, and then assist the student in integrating all of the senses. For example, an instructor may access the kinesthetic or proprioceptive modality by using a hand-under-hand approach to provide instruction in the smooth movement of the X-Y table of a closed-circuit television system. To use this approach, the instructor sits behind the student and allows the student to place his or her hands on top of the instructor's hands as the instructor smoothly guides the X-Y table to expose the text on the monitor. This approach allows the student to attend to feedback received from the muscles, tendons, and joints and to integrate this information with the information received through the visual channel as the student views the monitor. It eliminates the need for verbal instructions that are often confusing or distracting. As the student gains confidence, the instructor gradually slides back his or her hands so that the student's hands are resting directly on the X-Y table. The instructor gradually fades physical assistance as the student integrates the movements necessary to control the visual display on the screen.

Occupational and physical therapists contribute to the development of a successful intervention by addressing the readiness of the student's neurological system to function. They can contribute techniques for improving readiness, posture, muscle coordination, muscle strength (including hand and finger strength), bilateral coordination, eye-hand coordination, and motor planning. The recommendations of these professionals are integrated into instructional strategies.

SENSORY SUBSTITUTIONS AND MODIFICATIONS

Members of the team consider the use of sensory substitutions and modifications for students. In some instances, the visual modality is not the most efficient means for completing a task. Visual instruction, visual environmental adaptations, or assistive devices using the visual modality may not be sufficient. Sensory substitutions may be necessary in such instances. These are best determined by the IEP team based on a range of assessment results, including findings from functional vision evaluations as well as from learning media assessments in which the frequency of use of various sense modalities—including auditory, olfactory, gustatory, tactile, and proprioceptive—to gather information is documented to identify primary channels of information gathering for an individual student (Koenig & Holbrook, 1995). Once primary sensory channels have been identified, an instructor can provide sensory substitutions directly or may acquaint students with their use and availability so that the student can choose an appropriate substitution. Sidebar 9.4 provides some suggestions about using sensory substitutions and modifications.

ASSISTIVE TECHNOLOGY

Assistive technology can enhance an individual's ability to perform basic life skills and, in turn, lead to greater independence and a higher quality of life. Assistive devices can range from a simple, brightly colored, circular on-off switch or a reading stand to sophisticated portable closed-circuit television systems. Assistive technology includes optical and nonoptical devices, adapted materials, and electronic devices (Lueck et al., 2001). Detailed information about assistive technology devices can be found elsewhere (Kapperman & Sticken, 2000; Wilkinson, 2000), and a list of manufacturers and suppliers of optical and nonoptical devices and supplies can be found in the Resources section at the end of this book.

Effective instruction for successful use of assistive technology devices in the school, home, community, and workplace must include a number of basic elements:

Sensory Substitutions and Modifications for Students with Low Vision

Students with low vision can benefit from sensory modifications illustrated in these examples:

Auditory

➤ Provide information verbally that students will likely miss because of low contrast such as facial expressions (e.g., "Jim looks angry").

➤ Provide verbal instruction and directions, but be certain to give student time to process information visually first.

➤ Teach students to record directions on audiotape (e.g., steps for completing an activity, and directions to friend's home, local theater, restaurant).

➤ Work toward increasing reading efficiency by visually following a text while it is being read aloud or on an audiotape.

➤ Use Recordings for the Blind and Dyslexic (see Resources) from the library to obtain audiotapes for lengthy assignments or pleasure reading.

➤ Use music to guide the pace of physical movements involved in completing a repetitive task.

➤ Use environmental sounds to guide safe travel (e.g., street crossings).

➤ Use talking software computer program.

➤ Use a prescription service that provides talking labels.

➤ Use a beeping liquid-level indicator.

➤ Use talking scales.

➤ Assist students in signing up for free operator assistance through their telephone provider.

Gustatory/Olfactory

➤ Encourage eating hard candy or eating crunchy snacks if this type of activity improves visual attention. Sometimes using one sensory channel helps people focus on another sensory channel (Williams & Shellenberg, 1996).

➤ Confirm identification of safe substances that appear similar visually (e.g., baking powder, baking soda, cornstarch, flour).

➤ Associate taste and texture of food items with visual information.

Olfactory

➤ Use consistent environmental odors to confirm location (e.g., smells from bakery, candy store, restaurant).

(continued on next page)

➤ Use scent to identify items earlier than by using vision (e.g., identifying a person by her perfume).

➤ Teach odors to be reported: fire, gas, burning food, chemicals.

Proprioceptive/Vestibular/Tactile

➤ Teach touch typing and touch calculating.

➤ Use a hand-under-hand approach to assist in instruction when appropriate.

➤ Create two-dimensional drawings of three-dimensional objects by tracing contours.

➤ Use assistive devices with kinesthetic feedback (e.g., self-threading needle).

➤ Place rubber bands around the barrel of a telescope to identify the part that is moved when focusing.

➤ Encourage tactile exploration of materials.

➤ Fold bills systematically (each denomination in a specific way) for easy identification.

➤ Use tactile marks for similar items in refrigerator (e.g., packaged meats, cheeses, pickles).

➤ Teach tactile search patterns.

➤ Identify buttons or keys on devices by using tactile marking on items with low contrast.

➤ Place a finger in the cup when pouring cold liquids to determine the level of the liquid.

➤ Identify clothes that are similar in color by marking with safety pins.

➤ Use sock clips to keep socks together in laundry and in drawers.

➤ Place a mark on the CCTV screen as a point of focus so students do not move their head to reduce sense of dizziness from the motion of the print across the screen.

➤ Collaboration and continuing communication among key members of the interdisciplinary team are crucial for success.

➤ Devices must be used within critical tasks related to goals and objectives targeted by the interdisciplinary team.

➤ Direct instruction in device use is implemented by the teacher of students with visual impairments, O&M instructor, or other professionals determined by the interdisciplinary team.

➤ Instruction is reinforced by other team members within naturally occurring, critical tasks for additional practice that serves to solidify skills (e.g., using a prescribed magnifier to read menus both during school and on family outings).

➤ Instruction includes learning to use and care for devices.

➤ Device use is generalized to other tasks once the student acquires basic skills.

Specific instructional sequences and procedures for teaching the use of telescopic devices, magnifiers, visual field enhancement devices, and electronic magnification systems are discussed in Chapter 10 in this book and elsewhere (Berg et al., 1983; Cowan & Shepler, 2000a, 2000b; D'Andrea, 2000; Freeman & Jose 1997; Lund & Watson, 1997; Smith & O'Donnell, 1992, Watson & Berg, 1983). Curriculum guides that include instruction in skills required to use distance and near magnification devices and recommendations for integrating use of these devices into daily classroom and home activities are available from the American Printing House for the Blind (Hotta & Kitchel, 2002; Kitchel & Scott, 2002). A quick reference guide for instruction in the use of telescopes with school age students can be found in Appendix 9.2. A quick reference guide for instruction in the use of video magnifiers (also called closed-circuit television systems or CCTVs) for school age students can be found in Appendix 9.3. Both of these

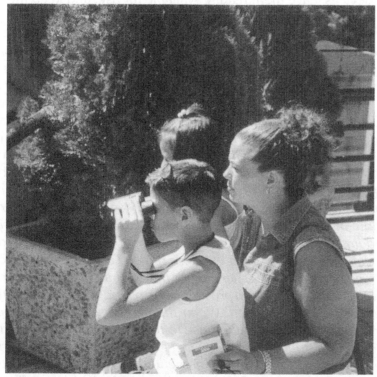

Reinforcing skills in a community setting. This student uses his new binoculars on a family outing to the zoo. His mother reports that this was the first time her son was not frightened by the animal sounds, and he looked at every animal through his binoculars. *(Irene Topor)*

guides can be used in conjunction with the detailed instructions provided in Chapter 10.

Successful enhancement of visual functioning through the use of optical devices requires an interdisciplinary approach. Teachers of students with visual impairments and/or orientation and mobility specialists must work collaboratively with low vision eye care specialists, the student, the family, and other members of the interdisciplinary team. Instruction in the use of optical devices is planned and initiated only after the student has received a low vision examination (Simmons & LaPolice, 2000). The low vision eye care specialist determines whether the student will benefit from optical devices and prescribes the power needed and the type of device appropriate to specified tasks. Some low vision eye care specialists provide initial training in device use in their offices or clinics, sometimes with the help of a low vision therapist, occupational therapist, or allied health staff trained in these techniques.

In the school setting, the teacher of students with visual impairments or O&M specialist designs and provides instruction leading to efficient device use within the critical tasks identified by the interdisciplinary team. Often this instruction is reinforced by other school professionals and by family members to ensure that instruction is integrated into meaningful activities. The student must be willing to use the devices, have them readily available for use, and keep them in good working order, as the following example illustrates:

A teacher of students with visual impairments recently noticed that Antonio, a sixth-grade student with low vision, has begun to look for other activities to do after reading for more than 10 minutes in his classroom. As a consequence, Antonio has not been completing his reading or workbook assignments. The teacher checks with other school staff, and they have also noticed this student's lack of interest in reading. She also checks with the boy's parents. They report noticing that their son has not been spending as much time on his homework as he used to. The teacher is wondering if this change in reading behavior is related to Antonio's vision. She notes that he is due for a low vision examination, and the boy's parents agree to schedule one.

The low vision evaluation findings indicate that Antonio would benefit from reading glasses at this time, since he is no longer able to accommodate for long periods of time at the close reading distance that he requires to read regular print. The teacher attends the examination with Antonio and his parents, and the low vision practitioner explains to the entire group how the eyeglasses are to be used. When the eyeglasses are prescribed, the teacher again demonstrates their use to the student, his parents, and the school staff. The student is more willing to wear his glasses at home, and now completes his homework assignments fully and on time. The teacher works carefully with the student to identify tasks for which he will wear his glasses in school (for example, completing math assignments and reading during free reading time). School staff are made aware of these tasks, and encourage Antonio to wear his eyeglasses during those times. The teacher of students with visual impairments monitors Antonio's use of his glasses carefully and encourages him to use them for more tasks over time.

Successful and frequent experiences tend to increase the rate of progress with optical devices. The instructor can assist the student, family, and school personnel in identifying situations in which a device may be helpful. To avoid frustration on the part of the student, the instructor must caution the student and team members not to expect use of a device in situations that require skills beyond those the student has already mastered or for tasks in which the device does not promote efficient task completion.

The instructor assesses the student's current skills in using prescribed optical devices for each of the critical tasks identified by the interdisciplinary team in which such devices might prove beneficial. Based on the student's current skills, the instructor then creates an instructional plan that builds on the skills the student has already mastered and reflects the student's visual abilities, learning style, and motivation.

As skills required for the efficient use of a device are mastered, the instructor shares this information with the rest of the team and works with team members to identify meaningful situations within which the device may be integrated. In this way, device use is generalized to other tasks with similar visual requirements. Three examples are provided here:

The instructor has designed an instructional sequence for a student to learn efficient telescope use in order to see items on a fast food menu. Each time the student has accomplished a step toward reaching this goal, the instructor informs the team members so that newly acquired skills can be reinforced by each team member when accompanying the student to a fast food restaurant and in other situations requiring similar telescope skills.

The general education science teacher is made aware that the student has mastered the skill of efficiently spotting a stationary target with a monocular telescope. The instructional ramifications of this skill within the science program have been explained. The science teacher might realize during a lesson that this skill can be applied, and asks the student to use the telescope to view the pieces of equipment the teacher has displayed on a table in the front of the classroom.

At the ticket purchase window at a movie theater, a student's father notices the posting of the movies and their show times and realizes that his daughter is probably not aware that this information is available. The father points out the listings and waits a few minutes for his daughter to use her telescope to read them.

If the student encounters difficulties using prescribed devices, the teacher of students with visual impairments or the O&M specialist consults with the low vision specialist and other professionals involved in device instruction. A follow-up examination may be required, or the low vision specialist may suggest a change in the type or power of a device. At the conclusion of instruction, the teacher of students with visual impairments or O&M specialist summarizes the student's progress in a written report. The report is made available to members of the interdisciplinary team, including the low vision specialist, following the school's policy regarding release of information.

PROMOTING VISUAL FUNCTIONING IN LITERACY ACTIVITIES

Literacy skills provide the foundation for many life activities including daily living, education, vocation, social emotional, and recreation and leisure pursuits. Especially for academically oriented school age students, promoting literacy in education is a major area of instructional need. The importance of literacy is becoming increasingly apparent for students with visual impairments. K. Wolffe (personal communication, 1999) indicates that a reading rate of 150 words/min is necessary to be competitive in the world of employment. School age students who have low vision need ample opportunity to receive instruction in literacy to achieve skill levels commensurate with the demands of the job market. Corn and Koenig (2002) have developed a framework for teaching literacy skills to students with low vision that identifies the following skills that need to be taught:

➤ Emergent literacy skills

➤ Integrated use of visual skills

➤ Use of optical devices for near and distant environments

➤ Beginning, intermediate, and advanced print literacy skills

➤ Literacy in dual media (print and braille)

➤ Braille literacy skills to supplement print skills

➤ Listening, aural reading, and live-reader skills

➤ Keyboarding and word-processing skills

➤ Technology skills.

This section will illustrate the implementation of compensatory methods related to vision functioning within this key area of the expanded core curriculum, focusing on literacy skills that have a major visual component. The following sections review basic visual skills for reading, early literacy instruction, selecting appropriate reading materials, methods to promote reading rate and comprehension, and the processing of information for reading.

Basic Visual Skills for Reading: Scanning and Fixation Time

Visual span is the amount of text that can be read at one glance (or fixation) before the eye moves on to the next set of characters. Readers with low vision may recognize fewer characters in one glance than readers who are not visually impaired. Readers with low vision whose visual spans are small must make more fixations as they read through text, resulting in slower rates of reading. Furthermore, fixation times on words or groups of words may be longer for readers with low vision (Legge, Ahn, & Klitz, 1997). These findings are based on laboratory testing procedures with adults that cannot be replicated easily in educational settings with children. It is not currently possible, therefore, outside of laboratory settings, to assess school-age students with low vision readily for visual span or fixation time. Nor is it known if instruction to improve scanning and fixation skills in reading tasks with children is effective. Because research is not available, practitioners must proceed with caution, carefully monitoring any instruction interventions to determine their effectiveness.

Symbol recognition exercises for children involve tracing lines of symbols, letters, words, sentences, and numbers. (Practice exercises that involve tracing symbols, letters, words, sentences, and numbers are available through Exceptional Teaching Aids; see the Resources section at the end of this book.) It is recommended that such exercises be attempted with students who have very slow reading speeds or who have recently experienced vision loss. Progress (i.e., change in speed and accuracy) should be documented and carefully monitored by instructors. If no progress is made over a designated period of time, then this instructional approach should be discontinued. If progress is made, then instruction should proceed as long as improvement is noted.

Early Literacy Instruction

Students with low vision need to receive specialized instruction in the perceptual and conceptual components of literacy in the preschool and kindergarten years. This will allow them to keep up with their peers in general education classrooms when reading instruction is emphasized in kindergarten and first grade. Developed visual skills need to be refined and applied systematically in early literacy activities. *The Program to Promote Visual Efficiency in Visual Functioning,* by Barraga and Morris (1980), contains many helpful exercises to promote these skills. Examples of some skills with visual components to be covered in early literacy programs include the following:

➤ Cutting along line

➤ Coloring within lines

➤ Identifying and matching colors

➤ Identifying pictures of different sizes

➤ Using a magnifier to see small details in pictures

➤ Tracing along lines

➤ Tracing shapes and letters

➤ Copying shapes and drawing them from memory

➤ Copying and drawing letters and numbers

➤ Visually following along a line, a line of pictures, and a line of letters

➤ Identifying and matching letters

➤ Identifying and matching numbers 0 to 10

➤ Counting objects 1 to 10

➤ Writing one's name

➤ Locating written and pictorial material on a page

The use of low vision optical devices, due to their reduced field of view, is not recommended in conjunction with the initial learning of decoding skills for reading. Research is not available to corroborate either positive or negative effects of this type of instruction on reading performance (Bevan et al., 2000; Jackson, 1983). Optical devices can, however, be incorporated into other appropriate early literacy activities (e.g., to see details in small pictures, to view items in the environment for concept development) to encourage their early acceptance and use. The team needs to consult with a low vision eye care practitioner to determine the most appropriate devices for a specific student.

Selecting Appropriate Reading Materials

Not all students with low vision will use print (regular print, large print, or print with the use of optical or electronic devices) as their primary or sole reading medium. Braille or auditory methods may be required, either alone or in conjunction with print reading. Selection of the appropriate reading medium is based on an evaluation of a variety of assessment data collected by the educational team, including the student, family, and caregivers. Methods for selecting appropriate learning media (i.e., a learning media assessment) have been described by Koenig and Holbrook (1995).

Once it has been determined that print is an appropriate reading medium for a student, reading material must be selected. Consideration needs to be given to print size, font preference, formatting requirements, contrast needs, lighting requirements, positioning of material, as well as nonelectronic or nonoptical adaptive reading devices, as reviewed in the following sections. All these factors must be applied to reading content that is appropriate in terms of a student's read-

SIDEBAR 9.5

Determining Appropriate Content for Reading

When attempting to select books of interest to a student, remember that when students know something about the subject area prior to reading a passage, they reportedly will read more fluently and have better comprehension than if the subject matter of the passage is completely new (Johns, 2001).

To determine the student's prior knowledge, administer informal reading inventories that include questions to survey what the student already knows about the passage. The *Basic Reading Inventory* (Johns, 2001) includes questions at the beginning of each passage at each grade level to explore the student's background knowledge of the subject area. Interviews are another way to discover what topics and areas of interest are most important to the student.

For help in motivating students to read, the *Accelerated Reader Program* (from Renaissance Learning) is a computer program that contains information on teaching children to focus their attention on the careful reading of books. This improves students' critical thinking skills and builds the intrinsic love of reading. Listening to books on tape from Reading for the Blind and Dyslexic, the National Library Service for the Blind and Physically Handicapped (see the Resources section), or a commercial publisher promotes listening skills for stories that students might not be able to access because their vocabulary and fluency are not yet at a high enough level to appreciate the content.

ing level and interests. A full discussion of reading content is outside the scope of this chapter; some information and references are provided in Sidebar 9.5.

PRINT SIZE

Print size is a critical issue for students with low vision. Selection of the most appropriate print size is based on the smallest size of print that permits the most efficient reading performance at a given distance.

Suchita, an 8-year-old child, can read 1M print but nothing smaller at her preferred viewing distance of 20 cm. By testing across a range of print sizes at 20 cm, it is determined that her reading performance (measured through reading speed) is best with 3M print or larger. While her reading performance was equally good with somewhat larger print sizes (e.g., 4M and 5M print), 3M print is selected for use at the 20 cm distance because it is the smallest size print that permits optimal reading performance at Suchita's viewing distance.

Several research groups have examined the relationship of print size and reading speed for students with low vision (Bailey et al., 2003; Lovie-Kitchin, Oliver, Bruce, Leighton, & Leighton, 1994; Lueck et al., 2003). The term *acuity reserve* has been used to express the relationship between the size of print a person intends to read and the size of the smallest print that that person can just read (Whittaker & Lovie-Kitchin, 1993). For best reading performance, we refer to the required or optimal acuity reserve: the ratio of the size of the smallest print that can be read with best efficiency to the size of the smallest print that can just be read at all. This has also been referred to as the critical print size (Legge, Ross, & Luebker, 1989). In the example just given, the smallest print size Suchita could read was 1M print (at 20 cm), but her reading performance peaked when 3M or larger print was made available. Therefore, Suchita's required acuity reserve was three times her threshold of 1M (3M/1M = 3).

It is important to remember that although the required print size varies depending on the viewing distance (also called working distance), the acuity reserve required by a given child will remain the same for a specific reading task. Thus, proportionally larger (or smaller) print will be required at longer (or shorter) viewing distances to allow the same ease of reading. An important exception to this is if the child lacks sufficient accommodation to maintain good focus on the reading material as the viewing distance decreases.

If Suchita were reading at 40 cm (twice the distance of 20 cm), for example, 6M print (twice the print size or $2 \times 3M$) would be advised. If she were reading at 10 cm (1/2 the distance of 20 cm), and it were determined that she could use her accommodation to maintain good focus at this short distance, then 1.5M print (1/2 the print size or $3M \div 2$) would be recommended. At 40 cm, the visual threshold (the smallest print size read) would be 2M (twice the visual threshold at 20 cm or $2 \times 1M$); at 10 cm the visual threshold would be 1.5M (1/2 the visual threshold at 20 cm or $1M \div 2$). At all distances, the optimal acuity reserve is the same: 3 (3/1 at 20 cm, 6/2 at 40 cm; 1.5/0.5 at 10 cm).

It is recommended that an acuity reserve of from 2 to 5 be maintained to achieve the most efficient reading speed for most students with low vision; the exact measure should be based on individualized evaluation. Determining a student's visual acuity threshold and required acuity reserve can help in determining the most appropriate print size to provide at a given working distance. Chapter 6 provides a more detailed explanation of print size notations, including M notation as well as visual reserve. Discussion here is limited to the use of regular and large print, since acuity reserve with respect to magnification devices requires more investigation before precise recommendations can be made.

FONT DESIGN

With the availability of texts on computer disk and the increased use of personal computers, the style of font can be varied to suit the needs of individual readers. A discussion of issues in font selection can be found in Appendix 9.4.

FOLLOWING A LINE OF PRINT

Some students with low vision may have difficulty following a line of print due to issues including oculomotor control or central scotomas. There are methods to promote ease of reading for these students.

A typoscope is a black piece of cardboard or other material with a window cut in it equal to the width of one to three lines of print. It is placed over the text on a page where the reader wishes to focus and helps the student maintain focus on the line of print being read by blocking out other print on the page. Typoscopes increase the contrast of the print within the window due to the black border, and reduce the amount of glare on the print since the black border also absorbs light. Typoscopes can be obtained commercially at a precut size, or they can be cut to fit the specific size of print, the number of lines to appear in the window, and the specific page size. A typoscope may be recommended for a student if the number of lines of print he or she skips while reading decreases or his or her rate of reading increases when using the typoscope.

Students can use a line marker (e.g., a ruler) above or below a line of print to keep their place. A line marker may be useful for students who skip lines of print as they read or who experience difficulty tracing along a line of print. Some people cut line markers in the shape of an *L* out of black cardstock to fit the exact page size. The long stroke of the *L* is placed under the line of print, so that the short stroke aligns with the left margin to help the student locate the beginning of each line.

A reference or anchor line can be placed at the left hand side of continuous text to help students locate the beginning of the next line. The line can be the same color as the text or of a contrasting color.

Some students use a finger to follow a line of print as they read. This can decrease the amount of attention they pay to extraneous stimuli on the page and guide their eyes along the line of print and to the next appropriate spot on the page.

LOCATING KEY VISUAL VARIABLES

Students with low vision may have difficulty locating material on a page, especially pages with complex formats or with very small print. Some students with attention deficits may not be able to take the time to scan a page and locate critical items on it. Enlarging material may not make it easier for students to negotiate around complex formats if the enlarged items are so large that the student cannot readily discern a visual pattern to them. There are several methods that instructors can use to encourage students to locate visual variables on a page.

Instructors can review page formats with students so that they are aware of page layouts and can anticipate where to find specific items on a page. For example, a particular spelling workbook may always list word definitions at the bottom of a page and a word list on the left hand side of a page; a dictionary always has words at the top of each page to indicate the page's contents.

Color coding key elements on a page for students who have intact color perception may help them to locate items more quickly. This can be used for reading complex formats or for finding items in study notes, for example.

For students with low vision who cannot scan pages easily for visual information due to oculomotor issues, central scotomas, or inability to maintain attention on a complex scanning task, assistance in isolating visual variables can lead to increased performance and comfort. Holbrook and Koenig (2000, p. 183) offer several methods to accomplish this:

➤ Students can use their hands to cover extraneous material.

➤ Colored overlays to isolate certain pieces of information can be used to block out unneeded material and systematically show important information.

➤ Simplifying visual information by reducing unnecessary text or picture complexity may prove helpful. (This is especially important for students with cortical [cerebral] visual impairment; see Chap. 8.) For example, in a lesson about the letter "c", a picture of a cow in a complex barnyard scene could be simplified to depict only the cow.

Students with low vision and visual-perceptual and visual-spatial disabilities may require varied approaches in reading instruction. If simplification of presentation does not promote reading that is fast and efficient enough to keep up with peers in class assignments, alternative reading media may be required. In a pilot study of children with cortical visual impairment due to periventricular leukomalacia (who had a reduction in visual-perceptual and visual-spatial abilities), Ek, Jacobson, Ygge, Fellenius, and Flodmark (2000), suggested that a sequential processing method such as braille be considered for children who experience difficulty deciphering letters crowded together, as occurs in reading tasks. They recommend the flexible use of assistive technology and instructional strategies for reading for this population. More research is needed to identify effective instructional approaches for children with low vision and visual-perceptual disabilities.

OPTIMIZING CONTRAST

If a student's contrast sensitivity is reduced, several adaptations may improve his or her reading performance. It is necessary to determine which adaptations are most appropriate on an individual basis, including the following suggestions:

➤ Absorptive lenses may improve the perceived contrast to some students. (This should be determined in conjunction with an eye care specialist).

➤ Colored overlays with a matte finish may improve the perceived contrast for some students. This is most effective when used over materials that are less than optimal contrast (i.e., red print on a pink background, as on some forms). Most students who use this method find a deep yellow overlay to be helpful. Other colors can be tried to determine the most effective color. Colored overlays and tinted lenses do not change the actual contrast, but may make the contrast differences in viewed material appear bolder.

➤ Darker paper placed under or around the reading task may serve to make the reading material appear brighter.

➤ Use of a dark fiber-tip pen on highly contrasting paper when writing can be useful.

➤ Provision of reading materials of the highest contrast (black on white is the highest contrast) on matte paper to reduce glare is another method.

➤ When using CCTV magnification systems, it is possible to change the color of the print and background as well as polarity of the presentation (dark print on light background or light print on dark background). Determine, for each student, the best colors and polarity to use.

OPTIMIZING LIGHTING

Some students require increased or decreased lighting for increased reading efficiency. Proper lighting is crucial to foster relaxed and comfortable reading rates.

An adjustable, directional lamp may enhance reading efficiency for some students. The light should be positioned so that it shines at an angle to the task (see Figure 6.8 in Chap. 6). Adjusting the arm of the lamp can reduce shadows. Always avoid shining the light directly into the student's eyes. As the lamp is moved away from the task, the amount of light will be reduced accordingly. Students should adjust the lamp to the optimal distance for each task to meet individual lighting needs.

Students with low vision may prefer a particular type of lighting (e.g., full spectrum, incandescent, xenon, or fluorescent). Give students the opportunity to select the type of lighting that makes images look best for them. Usually low wattage bulbs (40 to 60 watts) will suffice and can be positioned as close to the task as is necessary for best reading efficiency. High gloss desktops and work surfaces that cause glare can be covered with a dark blotter. Position students in the classroom so that glare is reduced (e.g., facing away from windows).

POSITIONING MATERIAL

Optimal placement of reading materials for a specific student is determined through a functional visual evaluation. Material may require careful positioning to reduce muscle strain from reading closely or at an angle, to reduce glare, to assist in maintaining the null point of nystagmus (see Chap. 2), or to maximize available visual fields.

The distance between the eye and the page is called the working distance. Students with low vision often read material at unusually close working distances. This behavior should be discussed with the student's eye care specialist and usually should not be discouraged. Bringing material closer enlarges the image of the reading material received by the eyes. The lens of each eye makes adjustments to keep these images in focus. Young children's lenses usually adjust easily to accommodate material at closer working distances, and the viewed material remains in focus. As people age, lenses become less flexible, and reading glasses are needed to keep near images in best focus (see Chap. 2 for a discussion of accommodation). For some school age students with low vision, reading glasses may be necessary either because the lens may not be able to make sufficient adjustments to keep the image in best focus at the needed working distance, or because the working distance is so close that it strains a student's eye mechanisms to maintain best focus over a long period of time. The need for reading glasses should be determined by an eye care specialist.

A reading stand allows the user to sustain a close working distance without experiencing strain in the neck, back, or arm muscles. Some reading stands incorporate a gooseneck lamp that enables the user to choose from a variety of lighting positions (Zimmerman, 1996). The angle of some reading stands can be adjusted to suit individual needs.

For some students with nystagmus (see Chap. 2), holding material while reading may not be as effective as placing material on a desktop or reading stand to allow them to maintain the null point of nystagmus. Based on the results of a functional vision evaluation and consultation with an eye care specialist, determine the direction in which the student holds his or her head and eye to use the null point gaze. The reading material may be placed off center, opposite the direction that the head turns. For other students, holding the material at an angle will reduce glare or allow the student to access the material at an angle or distance that cannot be achieved with a reading stand.

For students with right hemianopias (see Chap. 2), positioning reading material at an angle so that words are read from bottom to top, instead of right to left, may be beneficial. In this way, the student is not reading in the direction of the field loss. The amount of angle to turn the page of print should be determined on an individual basis in consultation with the student's eye care specialist.

Reading Rate

Reading rates for students with typical vision have been shown to vary depending on the reading goal (e.g., Carver, 1990). For example, skimming an expository text for information will take less time than reading the same text for detailed information. Silent reading rates for students with unimpaired vision can range from 80 words per minute for first graders to 174 words per minute for sixth graders. By the time a student reaches college age, typical silent reading rates range from 256 to over 333 words per minute (Koenig & Holbrook, 1995). In contrast, students with visual impairments reading standard print, large print, or standard print with optical devices are not likely to approach these reading rates (Corn et al., 2002; Gompel, Van Bon, Schreuder, Adriaansen, 2002; Lovie-Kitchin et al., 1994; Lueck et al., 2003). In work with adults, Legge, Rubin, Pelli, & Schleske, 1984 noted that reading was generally slower for low vision groups than in those with unimpaired vision. Reading has been shown to be slower for adults with low vision whose visual conditions involved central field losses than for those with intact central fields (Legge et al., 1988). Both central and peripheral visual field losses were found to be associated with reduced word-decoding performance by students with low vision in grades 1 to 6 (Gompel, Van Bon, Schreuder, & Adriaansen, 2002), although the reasons underlying the reduced reading performance may be different for students with central field losses than for those with peripheral field losses.

Print size has been related to reading rate for students with low vision when reading unrelated words and simple text (Lueck et al., 2003). Instructors must be certain that the print size used in reading tasks is within the optimal size range to promote maximum reading speed. This can be accomplished through the use of optical devices, screen enlargement programs, CCTV magnifiers, or enlarged print. Some of the benefits and drawbacks of each of these methods have been described by Corn, Wall, and Bell (2000) and by D'Andrea and Farrenkopf (2000). Print should be three to five times a student's visual acuity threshold (see the previous section on selecting appropriate print size). If the print is too small or too large, reading speed is affected. When characters are too small, they cannot be readily deciphered. When characters are too large, the number of characters that can be read at one visual fixation decreases, more fixations per line are needed, and reading speed is decreased as a consequence.

The effectiveness of reading instruction in increasing reading speed and comprehension for school age students with low vision has not received much attention in the research literature. Layton and Koenig (1998) showed that the use of an instructional method involving repeated reading of short passages of text resulted in moderate to large increases in reading rate for four subjects aged 7 to 11 years who had low vision, and that this generalized to classroom activities. Bevan et al. (2000) found that reading rates of children with low vision at high acuity reserves (two to three times larger than threshold) were significantly faster when magnification was provided by large print than by decreased working distances with optical devices. However, Corn, Wall, and Bell (2000) and Corn et al. (2002) offer preliminary data indicating that students with visual impairments receiving instruction in the use of optical devices with standard print are increasing their reading rates and becoming more efficient readers.

Reading material should be adapted to increase fluency and rate of reading as required by individual students. Koenig et al. (1992) stressed that individual assessments are necessary to determine appropriate learning media and instructional interventions for reading for students with low vision. A team using objective and systematic methods for collecting reading rate data and comprehension information should conduct these assessments.

Koenig and Holbrook (2000), and Koenig and Holbrook (2001) have delineated in detail a number of methods to promote reading fluency, including the following:

➤ Repeated readings: The student reads and rereads a short passage until a predetermined criterion for reading rate has been met.

➤ Paired readings: A student is teamed with a proficient reader as a reading model, with the proficient reader reading aloud first as the student reads along silently, followed by the student reading aloud the same passage.

➤ Radio reading: The student acts as a radio announcer using a script and having one or more listeners.

➤ Echo reading: The student reads along with an instructor who sets the pace to increase the student's reading rate and confidence.

Fridal, Jansen, and Klindt (1981) experimented with speed-reading methods with adults with low vision and showed dramatically increased reading speeds over a number of weeks. The authors used varied methods involving a card that was moved down the text as fast as possible; the goal was to increase speed without decreasing comprehension. In addition, they taught the adults about the purpose of reading, and provided information about the reading process (e.g., eye movement, regression, fixations). These methods have not been explored with school age students with low vision, and it is recommended they be attempted only after students have acquired efficient decoding and comprehension skills.

Processing Information for Reading

Corley and Pring (1993a, 1993b) suggest that phonics-based programs are effective in teaching reading to students with low vision, who may need more time to process pictorial material than students with unimpaired sight. On some tasks, students with low vision may have more difficulty integrating visual and verbal material presented in quick succession. Accompanying verbal explanations may be confusing to a student if his or her attention is redirected too soon or follows too quickly after visual inspection. He or she may need time to inspect a picture and retain visual images of the picture before the instructor offers verbal elaborations.

Koenig and Holbrook (2001) suggest several comprehension strategies that can be used with students with low vision to improve their understanding of reading passages.

➤ Cloze procedure: In the cloze procedure, a student reads a story with selected words omitted and tries to fill in each blank with a word that makes sense in the context of that story. Students learn to use contextual cues by suggesting replacements for words that have been systematically omitted from sentences.

➤ Text preview: This technique builds background knowledge before reading, provides motivation, and introduces an organizational framework for comprehending narrative or expository texts for students in upper elementary through high school grades.

➤ Generating interactions between schemata and text (GIST): The student learns to comprehend the gist of paragraphs, by writing 15-word summaries of several paragraphs or 20-word summaries of short passages.

➤ Possible sentences: Students learn new vocabulary prior to reading texts and generate sentences using the new words. Students then read the text selection and check the accuracy of their sentences, revising them if necessary.

Handwriting

Students with low vision may have special needs with regard to handwriting and may require additional instruction to perfect their handwriting skills (Tapp, Wilhelm, & Loveless, 1991; Koenig & Rex, 1996). For some students, handwriting may not be the best method for completing assignments; word-processing methods should be considered. Many students with low vision have more difficulty reading cursive lettering than print lettering, causing additional concerns as they enter third grade, when cursive handwriting is generally taught. Although print letters may be easier to read for students with low vision due to the spacing of the letters, they may be more difficult to produce since the writing implement must be repeatedly lifted off and lowered onto the page. Cursive writing is more difficult to read because the letters are not separated, yet it is easier to write because letters flow into one another (Hoffer, 1979). Some students may not be able to read handwriting that is the size usually required in handwriting lessons in general education classrooms. Students with low vision may also need to write with darker, thicker lines using fiber-tip pens or use bold-lined paper to see the lines when they are learning to write (Koenig & Rex, 1996). Instructors can work with a low vision eye care specialist to determine if any low vision optical devices can assist with this task. An assessment of handwriting skills is provided by Koenig et al. (2000, p. 161). A systematic approach to handwriting instruction, from readiness to cursive, is provided in *Handwriting Without Tears* (Olsen, 2001).

Hoffer (1979) describes four visual levels for a given individual's handwriting:

1. Writes primarily by touch, although may be able to see hand movement.

2. Uses vision to guide writing along the line. Cannot read own writing.

3. Sees the line as a writing guide, and can read back own handwriting.

4. Can read fine detail in handwriting (to dot *i's* and cross the *t's*), and can fill out forms.

It is important for teachers to evaluate students' needs and to determine the most appropriate individualized handwriting program for students with low vision. Teachers of student with visual impairments need to collaborate with general education teachers to explain handwriting requirements and to determine accommodations to meet students' individual handwriting needs. The following questions need to be addressed:

➤ Does the student require additional instruction to improve his or her hand-writing skills that address eye-hand coordination, such as staying on the line or related to the size and formation of letters?

➤ What assistive devices can facilitate handwriting skills (e.g., fiber-tip pen, bold-lined paper, line-writing guides, raised-line paper, closed-circuit television)?

➤ What is the student's preferred handwriting size? (I.e., what size script does the student naturally use and prefer to read back?) Is this size functional in the school setting or in work settings?

➤ What is the acceptable size of the student's handwriting for classroom assign-ments? Can the student read this size print to proofread his or her completed assignments?

➤ Does the student perform better using print or cursive writing?

➤ Should the student write primarily in print or cursive letters, or is the student able to use both? Have the student's general education teachers been made aware of this?

➤ What is the size and form of writing (print or cursive) required for notes to the student that will be written by teachers and peers?

➤ What assistive devices can the student use to read the handwriting of others (optical devices, closed-circuit television)?

➤ Should the student be encouraged to learn keyboarding and word-processing skills in order to complete written assignments?

Keyboarding Skills

Learning to use the keyboard for typing, word-processing skills, and other com-puter use is an essential part of literacy programs for students with low vision. These skills should be introduced in the first, second, or third grades (Koenig & Holbrook, 2000). Some instructors start teaching these skills to children in kinder-garten. *Type to Learn* (Wheeler & Wheeler, 1985) is an instructional program often used with students with low vision. The American Printing House for the Blind (see the Research section) has several computer programs designed to teach keyboarding skills to individuals with visual impairments.

When students are reading instructions from a textbook or paper while con-currently keyboarding, they constantly shift gaze from the computer screen to the paper copy, finding their place on each with each shift of gaze. This process can be difficult for some students with low vision. The following suggestions may help to facilitate the process:

➤ Give the student sufficient time to complete the lesson. It may take more time because the visual demands of such tasks are high.

➤ Make sure the reading material on the computer screen and hard copy is optimized for size and contrast for the individual student.

➤ Provide sufficient task lighting on the hard copy.

➤ Be certain that glare is reduced on the computer screen.

➤ Place the hard copy on a reading stand so that the material is at a comfortable reading distance and angle for the student.

➤ Be certain that the computer screen is at the optimal distance from the student. (See the section in Appendix 9.3 on Determining Optimal Magnification.)

➤ If a student consistently loses his or her place on the hard copy, attach a line marker to the hard copy that can be moved down the page by the student as the lesson progresses.

➤ Use a screen enlargement program with line marker capabilities for students who lose their place when reading material on computer screens.

➤ Provide instruction via auditory methods (audiotape, speech output) to reduce visual fatigue and potential errors.

Assistive Technology to Promote Literacy

Assistive devices of all kinds are increasing access to literacy materials for students with low vision (Lueck, Dote-Kwan, Senge, & Clark, 2001). Detailed instructional methods to promote use of assistive technology devices for literacy for school age students are provided by D'Andrea and Farrenkopf (2000). As with any assistive device, it is important to infuse instruction in using the technological devices into critical activities identified for each student.

CASE STUDIES

Instruction in methods to promote and facilitate the use of vision is required throughout the school career of students with low vision. As students gain skills and maturity, the techniques and tools available to promote vision use increase and become more complex. Students with low vision need to be made aware of the availability and use of these expanding options as their life goals evolve and become more defined over time. Students with low vision need to be guided to assess for themselves how various techniques and methods fit their needs so that they can make informed and independent choices about which techniques they will use for various life activities as they move into adulthood.

The two case studies presented in the following sections illustrate the application of the methods discussed in this chapter. In particular, they show how skills are best taught in the context of the critical tasks that the individual student needs to be able to perform.

Melissa Fong

Melissa Fong, a 5-year-old preschool student, is currently attending a half-day program in a small rural town. A teacher of students with visual impairments has provided consultative services to the preschool teacher and to Melissa's family. Melissa will be entering kindergarten next year.

Twice a year Melissa sees an ophthalmologist for comprehensive eye examinations. Her diagnoses include microphthalmia in the right eye and severe myopia and nystagmus in the left. She has undergone cataract surgery on her right eye. As reported by the ophthalmologist, Melissa's distance visual acuities with her current glasses were light projection in the right eye and 20/400 in the left. Her near visual acuity was not reported. The ophthalmologist has recommended surgery to bring the left eye into alignment. Melissa has also been evaluated by a low vision eye care practitioner. After determining critical tasks for Melissa with her teacher and parents, the low vision eye care practitioner prescribed the following:

1. A 4×12 monocular telescope for seeing objects at a distance (see Chap. 3 for an explanation of telescopes)

2. A 16-diopter paperweight-style magnifier used in combination with her glasses, which allows Melissa to read 0.5 M print from a working distance of 20 cm (0.20/0.5M)

3. NoIR 10 percent amber wraparound sun shields, which have improved Melissa's visual skills outdoors

Methods of instruction with the optical devices were discussed with the low vision specialist, and the teacher incorporated them into the critical tasks identified for Melissa. Through dialogue with Melissa's mother, her current preschool teacher and aide, and the kindergarten teacher at the elementary school Melissa will be attending next year, critical tasks were identified. Based on an analysis of the visual components of each task and Melissa's visual capacities, the team, including the low vision eye care practitioner, selected the compensatory methods Melissa will learn to use to meet the visual demands of each task. The critical tasks identified for Melissa, the environments in which they are carried out, and the compensatory methods to be taught for each are detailed in the following sections.

GOAL 1 (HOME, SCHOOL, AND COMMUNITY): IDENTIFY OBJECTS, ANIMALS, AND PEOPLE AT A DISTANCE

➤ **Visual environmental adaptations:** Use tinted lenses and cap when outdoors.

➤ **Visual skills instruction:** Learn to identify objects, animals, and people based on their critical features, (e.g. color of hair and skin, height, weight).

➤ **Assistive devices:** Learn to use a telescope to view details of objects, animals, and people when they are too far away to see without assistance.

GOAL 2 (HOME AND SCHOOL): LOCATE TOYS AND MATERIALS AND PUT THEM AWAY

➤ **Visual environmental adaptations:**

- Melissa's parents will replace the patterned carpeting in her bedroom and closet with solid colored carpeting that contrasts with most of her clothes and toys.

- Melissa's teacher will line the back of each shelf where toys and materials are stored with contrasting colored paper such as construction paper or adhesive-backed paper.

➤ **Visual skills instruction:**

- Learn to scan to locate empty spaces on toy/material shelves where toys may need to be returned.

- Tape a photograph of each toy or material to the edge of the shelf so that Melissa can match the object itself to the picture with adult assistance.

GOAL 3 (SCHOOL): WRITE THE ALPHABET

➤ **Visual environmental adaptations:** Melissa will use bold-lined paper, soft pencils, task lighting, and a slant board.

➤ **Visual skills instruction:**

- Provide systematic instruction to identify, copy, and match letters.

- Provide systematic writing program.

GOAL 4 (HOME, SCHOOL, AND COMMUNITY): LOCATE BIRTHDAYS, HOLIDAYS, AND SPECIAL EVENTS ON A CALENDAR

➤ **Vision training for literacy skills:**

- Learn to scan from left to right to locate a special event.

- Learn to interpret symbols visually that represent special events, such as a picture of a birthday cake, or a bus to represent a field trip.

➤ **Assistive devices:**

- Learn to use telescope to locate events on calendar during circle time.

- Learn to use magnifier to locate events on a desk calendar.

GOAL 5 (HOME AND SCHOOL): DEMONSTRATE PROGRESS IN MANIPULATIVE BALL SKILLS (E.G., THROWING, KICKING, AND CATCHING)

➤ **Visual environmental adaptations:**

- Use balls of color and size determined after vision instruction with them.

- Control glare with tinted lenses and cap when outdoors.

➤ **Visual skills instruction:** Use large, brightly colored balls, and gradually change to balls of smaller size and less vivid colors.

➤ **Sensory substitutions and modifications:** Use balls with sound source to direct her vision with auditory cues.

GOAL 6 (HOME, SCHOOL, AND WORKPLACE): START UP AND SHUT DOWN COMPUTERS, TAPE RECORDERS, CASSETTE PLAYERS, AND VIDEOCASSETTE RECORDERS, AND USE THESE DEVICES TO COMPLETE A TASK

➤ **Visual environmental adaptations:** Use remote control devices with large and/or color-coded buttons.

➤ **Visual skills instruction:** Learn to locate critical features of devices visually.

➤ **Sensory substitutions and modifications:** Mark power on and power off buttons tactilely.

Roberta Sanchez

Roberta Sanchez is a high school senior who plans to major in clinical psychology in college with a minor in dancing. She is considering working as a counselor for children and incorporating dance into therapy. She has applied to a local community college with plans to transfer to a university in her junior year. Roberta receives eye care from a general ophthalmologist and a retinal specialist. Her diagnosis has changed over time. At 4 months of age, she was diagnosed with congenital nystagmus. This diagnosis was changed to Stargardt's disease at 4 years of age, and to rod-cone dystrophy during her sophomore year in high school. Roberta's vision has decreased significantly over time.

Currently her unaided distance visual acuity is OD 10/225 and OS 5/600; OU not given. Her near visual acuity is OU 0.20/8M. With refractive correction her results show OD −1.50 to 1.75 × 180; visual acuity 10/160; OS −1.50 to 2.00 × 170; visual acuity 10/100. With a +4.50 add OU, her near visual acuity is 0.67M at 3 in. Her contrast sensitivity is severely reduced, peripheral visual fields are full, but central scotomas were noted in both eyes when tested with an Amsler grid.

Roberta began using a video magnifier system when she was 14. The low vision specialist prescribed a 10× monocular telescope to read low glare store signs and some street signs. A 40-diopter handheld illuminated magnifier was also prescribed so that Roberta could read price tags on items in stores. Roberta resisted the use of the video magnifier, but by her senior year in high school she was willing to use it in class. She took all notes on the video magnifier, did math problems, and used it to retrieve information from textbooks. Just before graduation, Roberta used the video magnifier to practice filling out forms, complete map work and job applications, and develop better handwriting skills. The teacher of students with visual impairments taught Roberta braille in her junior and senior years in high school because of her unstable visual prognosis. Although print is her primary reading medium, Roberta and the members of her educational team recognized the value of having a backup system to aid her in daily literacy tasks.

Through discussions with Roberta, selected teachers, and her mother, critical tasks were identified. Based on an analysis of the visual components of each task and Roberta's visual capacities, the team, including the low vision eye care practitioner, selected the compensatory methods Roberta will learn to use to meet the visual demands of each task. For older students like Roberta, the range of potential compensatory methods is greater than for younger students like Melissa. To illustrate this point, additional options that were considered but not selected by the team are presented as well.

GOAL 1 (TRANSITION GOAL): ACHIEVE A PASSING SCORE ON A STATE-MANDATED HIGH SCHOOL EXIT EXAMINATION

➤ **Visual environmental adaptations:** Use task lighting, a slant board, and possible reformatting of test to systematize the way answers are recorded.

➤ **Sensory substitutions and modifications:** Have reader give test orally to Roberta and record her answers, or have reader give test orally to Roberta who records answers on computer.

The team also considered but did not select the following methods upon consultation with Roberta:

➤ **Visual skills training:** Use systematic visual scanning to locate each question and answer on the instrument.

➤ **Assistive devices:**

● Use video magnifier for reading questions.

● Use reading spectacles or 40D illuminated handheld magnifier for spot-checking her answers.

GOAL 2 (HOME, COMMUNITY, SCHOOL, FUTURE WORKPLACE): ACCESS TEXT INCLUDING TEXTBOOKS, MAGAZINES, AND BOOKS

➤ **Vision training for literacy skills:**

● Through eccentric viewing training, learn to locate preferred retinal locus.

● Increase print reading efficiency through exposure to a variety of reading materials that are motivating to read.

● Learn mechanics of reading different kinds of literary material (e.g., horizontal, vertical, columns, graphics, and maps) using the video magnifier.

➤ **Assistive devices:**

● Use video magnifier and illuminated 40D handheld magnifier;

● Learn to use *VIP* computer software (from JBliss Imaging Systems; see Resources section of this book) to read books on CD, scan and read print, and send and receive e-mail.

The team considered but did not select the following additional methods:

➤ **Visual environmental adaptations:** Provide increased illumination, high-contrast condition on video magnifier, glare-free environment, and writing tools that give accessible feedback.

➤ **Sensory substitutions and modifications:**

● Use audiotapes as a supplemental media for gathering information.

● Use braille materials when these are available and effective.

● Learn hot keys on the computer.

GOAL 3 (COMMUNITY, SCHOOL, FUTURE WORKPLACE): DEMONSTRATE TECHNICAL AND ARTISTIC SKILLS IN DANCE CONSISTENTLY AND RELIABLY

➤ **Visual environmental adaptations:**

● Use colored tape (contrasting with color of floor) as visual cues for foot placement in dance.

● Arrange lesson and dance sequences so that Roberta keeps her back to windows on dance floor as much as possible to reduce glare.

● Add contrasting features to help identify critical environmental features (doorways, stairs, change in floor surfaces).

● Ask instructors to organize the environment to ensure Roberta's safety and ease of movement while she practices.

➤ **Sensory substitutions and modifications:**

● Listen to music on tape or compact disc before actual dance practice.

● Shadow a partner who demonstrates the steps for each type of dance.

● Watch a videocassette or digital video disk of individuals modeling different dance steps.

● Task analyze each dance step and learn in small increments.

The team also considered but did not select the following methods:

➤ **Assistive devices:** Use the 10× telescope to view demonstration dances in the community

GOAL 4 (COMMUNITY): SHOP INDEPENDENTLY AT A GROCERY STORE

➤ **Visual training for literacy skills:** Analyze most commonly purchased food items at close range, noting colors on labels and size, spacing, and style of print on packages so that Roberta knows what to look for when she is in the grocery store.

➤ **Assistive devices:**

- Use 40D handheld illuminated magnifier to read price tags.

- Uses 10× telescope to view and identify location of food items by aisle.

- Uses 10× telescope at an intermediate distance to scan shelves to locate food items.

The team also considered but did not select the following methods:

➤ **Visual environmental adaptations:**

- Orient to grocery store and the location of items in it with the assistance of the O&M instructor.

- Wear indoor glare-free lenses if the store lighting compromises visual functioning.

- Wear large fanny pack to carry magnification devices.

➤ **Sensory substitutions and modifications:**

- Use braille shopping list or audiotape of items.

- Bring a tactile or visual map of store with food items most frequently purchased identified on the map.

GOAL 5 (HOME): DO LAUNDRY INDEPENDENTLY

➤ **Visual environmental adaptations:**

- Adjust lighting in laundry area to decrease glare and increase overall light level, using illumination controls and a flexible-arm floor lamp.

- Mark switches and dials on washer and dryer with colored tape.

- Organize the laundry room so that cleaning agents are always on the same shelves.

- Identify bins where Roberta can consistently put her clean and dirty clothes.

➤ **Sensory substitutions and modifications:**

- Label bins with tactile symbols as needed.

The team also considered but did not select the following methods:

➤ **Sensory substitutions and modifications:** Mark common settings on washer and dryer with puff paint or braille.

GOAL 6 (WORKPLACE): WRITE FORMAL COMMUNICATIONS INCLUDING RESUME AND JOB APPLICATION

➤ **Visual training for literacy skills:** Refer to models of completed resumes and job applications for completing Roberta's own documents.

➤ **Assistive devices:**

- Use optical and electronic devices such as video magnifier and handheld magnifier.

- Scan documents into her computer and reads job application with a screen magnification program.

The team also considered but did not select the following methods:

➤ **Visual environmental adaptations:**

- Adjust lighting to increase visual efficiency.

- Use writing instruments that provide visual feedback to check the accuracy of work.

➤ **Sensory substitutions and modifications:**

- Listen to reader orally recite items on the job resume form. Reader records Roberta's answers in the correct place on the form.

- Use screen magnification speech output to read text on page.

GOAL 7 (SCHOOL, HOME): ACCESS THE INTERNET

➤ **Visual training for literacy skills:**

- Access all available visual information on computer monitor through continuing visual skill instruction.

- Use an Internet search engine.

- Bookmark her most commonly used Internet sites.

- Create folders and files to organize list of Internet sites.

➤ **Sensory substitutions and modifications:** Use speech option on screen magnification program for easier access to written material.

The team also considered but did not select the following methods for Roberta before making their final decision:

➤ **Visual environmental adaptations:**

- Use a 20–21-inch computer screen monitor to include more visual information on the screen.

- Position computer monitor to create a glare-free environment.

- Use non-glare computer screen.

- Select contrast features on monitor, using special software, to display the most efficient visual information depending on appearance of Internet site information.

- Use split-screen to decrease the need to go back and forth from Internet site to document on which Roberta is recording information.

- Learn hot keys to easily access computer functions.

➤ **Assistive devices:**

- Magnify images on computer monitor using screen magnification software.

REFERENCES

Bailey, I. L., Lueck, A. H., Greer, R., Tuan, K. M., Bailey, V. M., & Dornbusch, H. (2003). Understanding the relationships between print size and reading in low vision. *Journal of Visual Impairment & Blindness, 97*(6), 325–334.

Barraga, N. C., & Morris, J. E. (1980). *Program to develop efficiency in visual functioning.* Louisville. KY: American Printing House for the Blind.

Bevan, J., Lovie-Kitchin, J., Hein, B., Ting, E., Brand, P., Scott, M., & Fotkou, P. (2000). The effect of relative size magnification versus relative distance magnification on the reading performance of children with low vision. *EnVision. 5,* 2–3.

Berg, R. V., Jose, R. T., & Carter, K. (1983). Distance training techniques. In R. T. Jose (Ed.), *Understanding low vision* (pp. 277–316). New York: American Foundation for the Blind.

Carver, R. P. (1990). *Reading rate: A review of research and theory.* San Diego, CA: Academic Press, Inc.

Corley, G., & Pring, L. (1993a, September). *Partially sighted children: The visual processing of words and pictures.* Paper presented at the British Educational Research Association Conference, England.

Corley, G., & Pring, L. (1993b). The reading strategies of partially sighted children. *International Journal of Rehabilitation & Research, 16,* 209–220.

Corn, A. L. (1989). Instruction in the use of vision for children and adults with low vision. *RE:view, 21,* 26–38.

Corn, A. L., & Koenig, A. J. (2002). Literacy for students with low vision: A framework for delivering instruction. *Journal of Visual Impairment & Blindness, 96,* 305–321.

Corn, A., Wall, R., & Bell, J. (2000). Impact of optical devices on reading rates and expectations for visual functioning of school-age children and youth with low vision. *Visual Impairment Research, 2,* 33–41.

Corn, A. L., Wall, R. S., Joe, R. T., Bell, J. K., Wilcom, K., & Perez, A. (2002). An initial study of reading and comprehension rates for students who received optical devices. *Journal of Visual Impairment & Blindness, 96*(5), 322–334.

Covey, S. R. (1989). *The seven habits of highly effective people.* New York: Simon & Schuster.

Cowan, C., & Shepler, R. (2000a). Activities and games for teaching children to use magnifiers. In F. M. D'Andrea & C. Farrenkopf (Eds.), *Looking to learn: Promoting literacy for students with low vision* (pp. 167–188). New York: AFB.

Cowan, C., & Shepler, R. (2000b). Activities and games for teaching children to use monocular telescopes. In F. M. D'Andrea & C. Farrenkopf (Eds.), *Looking to learn: Promoting literacy for students with low vision* (pp. 137–166). New York: AFB.

Crisp, R. K. (1994). The relationship between the restricted functional near visual field of partially sighted children and reading problems. In A. C. Kooijman, P. L. Looijestijn, J. A. Welling, & G. J. Van Der Wildt (Eds.), *Low vision: Research and new developments in rehabilitation.* (pp. 307–315). Amsterdam, The Netherlands: IOS Press.

D'Andrea, F. M. (2000). Activities and games for teaching children to use a CCTV. In F. M. D'Andrea & C. Farrenkopf (Eds.), *Looking to learn: Promoting literacy for students with low vision* (pp. 189–214). New York: AFB.

D'Andrea, F. M., & Farrenkopf, C. (Eds.). (2000). *Looking to Learn: promoting literacy for students with low vision.* New York: AFB Press.

Ek, U., Jacobson, L., Ygge, J., Fellenius, K., & Flodmark, O. (2000). Visual and cognitive development and reading achievement in four children with visual impairment due to periventricular leukomalacia. *Visual Impairment Research, 2,* 3–16.

Erin, J. N., & Paul, B., (1996). Functional vision assessment and instruction of children and youths in academic programs. In Corn, A. L., & Koenig, A. J., (Eds.), *Foundations of low vision: Clinical and functional perspectives* (pp. 221–245). New York: AFB Press.

Freeman, P. B., & Jose, R. T. (1997). *The art and practice of low vision,* (2nd ed.). Newton, MA: Butterworth-Heinemann.

Fridal, G., Jansen, L., & Klindt, M. (1981). Courses in reading development for partially sighted students. *Journal of Visual Impairment & Blindness, 66,* 4–7.

Goempel, M., Van Bon, W. H. J., Schreuder, R., & Adriaansen, J. J. M. (2002). Reading and spelling competence of Dutch children with low vision *Journal of Visual Impairment & Blindness, 96,* 435–447.

Hatlen, P. (1996). The core curriculum for blind and visually impaired students, including those with additional disabilities. *RE:view, 28,* 25–32.

Hoffer, D. (1979). The handwriting visual aid. *Review of Optometry, September,* 63–65.

Holbrook, C. M., & Koenig, A. J. (2000). Basic techniques for modifying instruction. In A. J. Koenig & M. C. Holbrook, (Eds.) *Foundations of education* (2nd ed.): *Vol. II. Instructional strategies for teaching children and youths with visual impairments* (pp. 173–195). New York: AFB Press.

Hotta, C., & Kitchel, E. (2002). *ENVISION I: Vision enhancement program using distance devices.* Louisville, KY: American Printing House for the Blind.

Jackson, R. M. (1983). Early educational use of optical aids: A cautionary note. *Education of the Visually Handicapped, 40,* 20–29.

Johns, J. (2001). *Basic reading inventory: Pre-primer through grade twelve and early literacy assessments.* Dubuque, IA: Kendall/Hunt Publishing Co.

Kapperman, G., & Sticken, J. (2000). Assistive technology. In A. J. Koenig, & M. C. Holbrook (Eds.), *Foundations of education* (2nd ed.): *Volume II. Instructional strategies for teaching children and youths with visual impairments* (pp. 500–528). New York: AFB Press.

Kitchel, E., & Scott, K. (2002). *ENVISION II: Vision enhancement program using near magnification devices.* Louisville, KY: American Printing House for the Blind.

Koenig. A. J., & Holbrook, C. M., (1995). *Learning media assessment* (2nd ed.). Austin: Texas School for the Blind and Visually Impaired.

Koenig, A. J., & Holbrook, C. M. (2000). Literacy skills. In A. J. Koenig & M. C. Holbrook (Eds.), *Foundations of education* (2nd ed.): *Volume II. Instructional strategies for teaching children and youths with visual impairments* (pp. 216–324). New York: AFB Press.

Koenig, A. J., Holbrook, C. M., Corn, A. L., DePriest, L. B., Erin, J., & Presley, I. (2000). Specialized assessments for students with visual impairments. In A. J. Koenig & M. C. Holbrook (Eds.), *Foundations of education* (2nd ed.): *Volume II. Instructional strategies for teaching children and youths with visual impairments* (pp. 103–172). New York: AFB Press.

Koenig, A. J., Holbrook, M. C. (2001). *Fluency and comprehension strategies for students with low vision.* Paper presented at Texas Focus 2001 Conference: Looking at Low Vision, Ft. Worth, TX.

Koenig, A. J., Layton, C. A., & Ross, D. B. (1992). The relative effectiveness of reading in large print and with low vision devices for students with low vision. *Journal of Visual Impairment & Blindness, 86,* 48–53.

Koenig, A. J & Rex, E. J., (1996). Instruction of literacy skills to children and youths with low vision. In A. L. Corn & A. J. Koenig (Eds.), *Foundations of low vision: Clinical and functional perspectives* (pp. 280–305). New York: AFB Press.

Layton, C. A. & Koenig, A. J. (1998). Increasing fluency in elementary students with low vision through repeated readings. *Journal of Visual Impairment and Blindness, 92,* 276–292.

Lazear, D. (1991). *Seven ways of knowing: Teaching for multiple intelligences.* Palatine, IL: Skylight Publishers.

Legge, G. E., Ahn, S., & Klitz, T. S. (1997). Psychophysics of reading: XVI. The visual span in normal and low vision. *Vision Research, 37,* 1999–2010.

Legge, G. E., Ross, J. A., & Luebker, A. (1989). Psychophysics of reading: VIII. The Minnesota low-vision reading test. *Optometry & Visual Science, 66,* 843–851.

Legge, G. E., Rubin, G. S. Pelli, D. G., & Schleske, M. M. (1984). Psychophysics of reading—II. Low vision. *Vision Research, 25,* 253–266.

Legge, G. E., Rubin, G. S., Pelli, D. G., Schleske, M. M., Luebker, J. A., & Ross, J. A. (1988). Understanding low vision reading. *Journal of Visual Impairment & Blindness, 82,* 54–59.

Lewis, S., & Allman, C. B. (2000). Educational programming. In M. C. Holbrook & A. J. Koenig, (Eds.), *Foundations of Education* (2nd ed.): *Volume I. History and theory of teaching children and youth with visual impairments* (pp. 218–259). New York: AFB Press.

Lovie-Kitchin, J. E., Oliver, N. J., Bruce, A., Leighton, M. S., & Leighton, W. K. (1994). The effect of print size on reading rate for adults and children. *Clinical & Experimental Optometry, 77,* 1.

Lueck A. H. (1999). Setting curricular priorities for students with visual impairments. *RE:view, 31,* 54–66.

Lueck, A. H. (2001, June). *Compensatory instruction to promote vision use for students with visual impairments.* Paper presented at the Texas Focus Conference, Dallas, TX.

Lueck, A. H., Bailey, I. L., Greer, R., Tuan, K. M., Bailey, V. M., & Dornbusch, H. (2003). Exploring print size requirements and reading for students with low vision. *Journal of Visual Impairment & Blindness, 97*(6), 335–354.

Lueck, A. H., Dote-Kwan, J., Senge, J., & Clark, L. (2001). Going beyond the tools for literacy. Establishing priorities for instructional technology based upon curricular needs. *RE:view, 33,* 21–33.

Lund, R., & Watson, G.R. (1997). *The CCTV book: Habilitation and rehabilitation with closed circuit television systems.* Lillesand, Norway: Synsforum and Frolund.

McBiles, J. L. (1998). *Performance-based teaching, learning, and assessment model.* Phoenix: Bureau of Educational Research. College of Education, Arizona State University.

Olsen, J. Z. (2001). *Handwriting without tears method.* Cabin John, MD: Handwriting Without Tears.

Simmons, B., & LaPolice, D. J. (2000). Working effectively with a low vision clinic. In F. M. D'Andrea & C. Farrenkopf (Eds.), *Looking to learn: Promoting literacy for students with low vision* (pp. 84–116). New York: AFB Press.

Smith, A. J., & O'Donnell, L. M. (1992). *Beyond arm's reach: Enhancing distance vision.* Philadelphia: Pennsylvania College of Optometry Press.

Tapp, K. L., Wilhelm, J. G., & Loveless, L. J. (1991). A guide to curriculum planning for visually impaired students. Madison: Wisconsin Department of Public Instruction.

Topor, I., & Erin, J. (2000). Educational assessment of vision function in infants and children. In B. Silverstone, M. A. Lang, B. P. Rosenthal, & E. E. Faye (Eds.), *The Lighthouse handbook on vision impairment and vision rehabilitation, Vol. 2.* New York: Oxford University Press.

Watson, G. & Berg, R. V. (1983). Near training techniques. In Jose, R. T. (Ed.), *Understanding low vision* (pp. 317–362). New York: American Foundation for the Blind.

Wheeler, J., & Wheeler, K. (1985). *Type to learn.* Pleasantville, NY: Sunburst Communications.

Whittaker, S. G., & Lovie-Kitchin, J. (1993). Visual requirements for reading. *Optometry & Visual Science, 70*(1), 54–65.

Wiggins, G., & McTighe, J. (1998). *Understanding by design.* Alexandria, VA: Council for Exceptional Children: Association for Supervision and Curriculum Development.

Wilkinson, M. (2000). Low vision devices: An overview. In F. M. D'Andrea, & C. Farrenkopf, (Eds.), *Looking to learn: Promoting literacy for students with low vision* (pp. 117–136). New York: AFB Press.

Williams, M. S., & Shellenberger, S. (1996). *How does your engine run? A leader's guide to the alert program for self-regulation.* Albuquerque: Therapy Works, Inc.

Zimmerman, G. J. (1996). Optics and low vision devices. In A. L. Corn, & A. J. Koenig (Eds.), *Foundations of low vision: Clinical and functional perspectives* (pp. 115–142). New York: AFB Press.

Roles of Team Members in Educational Programming to Promote Vision Functioning

Each member of the interdisciplinary team plays a crucial role in determining programming to promote vision functioning for students with low vision. The following sections list the most common team members and their contributions.

Student

➤ Provides information about frequently occurring tasks at home, in the community, at school, and in the workplace (e.g., hobbies and favorite leisure-time activities; family activities; chores; school schedule; extracurricular activities and clubs; and job duties and environment).

➤ Provides information about how tasks are currently completed and which ones are visually difficult.

➤ Provides information about vision in functional terms (e.g., changes in vision; distances at which objects and people can be identified; preferred print size; and reading speed).

➤ Provides information about compensatory methods currently used as well as those tried previously but rejected.

➤ Provides information about future goals.

Parents

➤ Provides information about the child's present level of performance by sharing his or her vision history, vision capabilities, and difficulties.

➤ Ensures child receives eye exams at the frequency recommended by the eye care specialist and provides team with access to eye reports.

➤ Provides information about vision goals.

➤ Follows up recommendations in a timely manner so that the IEP can be fully implemented (e.g., getting prescriptions filled, keeping glasses adjusted, and maintaining optical devices and other equipment).

➤ Identifies activities that occur frequently in the child's home and community.

➤ Integrates vision goals into home and community environments (e.g., encouraging their child to use acquired skills and teaching him or her to keep environmental adaptations and assistive devices in places where they will be accessed, for example, by taking a telescope and pocket magnifier on a family outing to play miniature golf).

➤ Reinforces use of vision when child is out of school (e.g., drawing their child's attention to objects or people in the environment that may be overlooked, for example, by pointing out the location of an airplane in the sky using the concept of a clock or showing the child the send button on the drive-through bank teller window).

➤ Maintains a portfolio of the child's work for evidence of change in performance.

➤ Converses with their child about future dreams, current achievements, and social and emotional issues concerning visual impairment and emphasize what he or she has achieved (e.g., feelings, eye condition, functional vision skills).

➤ Participates in support groups and share information obtained there with team members.

➤ Shares techniques that they have discovered that assist child in using vision efficiently or ways to motivate child.

Teacher of Students with Visual Impairments

➤ Usually serves as the case manager for a student with visual impairments and provides links with other service providers (e.g., reviews records from eye care specialists and related service providers.)

➤ Provides information about the student's vision in layperson's language to IEP team members.

➤ Provides information about the student's present level of performance through:

- functional assessment of visual abilities for tasks critical to the student's success now and in the future.

- learning media assessment.

- environmental assessment.

➤ Works collaboratively with team members to develop a plan for vision instruction that infuses the use of visual skills, environmental adaptations, and assistive devices into frequently occurring tasks.

➤ Works collaboratively with team members to implement vision-related portions of the IEP by providing direct instruction, providing appropriate materials, and instructing other team members in ways to implement vision goals.

➤ Monitors the implementation of vision-related portions of the IEP and evaluates progress.

Orientation and Mobility Specialist

➤ Provides information about the student's present level of performance through a functional assessment of vision related to the ability to orient and move safely through space.

➤ Works collaboratively with team members through an interdisciplinary approach to develop a plan for mobility instruction that integrates the teaching of compensatory methods related to vision into frequently occurring tasks.

➤ Works collaboratively with team members to implement vision-related portions of the IEP by providing direct instruction, providing appropriate materials, and instructing other team members in ways to implement vision goals safely within specific mobility tasks.

(continued on next page)

General Education Teacher

➤ Provides the context in which visual skills will be infused, including information about the

- general curriculum.

- classroom and school environment.

- student's daily and weekly schedule, including transitions between activities, classes, and environments.

- student's social interaction with peers, both nondisabled and disabled.

➤ Provides information about assessment needs in relation to the general education curriculum (e.g., assessment tools utilized by the teacher or state-mandated testing for which individual modifications may need to be considered).

➤ Maintains a portfolio of the student's work for assessment.

➤ Works with the teacher of students with visual impairments and related service personnel to infuse compensatory instruction related to vision into meaningful activities.

Representative of the Local Education Agency or School Administrator

➤ Contributes information regarding the general curriculum.

➤ Provides information regarding the resources of the agency and locates personnel and funding to meet the IEP.

➤ Ensures that the IEP is implemented by providing or supervising the provision of instruction designed to meet the unique needs of the student with low vision.

➤ Encourages an interdisciplinary approach by providing time for staff to meet collaboratively and discuss IEP implementation throughout the school year.

Primary Eye Care Provider (Ophthalmologist or Optometrist)

➤ Provides information about the student's present level of performance through a clinical assessment of vision that includes:

- diagnosis of visual condition.

- prognosis of eye condition (i.e., stability of eye condition).

- results of a general vision assessment.

➤ Provides information about the potential to maximize the student's vision through medical, surgical, and/or optical means.

➤ Provides information about the eye condition to the student, the student's parents, and school personnel (with parental permission).

➤ Provides resources for additional information about the eye condition.

➤ Identifies a treatment plan (e.g., when eyeglasses are to be worn, and when to return to clinic).

➤ Refers students with low vision for a low vision examination and collaborates with the ophthalmologist or optometrist providing low vision services.

➤ Refers students for additional medical or educational services as appropriate.

Low Vision Specialist (Ophthalmologist or Optometrist)

➤ Provides information about the student's present level of performance through an assessment of vision and visual potential using specialized assessment instruments and procedures covering:

- health of the eye.
- refractive error.
- visual acuities.
- visual field.
- binocularity.
- eye motility, eccentric viewing positions, and null point of nystagmus.
- illumination and glare difficulties.
- contrast sensitivity.
- color vision.
- other areas as necessary.

➤ Provides information to parents, student, and team members regarding the functional implications of the student's eye condition and visual status.

➤ Provides information about the ocular effects of medications and systemic diseases.

➤ Helps to clarify appropriate visual goals.

➤ Contributes information that can be used to determine related services and supplementary aids to be provided to the student to maximize the student's functional vision (e.g., environmental modifications and nonoptical and optical devices).

➤ Prescribes eyeglasses, contact lenses, or low vision devices as appropriate and may provide some training in use of devices.

➤ Consults with the teacher of students with visual impairments and the orientation and mobility instructor in the implementation of educational programming.

➤ Refers the student for additional medical or educational services as appropriate.

Counselor or Psychologist

➤ Addresses social and psychological concerns of the student and family.

(continued on next page)

➤ Addresses motivational issues related to low vision and low vision instruction (e.g., fitting in with peers and concerns about the use of environmental modifications and assistive devices).

➤ Suggests referrals to local or national support groups for the student and family or introduction to adults with low vision who may serve as role models.

Physical and/or Occupational Therapist

➤ Contributes information about proper positioning to support efficient use of vision (e.g., relationship of chair to floor, chair to table, and elbow to table heights; and use of back supports).

➤ Contributes information for educational planning concerning integration of sensory systems, and development of visual-motor coordination skills.

➤ Collaborates in the determination of adaptive materials for students with visual and physical disabilities.

Transition Specialist, Vocational Rehabilitation Counselor, or Rehabilitation Teacher (Roles May Vary in Different Service Systems)

➤ Assists the student and his or her family in locating resources and obtaining materials to assist with visual functioning after graduation from high school.

➤ Provides vocational assessments and career guidance to the student to provide pre-vocational training prior to graduation to optimize vision capabilities on identified work tasks.

➤ Provides job and work site analyses, including analysis of visual environment and visual demands of employment tasks in jobs prior to graduation.

➤ Provides functional vision assessment including how an individual uses vision for tasks in the home, workplace, or community, and an environmental analysis (Wolffe, 1996).

References

Wolffe, K. E. (1996). Adults with low vision: Personal, social, and independent living needs. In A. L. Corn & A. J. Koenig, (Eds.), *Foundations of low vision: Clinical and functional perspectives* (pp. 115–142). New York: AFB Press.

Teaching Telescope Use for School Age Students

JANICE SMITH

Promoting Care of Telescopes

An important part of independent use of a telescope is its proper care and maintenance. The primary steps in proper care include the following:

➤ Unzip case and take out telescope.

➤ Take lens caps off the telescope and place into case; zip up case so that lens cap is not lost.

➤ Clean lenses with lint-free cloth or use small amount of rubbing alcohol and cotton-tipped applicator.

➤ Use wrist strap or neck strap.

➤ Keep telescope in holder on desk for easy access during classroom activities.

➤ Replace lens caps before putting telescope away.

➤ Wind strap around telescope, return to case, and zip up case.

➤ Report any problems or loss immediately to the instructor.

Determining Which Eye to Use

Some students may require assistance identifying the preferred eye for optimal viewing of targets.

➤ Encourage student to use the eye with better visual acuity.

➤ Student may prefer to use the eye with poorer acuity if he or she has restrictions in the visual field of the eye with better acuity.

➤ If both eyes are similar in acuity, check with student as to preferred eye.

➤ If unsure, ask student to look through a tube or in a kaleidoscope; observe several times and note preferred eye.

➤ If both eyes are used, have the student practice using the telescope with both eyes.

Holding the Telescope with Both Hands

Students who first learn to hold the telescope properly will have more success using it for critical tasks.

➤ Hold eye cup using thumb and index finger of hand on same side of body as eye.

➤ Hold barrel of telescope with opposite hand.

➤ Attach a grip to the telescope if student is physically unable to hold telescope.

(continued on next page)

➤ If student has motor control problems not overcome by practice:

- Use telescope with arms braced on table or chest.

- Mount telescope on a tripod or stand and prefocus for specific task

- Discuss problem with low vision practitioner who may prescribe a pair of binoculars, a heavier (larger) telescope, a lower power telescope with a larger viewing area, or a spectacle-mounted or clip-on monocular telescope (for comfort, attach a Velcro strap to spectacles to take weight off nose).

Finding the Target with Unaided Vision (without the Telescope)

Learning to find a target unaided will give students a reference point for orienting the telescope.

➤ Align nose with object to be viewed (if using eccentric viewing, point nose toward target and move eye to best viewing position).

➤ If the student has difficulty with alignment, have student point at the target with finger of hand used to hold barrel of the telescope.

➤ Work at closer distances initially and gradually move further away.

➤ Work indoors at first where lighting and glare can be controlled.

➤ Use adequate lighting and contrasting materials.

Maintaining Head and Eye Position

Learning to keep the head and eye position steady while keeping both hands on the telescope and smoothly bringing it up to the eye improves students' ability to view the target.

➤ Rest hand holding eye cup on facial structures to stabilize.

➤ Keep elbows and arms close to body.

➤ If the student has difficulty locating eye (e.g., brings telescope up to forehead or looks down at telescope instead of at target), have student massage area around eye or use object with larger opening for practice (e.g., paper tube).

➤ If student complains of movement or shaking, have him or her rest elbows on back of chair or high table or switch to lower power telescope for initial instruction and then back to prescribed power as he or she experiences success with its use.

Holding the Telescope as Close to the Eye as Possible

Holding the telescope close to the eye will give students a target with a greater field of view.

➤ Check to make sure hand holding eyecup is against face.

➤ If student wears glasses, turning back the rubber eye cup can increase the field of view, and gluing a piece of felt or rubber washer on the ring around the lens prevents scratching lens of glasses.

➤ If student reports seeing black, he or she is unable to find exit pupil. Try working in darkened room with brightly lit target, reposition telescope in front of eye, and check telescope to make sure it is not broken.

Keeping the Telescope on a Target

The most efficient use of the telescope is achieved when the student demonstrates no movement of the head or telescope while fixing on a stationary target.

➤ Initially work at a distance of 10 ft. and hold targets directly in front of student.

➤ Focus the telescope for the student.

➤ If student has difficulty at this distance, move in closer and refocus the telescope for the new distance.

➤ Require accuracy (aim for at least 90 percent) before moving on to new skills.

● Provide feedback but move toward having the student evaluate his or her own performance.

● If student was not on target (watch for movement of head or telescope), ask student to put down telescope, point nose toward target, and try again.

● If student was on target, let him or her know (students may enjoy inserting coins or tokens into container for each correct response and charting their performance over time).

➤ When successful, teach student to find targets above and below direct line of sight, and to align body with targets at the same distance but to the student's right or left.

Focusing a Telescope

Systematic instruction for viewing an image through a focused telescope will give the student more information about the target.

Concepts

➤ If the student does not understand the concept of a clear image, teach through analogies such as tuning a radio or focusing a slide projector, overhead projector, or closed-circuit television.

➤ Teach the student that once the telescope has been correctly focused for targets at a given distance, refocusing will not provide a clearer image (if the instructor has confirmed that the telescope is in focus, attempts by the student to refocus are an indication that the target is too small).

➤ Teach concept of depth of focus (the range of distances at which it is possible to focus the telescope).

Procedure

➤ Turn housing until it is all the way out so that the barrel of the telescope is fully extended.

(continued on next page)

➤ Then, *slowly* turn the housing in the opposite direction until the image is clear.

➤ Continue turning the housing in the same direction until the image begins to blur.

➤ Finally, turn housing in opposite direction until image is the clearest possible.

Using Telescopes Efficiently

Students need systematic instruction to determine the focusing capabilities of a telescope.

➤ If the image is not clear after the student has used standard focusing procedures, the size of the target may be too large. If the student can identify the target, then greater clarity of target may not be necessary.

➤ Ask student to refocus telescope as you move target closer and note closest distance at which the student can obtain a clear image.

➤ Teach the student to step back and then refocus when he or she is trying to view an object that is too close.

➤ Teach student that if he or she has focused on a target at 20 ft, targets farther away will also be in focus. If the student cannot see a target at a greater distance clearly, teach the student to move closer and refocus.

➤ Provide student sufficient practice in focusing the telescope to view objects at a variety of distances (check focus intermittently).

➤ Identify the most critical tasks for telescope use. Focus the telescope for one of the tasks and paint a contrasting colored line along the entire length of the housing. Teach the student to turn the housing to match the colored line in order to focus the telescope for that task. Such lines can be marked in different colors for several common tasks (Berg, Jose, & Carter, 1983).

➤ If the student is unable to learn to focus accurately with consistent practice, consult with low vision practitioner, who may prescribe a fixed focus telescope.

➤ Students who wear eyeglasses will achieve a larger field of view if they remove their eyeglasses and use their telescope directly, provided the telescope has a good range of focus adjustability. However, for most handheld telescopes, it is difficult or impossible to incorporate a correction for astigmatism. If a student has astigmatism and takes off his or her eyeglasses, the image will be somewhat blurred and taking off eyeglasses may not be advisable. It is best to consult with a low vision practitioner to determine whether or not a student should use a telescope with or without eyeglasses.

Reading Words and Signs

Reading words on signs in the environment (e.g., finding the correct bus stop or identifying a business address) is important for independent travel in the community.

➤ First present individual letters that are symmetrical (*x, i, o*).

➤ Increase complexity gradually from two-letter words to four- and five-letter words.

➤ Ask student to read one letter at a time after centering each in the telescope and then to identify the word (l–o–o–k, look).

➤ The first and last letters in the word are easier to read than reading the middle letters. If the student has difficulty, try covering the letters before and after the letter the student is trying to read. If the student is still unable to read the letters in the middle of a word, use larger letters or move closer.

Tracing

Efficient movement of the head and telescope as a unit for tracing along a stationary line will improve the student's ability to find the intended target.

➤ Trace along an edge that is perpendicular to student (e.g., bulletin board, tracing along a geometric shape during math class).

➤ Change the focus of the telescope while tracing a line which projects away from the student or toward the student (e.g., tracing along a baseball diamond).

➤ Encourage student to trace slowly and accurately.

➤ Practice tracing along lines in the environment to find a target (e.g., tracing the line for a pedestrian crosswalk across the street to find the corner prior to scanning for the pole for a street sign).

Tracking

Efficient movements of the head and telescope as a unit for tracking will improve the student's ability to follow, or track, a moving target.

➤ Track a target that is perpendicular to the student and moving horizontally.

➤ Track a target that is perpendicular to the student and moving vertically.

➤ Track a target that is moving diagonally away from the student.

➤ Track a target that is moving diagonally toward the student.

➤ Track a target moving toward and parallel to the student.

➤ Track a target moving in curved paths.

➤ Begin with slow-moving objects.

➤ Gradually increase rate of movement of objects.

➤ Always put the telescope down before walking.

Aligning the Body Directly in Front of a Target

A better field of view for the target is achieved when one is aligned with it.

➤ Teach safety (e.g., the student should not stand in street or parking lot to align with a target).

➤ Teach student to reduce glare off surfaces by stepping slightly to one side of the surface.

(continued on next page)

Appropriate Scanning of Patterns

The student needs to know where the target physically exists in the environment before the telescope can be used efficiently to locate objects not seen with unaided vision.

➤ Use horizontal scanning pattern to locate vertical objects.

➤ Use vertical scanning pattern to locate horizontal objects.

➤ Teach student to move telescope, head, and body as one unit.

➤ Teach students typical location of objects (e.g., house numbers near doorways, airline departure and arrival times on screens hanging from airport terminal ceiling).

Spotting Stationary Objects When Moving

When traveling in a bus or car, the student learns to recognize visual landmarks for location of destinations and orientation in a new environment.

➤ Allow students to sit in front passenger seat where they have an unobstructed view.

➤ Teach students to spot stationary targets far ahead, refocusing the telescope while moving closer (e.g., billboards, buildings, major street signs, speed limit signs).

➤ Students will experience dizziness if attempting to view objects out of car's side windows using a telescope.

➤ Teach students to spot moving objects while moving (seated in a car, bus, etc.).

Reference

Berg, R. V., Jose, R. T., & Carter, K. (1983). Distance training technique. In R. T. Jose (Ed.), *Understanding low vision* (pp. 277–316). New York: American Foundation for the Blind.

Teaching Video Magnifier Use for School Age Students

IRENE TOPOR AND IKE PRESLEY

Selecting the Appropriate Video Magnifier

Several models of video magnifiers are available to learners, and the type selected should match the requirements of the individual student's school, home, and work tasks.

Types of Systems

Desktop or Stand-Alone Units

Stand-alone systems include in-line viewing (the monitor is placed above camera on stand), separate camera, and television-based systems. These systems have a fixed camera, X-Y table, and a monitor located on top of or to the side of the camera. The material to be viewed is placed on the X-Y table and is shown on the monitor.

Portable Systems

The camera of portable systems is built into a small plastic case. The camera is rolled across surfaces of text and the image is displayed on a monitor. Since the camera is portable, labels and text on uneven surfaces, such as cylinder-shaped containers, can be read. This type of model is not easily used for writing unless a stand is provided for the camera.

Head-Mounted Systems

Head-mounted systems allow learners to use their hands because the camera is mounted at eye level and the monitor is built into the headgear. Some systems have autofocus. Learners who have excellent eye-hand coordination may find this system most appealing. As these systems become less expensive and cosmetically more attractive to students, more of these may be used in classrooms.

Factors in Selecting a System

Type of Task

For sustained reading, a desktop model might work most easily, while a portable model is better for short reading assignments or for locating a city, state, or country on a map. Television monitors have lower resolution than video monitors and may be less desirable for some learners engaged in sustained reading tasks. If writing is the primary purpose for using the video magnifier, the learner may want a desktop system with stand-alone or in-line monitors. If a learner attends different classes throughout the day and uses the video magnifier for many subject areas, a portable system may be more advantageous. When purchasing a video magnifier, a black and white or color monitor is a choice. If cost is not a factor in this decision, determine the kinds of information in color the learner will access to help decide if a color monitor is necessary.

(continued on next page)

Space Available

CCTVs with separate monitors tend to be less expensive than stand-alone types, but they require a compatible monitor to view the enlarged image. D'Andrea (2000) notes that larger monitors take up more space and may not fit easily on a table or desk.

Expense

Desktop and handheld cameras are less expensive than head-mounted systems, although the price of the head-mounted systems is decreasing.

Students' Motor Ability

The team should note if the learner has any fine or gross motor involvement that will limit his or her ability to move the X-Y tray. If so, other systems may be more desirable.

Teaching Video Magnifier Use

Getting the Learner Interested

Before instruction begins, a primary goal of the teacher should be the learner's motivation to use a new system. The learner will discover the benefits of a video magnifier by using it to view familiar two- or three-dimensional objects.

For learners with compromised motor or cognitive skills, magnification may be confusing because they are seeing part of the image and not the whole. Make sure that the learner understands that, for example, the nose of a dog is just a part of the picture. The learner will be instructed to move the mouse up, down, to the right or to the left to see the rest of the dog. Students are more easily motivated by viewing objects they bring from home:

➤ These include material of special interest to the learner and the class. For example, one young learner had pet worms that she watched on her monitor. The worms had hairs all over their bodies. These delicate hairs were visible to all as the entire class gathered around the monitor to watch them.

➤ Family photographs to view detail in faces of grandparents, sisters, brothers, parents, and friends.

➤ Photographs of favorite baseball or rock stars on trading cards or in teen magazines.

➤ Favorite pictures in books or magazines for details previously difficult to see.

➤ Athletic records of favorite athletes or teams.

➤ Finger scrapes, cuts, and sores are a viewing attraction for young children.

➤ Images from learner's personal collection of photographs, pictures, or drawings.

Familiarizing Students with the Video Magnifier

To begin familiarizing the student with the video magnifier, follow these steps:

➤ Lock the X-Y table, friction brake, and margin stops for the student.

➤ Ask him or her to identify an image at the smallest magnification.

➤ Slowly increase the size until the learner can identify it.

➤ Encourage the learner to maintain a comfortable viewing distance. This can be determined based on vision evaluation results and learner preference. Many students choose to view within a range of 10 to 15 in.

➤ Ask the learner to identify details and then slowly increase the size until the viewer can identify them easily.

Essential Video Magnifier Functions

For video magnifiers that have manual focus, the learner needs to master four functions to operate them effectively. In teaching these steps, the instructor does not lock the X-Y table, friction brake, or margin stops or prefocus the camera.

1. Operate the power switch.

2. Use size and focus functions to allow viewer to adjust magnification and focus.

3. Learn brightness and contrast functions. The teacher can demonstrate the effects these controls have on the image being viewed. Allow the user to manipulate these controls with line drawings, photographs, and objects. Point out how these controls may need to be adjusted for the different images being viewed.

4. Operate color and polarity functions. The teacher can demonstrate the effect these controls have on the image being viewed. Allow the user to manipulate these controls with line drawings, photographs, and objects. Point out how these controls may need to be adjusted for the different images being viewed. Note that the learner may prefer different settings for line drawings, photographs, and three-dimensional objects.

Promoting Care of the Equipment

In addition to learning how to use the video magnifier system, the learner needs to keep the system free of debris and glare and know what to do if the system is not operating correctly.

➤ Remove items on and around the video magnifier that are not necessary for current use. Ample space should be available for system and needed materials.

➤ Check position of video magnifier for glare on monitor. Reposition monitor if necessary. Monitor should be away from and perpendicular to windows.

➤ Check for cleanliness of monitor. If necessary, clean with lint-free cloth or a small amount of rubbing alcohol on a cloth to wipe smudges or prints off the monitor.

➤ Use dust cover to protect monitor when not in use.

➤ Report any problems or loss immediately to instructor.

Preparing the Environment

The student who learns to prepare the video magnifier environment will have greater success and opportunity to use the electronic projection system.

(continued on next page)

➤ Learn location and function of knobs on the video magnifier to turn on and off, lock and unlock the X-Y table, set polarity, and adjust focus.

➤ Lock X-Y table, friction brake, and margin stops.

➤ Adjust supplemental lighting so that there is ample light to see the monitor image while not producing glare on the monitor.

➤ Position chair so that student's feet are flat on the floor and his or her back is straight. Smaller students can use a foot cushion if needed.

➤ Move chair or video magnifier to the appropriate viewing distance as determined by results of the low vision evaluation or functional vision evaluation.

➤ Materials to be used with video magnifier should be within arm's reach before instruction begins.

➤ Note preference for black-on-white or white-on-black image. Differentiate between graphics and text.

➤ Note preferences for various color combinations of the image being enlarged.

➤ Use tempered glass over reading material if necessary to keep it relatively flat.

Focusing Two- and Three-Dimensional Objects

Students who can independently focus the video magnifier will experience increased clarity in viewing objects, pictures, or words.

➤ Determine if the video magnifier is autofocus or manual focus. If the video magnifier is autofocus, three-dimensional objects may be more difficult to bring into focus for detail.

➤ Place a full page of names and phone numbers from a telephone directory on the X-Y table. If the video magnifier is manual focus, turn knob in the direction that increases the size of the image.

➤ Focus the print at the largest size using the focus knob. Once the image is focused, it will not be necessary to refocus unless reading material is placed closer to or further away from the camera.

➤ Adjust the print to preferred size by turning the size knob. Do not touch the focus knob. If the material is no longer in focus when the print sizes change, repeat focusing at the largest size setting. If focus still is not maintained when sizes change, the video magnifier may need to be repaired.

➤ Check all sides of the paper on the screen to ensure that all written text or graphics are within view.

Determining Optimal Magnification

Students will benefit most by using the size print necessary at a comfortable viewing distance to sustain reading for the desired task.

➤ For learners who are unable to appreciate print comfortably at a 10- to 15-in. reading distance, begin by having them view an image on screen at 6 in. from a 20- to 21-in. screen.

➤ Learners can then move to 8 to 10 in. away from the screen so that an entire line of print is in their field of view.

➤ Magnification should be determined for learners who are at a comfortable reading distance for a sustained period of time.

➤ Learners may choose a bigger monitor rather than increased screen magnification. A bigger screen is a more efficient way for some learners to see the image without having to navigate around the screen.

➤ Learners' reading rate and comfort can be determined at a given working distance with varying print sizes to determine the best print sizes at this distance. It is best to determine optimal print size and working distance in consultation with an eye care specialist.

➤ The following suggestions may be useful for learners who may need more magnification than is available on the video magnifier:

- Use the zoom capability on recent Windows programs. The learner can zoom to 500 percent; however after 3× to 4× enlargements, pixels on these magnification programs become visible. If this is distracting to the learner, a software magnification program may be necessary.

- Use screen magnification software with color and contrast features. Enlargement of the image beyond 3× or 4× may be easier to see if the program has a smoothing feature. These programs enable the learner to enlarge one line of text at a time and also have a magnifier "lens" feature.

- A speech feature accompanying the visual information allows the learner to confirm what is seen on screen.

Adjusting the Reading Table

Proper adjustment of the X-Y table will allow for increased concentration on the reading task.

➤ Tighten the drag knob so that the table moves smoothly.

➤ Tighten the drag knob the entire way and move margin stops into the center to tighten if task can best be done on a stable table.

➤ Set margin stops at the left and right margins for long-term reading.

➤ Set friction brake for controlled up and down movement of the X-Y table.

Other Useful Activities

Learners need instruction specific to the mechanics of the video magnifier to ensure their successful use of it.

➤ Horizontal tracking (left to right, one row). Lock friction brake and adjust margin stops. Start with simple activities in which the viewer moves the table horizontally (see activities in *Ann Arbor Tracking Program*, available from http://www.annarbor.co.uk.

(continued on next page)

➤ Vertical tracking (top to bottom). This includes moving horizontally and vertically using mazes and matching activities.

➤ Searching for items on the screen. This can be done using "what's missing" and "what's wrong" pictures such as those in *Highlights* magazine for children (http://www.highlights.com); and horizontal tracking in multiple rows using, for example, the *Ann Arbor Tracking Program* (available from http://www.annarbor.co.uk) and the activities suggested by D'Andrea (2000).

Learning to Read More Efficiently

Strategies to facilitate reading and looking include using the shapes of words and context to predict words (ascenders, descenders, wide letters); reading sentences that fit on one line; and setting margin stops and friction brake. A learner can also use double, triple, or greater spacing between lines, and look away after reading to decrease fatigue.

Some CCTV users may experience motion sickness when first learning to read magnified text. Lund and Watson (1997) suggest ways to reduce feelings of nausea or dizziness while reading:

➤ Eat a soda cracker before the session begins.

➤ Expose one line at a time with an electronic line marker.

➤ Slowly increase reading speed.

Writing More Efficiently

Learners need specialized instruction to write efficiently using the video magnifier. Try the following strategies:

➤ Lock the X-Y table.

➤ Work in two planes (learner writes on paper placed on horizontal X-Y table but looks at monitor on vertical plane).

➤ For eye-hand coordination, trace stencils and templates, complete activities connecting dots, match like figures, search for words, complete crossword puzzles, write using lined and unlined paper.

Additional References

D'Andrea, F. M. (2000). Activities for teaching the use of the CCTV for reading. In D'Andrea & C. Farrenkopf (Eds.), *Looking to learn: Promoting literacy for students with low vision* (pp. 210–212). New York: AFB Press.

Lund, R., & Watson, G. R. (1997). *The CCTV book: Habilitation and rehabilitation with closed circuit television systems.* Lillesand, Norway: Synsforum and Froland.

McCall, K. (2002). *The box came today . . . now what do I do? A resource for CCTV assessment and training.* Toronto: Karlen Communications.

Presley, I. (2001). Instructional strategies for using video magnifiers (CCTVs) to facilitate literacy. Paper presented at Getting in Touch with Literacy Conference, Philadelphia, PA.

Selecting Fonts for Readers with Low Vision

ARIES ARDITI

People with low vision are often unsatisfied with the size and style of fonts used for printed material. This is not surprising, since low vision readers are often reading at their acuity limit, where subtle variations in typeface and layout may make the critical difference between their being able to read and not. As a result, the relationship between typographic variables and legibility has practical consequences for the low vision reader.

Commercially available fonts vary along many dimensions, making it difficult to study font characteristics individually. Using fonts that are defined parametrically (i.e., by assigning parameter values to font features, such as stroke width) and generated by a computer program, however, typographic variables can be studied in relative isolation. The results of studies of font parameters and legibility are summarized below.

Point Size

Point size affects the overall size of letters, but this measure usually gauges only the vertical size of a font. Font point size strongly affects legibility, since, as is well-known, optical magnification and large print make print more readable; indeed, we often measure and the legibility of written materials based on minimum readable size (i.e., acuity). However, a font's point size is not a fixed or objective measure: different fonts may have very different letter form sizes even if they have the same nominal point size. Computer-designed typography is changing this somewhat. It is now fairly conventional in computer typography to use the point size to describe the sum of the height of the tallest (upper-case) letter and the lowest descender (i.e., the minimum vertical size needed to set the font without successive lines overlapping).

X-height

X-height is the height (in absolute measure, such as printer's points, or relative measure, such as a percentage of the point size of the font) of a lower-case x of a given font. It characterizes the height, and generally the size, of the body of most lower-case characters (Arditi et al., 1990).

Letter Aspect Ratio

Letter aspect ratio refers to the ratio of width to height of characters in a font, and should be measured using a symmetrical character like O. For fonts of any given (vertical) point size, fonts with different aspect ratios differ only in the width, or fatness, of the letter forms. Fonts with characters that are expanded horizontally are generally more legible (Arditi et al., 1995a) because such expansion is a form of (horizontal) magnification; however, like most things that enhance legibility, a large width-to-height ratio prints fewer characters on each line, and as a consequence, can increase printing costs.

(continued on next page)

Interletter Spacing

Spacing between letters has a significant impact on legibility, especially at small sizes relative to a person's visual acuity (Arditi et al., 1990). Since people with low vision are often reading close to their acuity limit (i.e., with little acuity *reserve*), adding additional space between letters is particularly advantageous to them. Again, printing costs may increase, because there are fewer characters on each line.

Proportionality of Spacing

Fixed- and variable-spaced (also called proportional) fonts differ in the amount of horizontal space occupied by each character. With variable spacing, characters generally take up only the amount required by the character form; for example, a lower-case *i* takes up far less space than an upper-case W. With fixed spacing, all characters take up the same amount of space, generally the width of the widest letter (usually the W). Fixed-space fonts are more legible at small character sizes (relative to acuity). However, it appears that it is not the proportionality of the font that is important: the legibility advantage can be fully accounted for by the fact that the average interletter spacing is greater in fixed than in variable-spaced fonts (Arditi et al., 1990).

Color and Contrast

A complete discussion of this topic is beyond the scope of this brief appendix (for more information see Arditi, 1999a) but, in general, using very dark (i.e., close to black, or black itself) against very light (i.e., close to white, or white itself) colors yields the most effective contrasts. For people with some types of low vision, light letters against a dark background are more effective than the reverse.

Stroke Width

Stroke width refers to the thickness of the strokes making up the letters. In general, bolder strokes are more legible than lighter ones (Arditi et al., 1995b). However, when strokes become too bold, the letter forms "fill in" and become less legible. In general, however, thin-stroked fonts are considerably less legible than thick-stroked fonts of the same size.

Outline vs. Filled

Outline fonts, in which the interior of letter strokes has been removed, are far less legible than filled fonts of the same size (Arditi et al., 1997), and should be avoided for use by the low vision reader.

Serifs

Serifs are the little "feet" that punctuate the ends of strokes on most lower-case and some upper-case letters of specific fonts. Our research (Arditi & Cho, 2000a) has recently shown that fonts with serifs have a minuscule advantage in legibility over sans-serif fonts, but that the advantage is wholly accounted for by the small increase in interletter spacing that fonts with serifs must have to avoid collisions with neighboring letters. This advantage is so small, however, as to have virtually no impact on the decision to select a serif or sans-serif font. Both can be highly legible.

Letter Case

Common wisdom, aesthetics, and some studies from cognitive science suggest that words composed of lower-case letters are more easily identified than those of upper-case letters, presumably because word shape in the former is more distinctive. Our recent results (Arditi & Cho, 2000b), however, indicate that upper-case characters are more legible than lower-case, for both readers with low vision and those with unimpaired vision, both in terms of minimum discriminable size (acuity) and reading speed. The reason is simple: when equated for point size, upper-case letters are simply bigger.

Familiarity

Standard roman and sans-serif fonts are much more legible than ornate, nonstandard, or decorative fonts. Letter forms should be simple and easily recognizable, avoiding special effects such as drop-shadows and three-dimensional shading.

References

Arditi, A. (1996). Typography, print legibility, and low vision. In R. Cole & B. Rosenthal (Eds.), *Remediation and management of low vision* (pp. 237–248). St. Louis: Mosby.

Arditi, A. (1999a). *Effective color contrast: Designing for people with partial sight and color deficiencies.* New York: Arlene R. Gordon Research Institute, Lighthouse International.

Arditi, A. (1999b). *Making text legible: Designing for people with partial sight.* New York: Arlene R. Gordon Research Institute, Lighthouse International.

Arditi, A., Knoblauch, K. and Grunwald, I. (1990). Reading with fixed and variable character pitch. *Journal of the Optical Society of America A, 7,* 2011–2015.

Arditi, A., Cagenello, R. and Jacobs B. (1995a). Effects of aspect ratio and spacing on legibility of small letters. *Supplement to Investigative Ophthalmology and Visual Science, 36*(4), S671.

Arditi, A., Cagnello, R. and Jacobs B. (1995b). Letter stroke width, spacing and legibility. In: *Vision Science and its Applications, 1,* 1995 OSA Technical Digest Series. Washington, D.C.: Optical Society of America, 324–327.

Arditi, A. & Cho, J. (2000a). Do serifs enhance or diminish text legibility? *Investigative Ophthalmology and Visual Science* (Supplement) *41*(4), S437.

Arditi, A. and Cho, J. (2000). Letter case and text legibility. Supplement to *Perception, 29,* 45.

Arditi, A., Liu, L., and Lynn, W. (1997). Legibility of outline and solid fonts with wide and narrow spacing. In D. Yager (Ed.), *Trends in Optics and Photonics,* Vol. 11. Washington, D.C.: Optical Society of America.

Interventions for Adults with Visual Impairments

R. D. QUILLMAN AND GREGORY GOODRICH

E ffectively delivered vision rehabilitation services can transform people's ability to perform everyday tasks and, in turn, their lives. According to Rosenbloom (2000, p. 90), "low vision rehabilitation is a process comprising a range of services directed in a coordinated manner toward helping the person with low vision achieve fulfilling and realizable goals in those activities affected by vision loss." As previous chapters have shown, the goals of low vision services for children and adolescents may often focus on promoting growth and development and the ability to perform functional as well as academic tasks. For adults of working age, rehabilitation goals most often center around transition from school to work, career exploration and planning, employment, underemployment, and preparation for retirement (Leonard, 2000) in addition to daily living, independent travel, participation in the community, and psychosocial concerns. Crews (2000) highlights the need for coordinated, comprehensive services for elderly people with visual impairment that include social work, rehabilitation teaching, orientation and mobility (O&M), low vision, and peer support services to address health, psychosocial, travel, vocational, leisure, and daily living concerns. For all adults with low vision, an important part of these services is functional vision evaluation and intervention correlated with critical activities identified by the clients that promote their fullest possible integration in work, home, and community environments.

This chapter focuses primarily on three issues: (1) intervention methods related to optimizing the use of vision in near and distance tasks, (2) guidelines for the selection of environmental modifications that can be incorporated into key life tasks, and (3) instruction in the use of low vision devices that will be used in critical life tasks. An emphasis has been placed on instruction in the use of low vision optical devices for adults since detailed information about this type of training is not often readily available.

The compensatory methods discussed in this chapter can be incorporated into rehabilitation goals related to work and life skills for individuals with low vision. For example, instruction to improve the ability to trace down columns of visual data may be a critical skill for an engineer who needs to monitor daily performance logs for a particular device he has recently developed to improve productivity in a factory assembly line. Instruction in the use of a low vision optical device to read mail may be a major step toward increased independence and feelings of competence for a retiree who has experienced a recent loss of vision. Information about establishing comprehensive rehabilitation goals and rehabilitation plans for individuals with low vision is outside the scope of this chapter. However, the case studies at the end of the chapter illustrate how vision intervention goals are tied to tasks deemed important to the general life concerns of individuals with low vision. More information about comprehensive rehabilitation plans can be found in works by Wolffe (1996), Moore and Wolffe (1996), and Watson (1996).

BACKGROUND

History

Although instruction in the use of low vision devices for people with low vision was advocated by the noted optometrist William Feinbloom (1931), it was not until the late 1960s and early 1970s that the importance of training was recognized. Before 1970, most clinics or agencies—if they did anything at all for this group of clients—had an ophthalmologist or optometrist examine clients, prescribe new eyeglasses, and (on rare occasions) recommend use of a magnifier or a telescope. Teaching people how to use their vision or prescribing assistive devices was rarely considered. Traditional thinking seemed to be that since these people had vision, they must know how to use it, even though they had acquired a visual impairment.

It was not widely acknowledged that people with low vision needed to be shown how to use the available assistive devices or how to use their remaining vision more efficiently. Too often optical devices ended up in a dresser drawer or on a closet shelf. Too often the ophthalmologist or optometrist wondered why this was happening. And too often clients were left wondering if their eye care specialists knew what was best for them and whether the ophthalmologists or optometrists cared whether they were able to use their devices.

With increasing frequency, however, ophthalmologists, optometrists, and other professionals began to recognize the importance of offering people with low vision practical experience in using the devices. People were needed who could teach clients with low vision how exactly to use their vision in conjunction with low vision devices. Eye care practitioners turned to other professionals to conduct this training, usually those already working with people who were blind or visually impaired who were willing to add to their knowledge and increase their responsibilities. Thus, the early 1970s saw an increase in the number of people providing training or instruction to adults with low vision. As more and more professionals realized that low vision rehabilitation was becoming an established and acceptable discipline, the number of members in this new profession quickly grew. No longer was the emphasis on treating all people with visual impairment with techniques developed for people who were totally blind. The new emphasis focused on utilizing a person's available vision, and on ability rather than disability.

Professionals began clamoring for more information about low vision. In 1976, the American Association for Workers of the Blind (AAWB) (Goodrich & Bailey, 2000) formed a Low Vision Division with a primary focus on promoting continuing education in low vision. As other groups, including the American Academy of Optometry and the Low Vision Clinical Society, promoted continuing education, an increasing number of professionals gained knowledge of low vision rehabilitation techniques. These early continuing education offerings were highly successful, and there seemed never to be a lack of attendance at seminars and conferences devoted to low vision. Practitioners wanted to learn about low vision assessment and training, and how to apply that knowledge for each client with low vision. At this time professionals also realized that continued use of an assistive device by a client with low vision was related to the amount of training in its use that he or she received.

Rationale for Instruction

Today it is widely recognized that the success of a low vision program depends on the client using his or her residual vision and any prescribed optical or electronic devices efficiently. When a person's vision changes, he or she needs to become accustomed to altered visual capacities and learn to integrate and use these in the performance of visual tasks. As a result of vision changes, examinations by an ophthalmologist or an optometrist will be done and optical devices may be prescribed. "The importance of proper training in the use of low vision aids cannot be overemphasized for successful vision rehabilitation. Many low vision devices that are unused, are rejected because of inadequate training" (Mehr & Freid, 1975, p. 155).

One of the major concerns in the mid-1970s was making sure that optical device instruction was done under the guidance or consultation of an optometrist or ophthalmologist. That concern still exists, but more and more professionals have realized that all low vision work should be done in a collaborative setting. All professionals providing service to a client with low vision, including those performing low vision evaluations, functional vision evaluations, O&M instruction, counseling, or instruction in daily living skills, need to be in touch with each other and to be prepared to make modifications in instruction based on feedback from the client. Each professional needs to be free to provide expertise to the consumer but also needs to respect the work of the other team members.

Properly conducted and coordinated evaluation and consultation culminate in suggestions for procedures that will help a client to function more independently. Most of these methods involve training. Without instruction, the program may not progress to meaningful outcomes. A person given a computer without training might eventually figure out how to use it, but with training, the person is likely to have a much more positive experience with computers. Similarly, without training in using low vision and low vision devices, the experience is rarely as fulfilling.

It is important to determine that the client is profiting from the use of any prescribed devices. If he or she is not, it could be (1) a device problem—perhaps it is not strong enough, or it is too small to hold; (2) a client issue—perhaps the client is holding the device improperly, is not obtaining proper alignment, or is uncomfortable using the device in public; or (3) a combination of device and client issues. The practitioner must be able to assess these possibilities and suggest any necessary changes.

As with other groups of clients discussed throughout this book, it is crucial to incorporate training for adults in the use of low vision devices into the vocational and daily needs of each client. An individualized written rehabilitation program (IWRP) provides one structure for incorporating low vision objectives into broader life goals for each client (Moore & Wolffe, 1996; Watson, 1996).

Terminology

The term *practitioner* is used throughout this chapter and refers to the professional who conducts functional vision evaluations and provides vision and optical device instruction for adults. Practitioners can be a variety of professionals on the low vision care team, including the ophthalmologist or optometrist, but most often they will be low vision therapists (Watson et al., 1999), occupational therapists, rehabilitation teachers, O&M specialists, and allied health personnel such as nurses with training in low vision (see Chap. 1). It is important that any type of instruction should be done in conjunction with an ophthalmologist or optometrist who has knowledge of low vision and in a collaborative manner that coordinates feedback about the adequacy of the prescribed device for the individual and the effectiveness of training.

OPTIMIZING INSTRUCTIONAL OUTCOMES

People learn in different ways. The low vision practitioner must have an understanding of each client's learning needs in order to maximize his or her instructional outcomes. This includes understanding the unique characteristics of each client, including learning style as well as physical and cognitive capabilities. Methods to make learning relevant to each client's life situation are particularly important for adult learners. This includes attention to the particular needs of clients from culturally or linguistically diverse backgrounds (Merriam & Caffarella, 1999).

Many individuals with low vision require time to adjust to the effects of visual impairment on their lives and the lives of those around them. Recent vision loss may be emotionally draining for some time. It may affect the way an individual learns and the amount of information he or she can take in at one time. Instructional approaches in rehabilitation programs must conform to each client's current learning needs while the client is working through these adjustment issues. (For more information on addressing psychosocial concerns in the rehabilitation process, please see Chapter 1.)

Additional physical factors may also affect learning. Stroke, neurological impairments, and medications that may interfere with an individual's abilities need to be assessed as part of the planning for instruction.

Clinical experience suggests that there are commonalities in low vision intervention programs for adults of all ages, as well as some general training techniques that can help to facilitate positive outcomes for older individuals. These are presented in the sections that follow.

Pace the Introduction of New Ideas

Some people may need to have new information presented to them slowly, a few items at a time, for the reasons mentioned in the previous section. Some clients are more likely to grasp new skills or techniques if they are allowed to absorb a few points each day rather than a lot in one day. If there are five points to master in using a new device or technique, it is may be best to introduce two or three of them the first day and the others on the second or third.

The pace at which new ideas are presented may need to be varied, not only from client to client but also for the same client. Point 1 might be introduced at the beginning of training session one, but the client might not be ready to accept point 2 until the latter part of that training session.

Take Learning Style into Account

It is necessary to ascertain how a client receives and processes information. Some people need material presented to them sequentially (step 1 followed by step 2 followed by step 3, and so on). They may be unable to go from step 1 to step 3 without going through step 2. For one client, the practitioner needs to discover that early and present the information appropriately. Information presented any way other than sequentially will be useless for that client. Conversely, another client B might be presented with step 1 followed by step 5 and grasp steps 2, 3, and 4 intuitively, without explanation. If information is presented to this client in sequence, chances are good that he or she will be bored and reluctant to participate in the training program.

Address Issues of Acceptance

People often have preconceived notions of the effects of vision loss. For whatever reasons, they may have underlying thoughts that tend to revolve around the negative aspects of sight loss: "Why me?" or "I can't do anything now," or "Life is over as far as I am concerned." Sight loss does affect how one conducts oneself, but it is not the end of life. Many wonderful and productive years are left. A good low vision practitioner will work on issues of acceptance as well as the actual training as part of rehabilitation. The most powerful tool in the rehabilitation process is what is inside the client's head (Tuttle & Tuttle, 1996). Sometimes a referral to counseling or to support groups for people with low vision may be beneficial for the client and his or her family.

Dispel Myths About Visual Impairment

Many people believe that any and all visual diseases automatically lead to total blindness. It is necessary to help dispel those thoughts and replace them with accurate information. Such information bears frequent repetition. Reading, activities of daily living, enjoying family photos, many vocational tasks, and other important activities are often possible, while other activities (e.g., driving) may not be. Identifying the reality and dispelling the myths are important components of rehabilitation, but they also should not be overdone. Stating the facts a few times and making sure the client understands is good rehabilitation for people of all ages.

Suggest Functional Possibilities Positively

Giving clients a positive picture of their potential after rehabilitation is another important hurdle to overcome. Reading, for example, is a major area of concern for many clients with low vision who have a difficult time reading or can no longer read. Hearing that reading again is a good possibility, based on results from the low vision and functional vision examinations can be a big relief for a client. No assurances can be made, but stressing positive possibilities can be very productive. It is usually necessary to state that reading will not be done as it was before the vision loss occurred, but that being able to read is very likely.

Recent evidence is consistent with the view that with the proper prescription of a reading device such as a closed-circuit television and proper training, even older visually impaired individuals can read about as fast as age-matched individuals who are not visually impaired. In 2001 investigators from the Smith-Kettlewell Eye Research Foundation published data on the reading speeds of a large sample of elderly persons who were not visually impaired (Brabyn, Schneck, Haegerstrom-Portnoy, & Lott, 2001; Lott et al., 2001), measured using the Pepper Visual Skills for Reading Test (Watson, Whittaker, & Steciw, 1995). These data suggested that reading speeds were slower than previously assumed and decreased

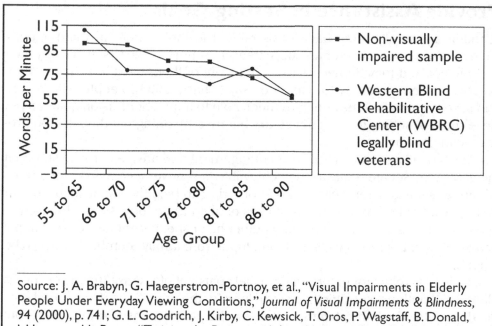

Source: J. A. Brabyn, G. Haegerstrom-Portnoy, et al., "Visual Impairments in Elderly People Under Everyday Viewing Conditions," *Journal of Visual Impairments & Blindness,* 94 (2000), p. 741; G. L. Goodrich, J. Kirby, C. Kewsick, T. Oros, P. Wagstaff, B. Donald, J. Hazen, and L. Peters, "Training the Patient with Low Vision to Read: Does It Significantly Improve Function?" In C. S. Stuen, A. Arditi, Eds., *Vision Rehabilitation: Assessment, Intervention, and Outcomes* (Exton, PA: Swets & Zeitlinger, 2000), p. 230; and L. A. Lott, M. E. Schenck, G. Haegerstrom-Portnoy, J. A. Brabyn, J. A. Gildengorin, and C. G. West, "Reading Performance in Older Adults with Good Acuity," *Optometry and Vision Science,* 78(5) (2001), p. 316.

Figure 10.1. Comparison of reading speeds of 186 legally blind veterans after low vision reading training with speeds reported for an age-matched, non-visually impaired population.

with age. Figure 10.1 compares these data with data from 186 legally blind patients of the Western Blind Rehabilitation Center reading continuous text fifth-grade comprehension materials (Goodrich et al., 2000b). The comparison is limited since the two projects used different measures of reading speed, but the comparison is nevertheless informative. It suggests that the appropriate device and training regimen can restore reading performance to a level that approximates that of elderly individuals who are not visually impaired.

However, if low vision and functional vision examination results indicate that the client does not have the capacity to read visually, that information needs to be conveyed in as positive a manner as possible. Letting clients know about optical character recognition (OCR) systems, for example, is a good approach. An OCR system can scan printed material and provide the contents of the page in synthetic speech (Leventhal & Earl, 2000; Singer, 1999), allowing even individuals who are totally blind access to printed materials. Some clients may also be interested in learning to read using braille.

Provide Assistance in Setting Goals

Working age adults often have goals related to their career in mind; elderly clients who are not actively pursuing careers may not be able to state clearly their specific goals. It may be necessary to draw out of them what it is they want to do and to listen carefully to what they say (Chase, 2000). People with recent and severe vision loss may not have been able to think about vision goals as yet. Nevertheless, setting goals is necessary before a meaningful rehabilitation program can commence.

Clients of all ages may require encouragement and advice to make sure that the goals they set are realistic and achievable. It is never a good idea for a practitioner to set a goal for a client; it is appropriate to help the client set his or her own goals. Find out what the client likes or liked to do, how he or she used to and now spends his or her time, or whether he or she has hobbies or vocational or avocational interests (Watson, 1996). Input from family members can also be helpful.

If a client is reluctant to formulate visual goals out of a sense that he or she "is blind," and nothing can alter that, it is helpful for the practitioner to acknowledge the degree to which the statement is true—the person is visually impaired—but also to suggest that the client's perception is only partially correct. Although the person cannot see as he or she once could, with the proper devices and training he or she may be able to see much better than at present (Defini & Burack-Weiss, 2000). Once goals are set, the practitioner is then able to design a training program to meet them.

Address Elderly Clients' Special Needs

As people advance through life, they may experience a variety of health conditions that may need to be taken into account during instruction. Because some elderly individuals may be experiencing physical or cognitive decline or dual sensory losses, it is very important that the training environment be made physically as well as emotionally comfortable for elderly clients who have special needs (Watson, 1996).

Some elderly people can be very sensitive to room temperature. Even though it might be 95 degrees outside and the air conditioner is barely cooling the room, many elderly people will feel chilled. Others will feel warm, even in cold temperatures, but this is not as common.

Many elderly people have a hearing loss in addition to a vision loss. In such cases, speaking into the ear with better hearing is necessary if the client's hearing is less impaired on one side. Slowing one's speaking rate also usually helps. Elderly people who have both hearing and vision losses may be slower to process information and may be emotionally affected by this combination of losses. It may be necessary to adjust the pace of training for such individuals. It is therefore especially important with older clients to avoid environmental distractions whenever possible. For example, presenting new information in a noisy hallway will be much less successful and much more frustrating than presenting that same information in a quiet room with the door closed.

VISUAL SKILLS AND VISION USE

Low vision training contributes to a client's successful performance of specific tasks that facilitate his or her rehabilitation goals. Results from low vision and functional vision evaluations help to determine the methods to be used to promote rehabilitation goals determined by each client. When these methods involve the use of functional vision, low vision training may be required as determined by the low vision care team.

Suppose a client needs to read daily reports as part of her job duties. The low vision care team determines, based on low vision and functional vision evaluation results, that visual reading is possible for this client, and the low vision eye care practitioner prescribes an optical device. The team recommends that visual skills training and optical device training be implemented to improve the client's use of vision and of the prescribed optical device. The goal is to maximize this client's performance on her work-related reading task with the help of low vision training.

For adults, low vision training is usually classified into three types: training in visual skills and use of vision, training in the use of visual environmental adaptations and sensory substitutions, and training with assistive devices. These training approaches can be used for both near and distance tasks. Table 10.1 offers examples of different interventions that can be taught using each type of training, each of which is discussed in the sections that follow.

For adults with acquired vision loss, low vision training most often involves visual skills instruction (i.e., learning to use basic visual skills such as eccentric viewing, tracing, tracking, scanning), and visually dependent task instruction (i.e., learning to apply visual skills in specific tasks such as reading). In most cases, if visual skills training is necessary, it is best done prior to any training on visually dependent tasks or training with assistive devices, since basic skills must be mastered before being applied to more complex tasks. In addition, once clients have had visual skills training, they are likely to be able to use assistive devices more efficiently if needed later. It is possible that visual skills training will allow a client to use less magnification than was originally thought necessary with an optical or electronic device. Eccentric viewing training should be completed prior to other visual skills training. For other visual skills discussed in this section, the recommended sequence of instruction is from tracing to tracking to scanning, starting with the simplest and working toward the most complex, although some practitioners will put scanning before tracking. Specific instructional strategies commonly used with adults are described in the sections that follow.

TABLE 10.1

Interventions in Types of Vision Instruction for Near and Distance Tasks

TYPE OF TASK	VISUAL SKILLS AND VISION USE	VISUAL ENVIRONMENTAL ADAPTATIONS AND SENSORY SUBSTITUTIONS	ASSISTIVE DEVICE INSTRUCTION
Distance tasks	Eccentric viewing Spotting Scanning Tracking	Environmental adaptations/ sensory substitutions	Field enhancement training Telescope training
Near tasks	Eccentric viewing Tracing Tracking Scanning Remedial reading skills Visual skills in reading tasks Visual skills in writing tasks	Environmental adaptations/ sensory substitutions Task lighting	Optical magnification device training Electronic magnification device training Nonoptical reading/writing device training

Eccentric Viewing

It is best to work on eccentric viewing techniques prior to any other training methods since eccentric viewing can be utilized with other skills and techniques to optimize effective use of vision. Eccentric viewing is useful for anyone who has a central scotoma (blind spot) and thus has difficulty seeing objects in the central part of the visual field. With a central scotoma, a person must use a non-foveal part of the retina to see objects as clearly as possible. The client will have to turn the eye up, down, left, right, or somewhere in between to position the visual image onto the area of the retina that serves as the area of best vision. This area varies from person to person.

All individuals with a central scotoma can benefit from eccentric viewing, but there is a great deal of variety in how readily individuals learn to do so. Some individuals appear to develop the ability spontaneously, while others benefit from formal training in eccentric viewing. Some people will be unable to grasp and, therefore, perform eccentric viewing. There is no way to know how a particular client will fare until the training begins. Not all individuals with a central scotoma will need eccentric viewing training, but the ability to view eccentrically will improve their performance in a wide variety of visual tasks.

It is prudent to assess new clients to see if they have developed effective eccentric viewing skills. The vast majority of clients with low vision find eccentric viewing training successful and thus function more efficiently in their daily lives. Eccentric viewing is applicable in every daily situation and will make functioning easier, quicker, and more expedient. Some clinicians use scanning laser ophthalmoscopes (SLO) to help determine the best area of the retina to train eccentric viewing (the preferred retinal locus, or PRL) and to train eccentric viewing (Fletcher, Schuchard, Livingstone, Crane, & Hu, 1994), however, relatively few low vision clinics use these devices. An SLO is not necessary for the majority of low vision services, and a variety of techniques have proven to be equally clinically effective (Goodrich & Quillman, 1977; Inde & Bäckman, 1975). One procedure that does not require specialized, expensive equipment is described in the following section.

DETERMINING THE AREA OF INTACT RETINA TO USE

In assessment and training, it is usually best to refer to the four cardinal directions (up, down, left, right) since it is easier to move the eye in one of those directions than it is to turn it toward, for example, a 2 o'clock position using clock hours.

In most cases, the part of intact retina closest to the macula is used for eccentric viewing. That point will have a better acuity than some point further away from the macula (Anstis, 1974). For any number of reasons, that closest point might not be the most productive: It might be surrounded by scotoma; it might be a small island of vision that is not really useful; or it might be easier for a client to move his or her eye in a different direction. In those cases, it is best to use the point that the client is most comfortable using.

It is best to have a good plot of the central visual field, showing the size and shape of the scotoma. By looking at that plot, a practitioner can choose the area of intact retina closest to the macula and to one of the four cardinal directions.

Assume that Client A has a central scotoma that extends 5 degrees below fixation and that all other parts of the scotoma extend out to 10 degrees. The client would use the point just below 5 degrees since that is closer to the macula than the other points just beyond the scotoma. If Client B's scotoma extends 10 degrees to the right but 15 degrees at all other points, that area just beyond the scotoma on the right would be the correct point to use.

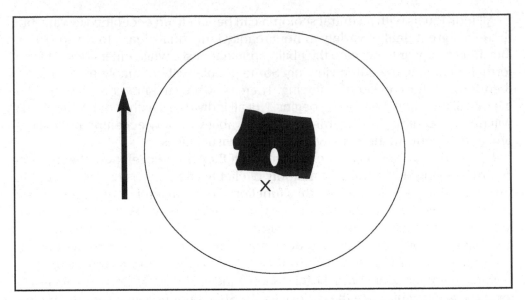

Figure 10.2. Using eccentric viewing with a central scotoma shown on a visual field plot of the right eye. The central oval represents the area of normal fixation (macula). The black area is the scotoma. The client must turn the eye up to place the eccentric viewing point (X) in line with the target by moving the scotoma out of the way.

MOVING THE EYE

The client needs to move the scotoma out of the way in order to see the target. To do so and to use the point closest to macula, the client needs to move the eccentric viewing point to fixate on the target. This moves the scotoma out of the way and allows intact retina to view the target. With Client A described above, we know that the point to use is just below the scotoma. Client A would move his eye up because in doing so he is moving the eccentric viewing point toward the position of fixation. That moves the scotoma out of the way and allows the target image to fall on usable retina (see Fig. 10.2).

If a visual field plot is not available, the instructor can use his or her face instead. Have the client sit facing the instructor and about 3 ft away. Direct the client to move his or her eye so that the instructor's face is covered by the scotoma. Then direct the client to look up until he or she sees the instructor's face and then return to covering the face with the scotoma. Do this two or three times so the client gets a lasting impression from looking up. Repeat this procedure, having the client look to the right, down, and to the left. After the client has repeated this looking in all four directions, ask the client which direction produced the best image of the instructor's face. If the client is unsure, repeat the movement in all four directions. If the client is still unsure, ask the client which direction felt the easiest: that will probably be the best direction. There are some cases in which the client's preference will prevail even though from the plot of the visual field the best eccentric viewing point might be another direction.

Having the use of an SLO can make this task very easy: This instrument can pinpoint exactly the best spot on the macula (Brilliant, 1999). However, as noted, SLOs are expensive, are rarely available to assist in training, and usually require a trained technician or clinician experienced in their use.

TRAINING SEQUENCE

Eccentric viewing training is most often done monocularly. The eye with the better acuity is usually used. However, the client might prefer using one eye over the other, or the dominant eye might be so powerful that the eye with the better acuity becomes secondary. The other eye is usually patched, but cupping the hand or using any kind of occluder is also effective. One eye is usually used for eccentric viewing training primarily because most people with low vision have one eye that is better than the other. The better eye will, in most cases, be used for reading and optical device training and it makes sense to train that eye.

Once the eye and the proper direction to turn that eye have been determined, the actual training can begin. It is usually better to start training at a distance of at least a few feet. The easiest method is to present cards with single letters and numbers on them. Present each card to the client, making sure the scotoma covers the letter. Then direct the client to turn the eye in the proper direction and indicate what the letter or number is. By covering the target with the scotoma and then moving the eye, the client learns that in order to see objects as clearly as possible, the eye must be moved. The movement of the eye away from center is usually not as great as the client expects it will be.

Since the practitioner is looking directly at the client's eye movement, it is easy to see if the technique is being done correctly and to provide immediate feedback. The letters or numbers on the cards should be of a size that will be fairly easily recognized by the client once the scotoma is moved out of the way. This can be determined based on the client's visual acuity. For example, if the client's acuity is 10/100 and the training is being done at 4 ft, the equivalent acuity is 4/40. The letters or numbers should therefore be larger, but not much larger than 40-ft letter size (see Chap. 6 for a further explanation of letter size and visual acuity).

Making the task easy during the initial training sequences is vital to success. As the training goes on, more difficult tasks are introduced by increasing the distance between the client and the targets and/or using letters or numbers that are smaller.

After the first card has been identified by the client, letters are presented in random order. The client should cover the letter with the scotoma and then move the scotoma out of the way to identify the letter. After going through single letters or numbers, the client progresses to two-, three-, and four-letter words. When the client has demonstrated proficiency moving the scotoma to identify the target, he or she will know how much to move the eye to see best.

Identifying targets without covering them first can commence once the practitioner thinks the client can demonstrate proficiency. Varying the distance between the client and the targets can help in this regard. Reminding clients to move the head and not both the head and eye is usually vital to good performance.

Keeping the eye in the eccentric viewing position and moving the head to find targets is the better way of functioning, since it involves one movement rather than two.

If a practitioner does not have available cards with numbers or letters on them, he or she can instruct the client to view eccentrically and follow an object with a straight edge. This should be done after the correct position has been determined. The lines should run horizontally initially: a table edge, a handrail on a wall, or a head board could be used. Later on, vertical eccentric viewing can be done. Monitoring progress in this task is somewhat more difficult, but it can be accomplished.

As previously noted, some clients develop an effective eccentric viewing angle without training. The amount of training required to teach effective eccentric viewing strategies to clients is not precisely known and may vary from client to client. The earliest study on training eccentric viewing (Holcomb & Goodrich, 1976) used 15 training sessions, but a more recent study by Nilsson and colleagues suggests that fewer training sessions may be equally effective (Nilsson, Frennesson, & Nilsson, 1998). In this study patients were trained to use eccentric viewing for reading, and reading performance was maximized with four to five hours of training. Although the Nilsson study was conducted on only six patients, the results are consistent with the authors' own clinical experience.

Tracing

Tracing involves following a line or lines visually. In everyday life, tracing can be a distance task at one moment and a near task the next moment. Hence, both types of tasks should be taught in the training program.

For example, vertically following a street light pole or telephone pole to locate a street sign is a distance tracing task. Another example is locating a house number by following the edge of the sidewalk to the house and then following the edge of the door frame to find the number. A near tracing task might involve reading across the line for the name, address, and telephone number of a particular person or business in a telephone directory. Another example might be following a map to a specified destination.

The easiest way to teach tracing is to draw straight lines on a blackboard or on a piece of paper and have the client follow them from one end to the other. To know if the client is doing it correctly, have him or her follow the line with a finger in conjunction with eye movements. This informs the practitioner about the client's eye-hand coordination, and indicates whether the tracing is smooth. This beginning task can be followed with practice in tasks of daily life that involve tracing.

Tracking

Tracking is following a moving object visually. For someone who is visually impaired, tracking can be rather difficult. Tracking has most often been thought of as a distance vision task, because following a moving object at near was rare before the widespread use of computers.

If a client needed to be sure of a bus number and to do so quickly, he or she would need to track the bus as it approaches. For a golfer, being able to follow a putt is a tracking task. Computer users must be able to follow cursors as they move along the screen and to follow print when scrolling up or down a page.

For training purposes, it is usually best to begin by having the client follow a slowly moving object. Since tracking can be difficult, the initial exercises should be easy. Have a client follow the instructor's finger as it moves horizontally. Doing this from left to right and from right to left is a good way to build skills. Following a person walking across the path is a more difficult step; the last one might be following a moving car.

For computer tasks, it is best to have the client learn to track a cursor. Using colored lines or colored lines of print that are in high contrast to the cursor may help. When using special large-print computer programs, it may be possible to highlight the lines of print as the cursor moves along. Using a colored cursor as a reference point in these special programs may also help when following moving print during scrolling. Following the movement of the mouse pointer (arrow) is another tracking task. Computer software programs that do not require the use of a cursor or other visual cues may need to be used for some clients with low vision.

Scanning

Scanning involves making eye or head movements to search for and locate a target. Scanning done by people with unimpaired vision is often random and there is nothing wrong with that approach for them since there is no impediment in the visual system. For a person with a visual impairment such as a scotoma, however, the random approach no longer works well. A systematic approach works far better. Scanning is particularly important for people who have small visual fields. If they do not scan systematically, they will likely miss some information.

Scanning can be and is done by people with low vision in every environment imaginable. Tasks in which scanning is of critical importance include:

➤ Scanning an area systematically to locate a familiar landmark

➤ Scanning for the return address on an envelope

➤ Scanning the interior of a room looking for a particular person

➤ Scanning a page of printed material looking for a particular item

➤ Scanning the scoreboard looking for a team's score

Teaching good scanning technique is fairly easy. Scanning usually involves moving the eye or head horizontally, dropping down to the next lower horizontal plane, and repeating that procedure.

It is generally best to use a left-to-right sweep when scanning, and, if necessary, an up-and-down sweep. This can be illustrated using a clock face. The first horizontal sweep would be from the number 11 to the number 1. After dropping the gaze down to the number 2, the next sweep would be from 2 to 10. After dropping down to 9, the next sweep would be from 9 to 3. This pattern continues using 4 and 8, and 7 and 5 o'clock. The vertical sweeps can be thought of from 2 to 4, from 5 to 1, and so on.

Even though it might take more time to scan slowly and smoothly, it is worthwhile. Consider the numbers 1 through 10 arranged in a row. If a person with low vision sees 4, then 7, and finally 10, he or she has missed other numbers. If the information that he or she needs was in the range 2 to 3 or 8 to 9, fast scanning was not helpful. The individual now has to find 1 again and start again. Thus, slow, methodical eye movements are best. Warren (1996) has developed a program with specific exercises to improve scanning performance for people with macula scotomas who have visual acuities up to 20/200.

Reading Tasks

For clients who experience difficulty putting letters together to form words, reading will be laborious. They may have forgotten how to spell or what letters look like. They may be lacking in education or reading skills, or have experienced the effects of a stroke. With some preparatory work, however, many people with low vision can regain lost reading skills.

The Pepper test (Watson, Balsadare, & Whittaker, 1990) and the reading exercises in Quillman's *Low Vision Training Manual* (Quillman, 1980) are good tools to use for a client who has difficulty putting letters together to form words. In addition, the *Learn to Use Your Vision for Reading Workbook* (Watson, Wright, & De l'Aune, 1992; Wright & Watson, 1995) can be used independently by persons with macular degeneration to improve visual skills associated with reading. Other training materials and regimens have been created for optometric practices (Freeman & Jose, 1997) and for low vision clinics (Backman & Inde, 1979; Backman, 1998).

The Quillman exercises contain a page each of single letters, two-letter words, three-letter words, four- and five-letter words, words of six or more letters, and sentences. Each of those designations appears in four different print sizes: 3M, 2M, 1.5M, and 1M. The objective of the exercises is to assist the client in reading again or in learning to read again by reading larger print and/or short words and building visual skills in order to read normal size printed material.

The Pepper test is a series of cards with print of decreasing sizes on them. The cards have print that is larger than those in the Quillman series but do go down to 1M. Even though the Pepper test was devised as an assessment tool, it can be used for training purposes.

In the *Learn to Use Your Vision for Reading Workbook,* "Seeing Exercises" focus on eccentric viewing, maintaining steady fixation, and the scanning techniques used for reading. "Thinking Exercises" focus on cognition and comprehension for reading. "Practice Stories" allow readers to blend their visual and cognitive skills using material that gradually increases in difficulty. The training process for reading tasks involves a step-by-step approach in which clients first recognize single letters and do so correctly. Next clients recognize and read two-letter words, and they then progress to recognize and read three-letter words, four-letter words, and so on. Reading sentences and then paragraphs are the final steps in this process.

Many adults, especially elderly clients, may experience difficulty going from line to line while reading (Watson, 1996). Following the line just read back to the beginning of that line and dropping down to the next one is one way to help. Having them return using the space between lines of print is another way of helping. Dropping down at the end of a line to the next line (without missing a line due to a paragraph end) is another option.

Sometimes a client will have difficulty locating the first word in the next line of print. One possible solution is to use a typoscope or line guide (see Chap. 9). Another solution is to have the client place the left thumb directly under the line being read, return to the thumb after reading that line, and lower the thumb to expose the first words in the next line. This is continued for each successive line. Using the left index finger instead of the thumb can work also, but not as well.

Some clients have difficulty remaining on the line of print. Using a typoscope or a line guide can help to maintain orientation. Following the line just read back to its beginning, as described previously, can also help. (Additional information about promoting reading performance, including selection of an appropriate type font, can be found in Chapter 9.)

VISUAL ENVIRONMENTAL MODIFICATIONS AND SENSORY SUBSTITUTIONS

Modifying the environment does not usually involve great expense and can meet the needs of individual clients. Visual modifications can be classified into the following major categories described in the following sections:

➤ enhancing contrast

➤ using filters

➤ optimizing lighting

➤ increasing size

➤ changing distance

➤ using color cues

Visual adaptations are not the only tools that can be used by people with low vision to make their lives easier. It is important to consider auditory and tactile adaptations (sensory substitutions) as well as visual ones on a case-by-case basis.

Whatever adaptations are adopted, it is important that persons with low vision, especially older adults, learn safe techniques for moving around their environment. Without the confidence that comes with rehabilitation, many individuals, especially those who are elderly, may curtail travel. Some have advocated vision rehabilitation services as a likely means to help elderly persons who are visually impaired maintain good nutrition and exercise (Salive et al., 1994). Others have noted that severe visual impairments put the individual at increased risk for falls, with 18 percent of all hip fractures in the elderly attributed to a visual impairment (Dargent-Molina, et al., 1996). Whether to maintain healthy exercise or to prevent falls, good rehabilitation practices help people with low vision learn to use their vision and other senses effectively and to modify their environment to make it safe. A handout for clients and their families that provides examples of many environmental adaptations is provided in Appendix 10.1. Additional in-depth information on helpful adaptations for the home environment written for clients and their families can be found in *Making Life More Livable* (Duffy, 2002).

People with low vision do well in environments that are familiar to them. They know what to look for in familiar places, making their visual search strategies more effective. Therefore, family members should not move furniture in any room without first telling the person with low vision and then familiarizing him or her with the new arrangement. In new environments, many persons with low vision may benefit from introductory assistance from a co-worker, family member, friend, or professional, depending upon the specific circumstances.

Low vision practitioners can demonstrate to their clients the many types of visual environmental adaptations and sensory substitutions that can make the completion of daily tasks easier and often safer. The principles for the selection of the various adaptations are presented in the sections that follow and can be discussed with clients along with examples of each method. With this information, clients and their families often develop their own creative adaptations specific to the activities they encounter in their daily lives. Giving clients and their families information about adaptations to review on their own, like the information offered in Appendix 10.1, provides a way for them to learn about and to integrate the new information provided by the low vision practitioner.

Enhancing Contrast

Contrast describes the difference in brightness between two adjacent surfaces. Maximizing the differences between two surfaces makes each one more visible and can improve task performance for clients who have difficulty differentiating objects against a low-contrast background.

Suggestions for increasing contrast include the following:

➤ If a kitchen table top is dark, consider using light-colored place mats or dishes.

➤ If white dishes are used, encourage use of dark-colored placemats. The opposite is also helpful.

➤ Use a tablecloth that contrasts with tableware.

➤ Place light-colored food items on dark plates.

➤ Cut dark-colored foods on light-colored cutting boards.

➤ Circle the handle of a transparent plastic hairbrush with brightly colored electrical tape.

➤ Write with medium to wide fiber-tip pens on white paper.

➤ Put contrasting strips of tape on the bottom and top steps of a flight of stairs.

➤ Outline electrical outlets with masking tape of a contrasting color.

Using Filters

One of the best ways to promote more efficient functioning for some individuals is through the use of filters or sunglasses (Brabyn et al., 2000). Many people with low vision need the protection of a tinted lens indoors as well as outdoors. It is surprising how much this can improve performance. Being able to present different tints and light and dark shades gives the client more options for increasing his or her independence. The client should be given enough time to make the tint selection. Tint evaluation should be done in conjunction with the optometrist or ophthalmologist to maintain continuity of service and to be certain that medical issues in prescribing are properly addressed. Tints may also be essential in preventing further loss of vision from exposure to the sun. Practitioners routinely prescribe commercial filters (sunglasses) to help their clients cope with glare and bright light (Ludt, 1997). A new rating system, called the FUBI (fashion, ultraviolet, blue, and infrared) system has been proposed to aid in rating non-prescription eyewear for its ability to protect the eye against damage caused by the sun (Hall & Schultmeyer, 2002). This system rates the physical coverage of the lenses, as well as harmful portions of the solar spectrum (e.g., ultraviolet light) and provides a quantitative value for the protection provided by the eyewear. Use of filters may be preferred by some people with low vision since they give the impression that contrast has been improved. In actuality, the filters may make some color differences more exaggerated leading to the perception of increased contrast.

Optimizing Lighting

Determining the best amount and type of light (e.g., sunlight, fluorescent, incandescent) can be challenging, but achieving a good balance can increase the client's quality of life. The easiest task to use in making an accurate assessment of lighting needs is reading or a similar purely visual task (Cornelissen et al., 2000). During the assessment, the following suggestions may be helpful:

➤ Increasing the wattage of light bulbs used can improve some clients' functioning.

➤ For some clients, however, too much light can create problems.

➤ Window blinds that the client can set for his or her comfort are useful.

➤ Dimmers on light switches provide control over light levels.

➤ An adjustable, incandescent lamp with an opaque shade and an inner reflector can be useful for near work. The opaque shade ensures that light is emitted from only one direction, thereby concentrating the light beam. An inner reflector keeps heat away from the client. The adjustable arm allows the client to move the lamp into proper position to prevent glare and to illuminate the working material more precisely.

➤ Making sure that no window glare is hitting a television screen can enhance the client's television viewing. Similar care to minimize glare should be taken if he or she uses a computer monitor.

Increasing Size

Some ways to increase the size of items used everyday include the following:

➤ Use a large-print telephone dial.

➤ Mark contents of cans containing food using large letters.

➤ Use magnifying mirrors for applying makeup or shaving.

➤ Use large-print watches.

➤ Use large-print checks.

➤ Use large-print playing cards.

Changing the Distance

Many people have difficulty seeing the television. One way to overcome this is to sit closer to the screen, which effectively increases the size of the image on the retina and requires no additional expenditures for larger screen displays. Similarly, sitting in the front section in movies, theaters, and sporting events makes the show easier to see by effectively increasing the size of images.

Using Color Cues

Items can be color coded with high-contrast colors to assist in their identification. Some examples include the following:

➤ Mark the 350-degree mark on the oven dial with a piece of contrasting color tape or with an item the client can feel, such as Velcro. Two or three different colors can be used to indicate different temperatures.

➤ Use colored key covers to identify specific keys for different doors.

➤ Organize files using color-coded dividers or file markers.

ASSISTIVE DEVICES

One of the cardinal rules of successful low vision care is that the patient must demonstrate that he or she can use any prescribed assistive devices. This rule applies even in the case of the most simple nonoptical devices, such as typoscopes (a black card with a wide slit or window cut out that exposes one or more lines of print) (Mehr & Fried, 1975). Assistive devices for low vision are classified as nonoptical, optical, or electronic magnification devices.

Nonoptical Devices

Nonoptical devices, which do not involve lenses, can make the difference in allowing clients to perform crucial tasks. Some of the more common nonoptical devices used for reading are reading lamps, reading stands, and typoscopes. (Detailed information on the use of such devices for reading can be found in Chap. 9.) Other devices include large-print telephone dials, playing cards, and calendars as well as voice output devices such as talking scales or talking clocks. Catalogs of commercially made devices that address daily living, recreational, avocational, and vocational needs are available, and it is helpful to provide clients and their families with information about them. (A list of such catalogs can be found in the Resources section at the end of this book.) The low vision practitioner cannot possibly be aware of all the daily needs of each client. When clients and their families are given the opportunity to review these catalogs at their leisure, they often find items that address very specific daily needs. Clients can be encouraged to discuss these items with the practitioner before making any purchases since the practitioner is likely to be more familiar with the devices and can assist in determining how well they may meet an identified need. The practitioner may also recommend a specific course of instruction with certain devices prior to purchase (e.g., check-writing guides).

Many catalogs include long canes and low vision optical devices in their inventory. Long canes are used for safe and efficient travel and should be used only after a course of instruction with an orientation and mobility specialist. Low vision optical devices, which involve lenses of various kinds, need to be prescribed by an ophthalmologist or optometrist and clients should be advised that they not be purchased without a prescription. A low vision optical device purchased without a prescription may not be appropriate for the client's vision, and the client may be unable to use it. The client will have spent money unnecessarily and may end up with a false impression that low vision optical devices are not useful.

Optical Device Training

Clients require training in the proper use of any optical device that has been prescribed before they will be able to use it. In most low vision clinics, device training is limited to one session per device; this may not be enough for most people. Recent research on optical device use for reading by adult clients with central visual field loss indicates that reading speed reaches maximum levels after five training sessions, although a few people did well with fewer training sessions (Goodrich et al., 2000b). There may be training differences between people with different types of vision loss (Goodrich et al., 2000a). Although more research is needed to match training methods, optical device type, and visual conditions, it is important that practitioners provide their clients with sufficient training in the use of any prescribed device to ensure optimal performance. This requires careful monitoring of a client's performance to determine when performance levels plateau. There is no set sequence of optical device training. It depends on the client's goals and the devices prescribed or recommended, the client's motivation, and what the client wants to accomplish.

A discussion about training with optical devices requires a general understanding of basic optics and the optical characteristics of devices (see Chap. 3 for more detailed information).

MAGNIFICATION

There are four ways of achieving magnification: relative distance, relative size, angular magnification, and projection magnification. Relative distance magnification means getting closer to the object. If a client is viewing an object at 10 ft initially and then moves to 5 ft, two times magnification has been achieved ($10/5 = 2$). Relative size magnification refers to a larger object at the same distance. If the numbers and letters on a large print telephone dial are three times as large as on a regular dial, three times magnification has been achieved. Angular magnification is achieved by optical devices such as magnifiers and telescopes. It compares the size of the image created by the magnifier to the size of the object being viewed. (For more information on magnification with optical devices, see Chap. 3.) Projection magnification is achieved by projecting an image that is larger than the original one. The most common device is the closed-circuit television magnification system (CCTV), also called a video magnifier. Other devices in this category include the overhead projector and slide projector.

Whichever method of magnification is used, it needs to provide magnification above the patient's threshold in order to provide "reserve" magnification (more than necessary to just be able to see the print) (Whittaker & Lovie-Kitchen, 1993). This makes reading easier and less visually strenuous.

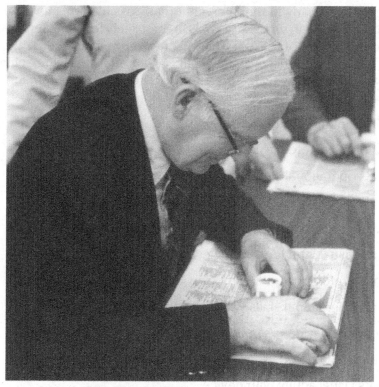

Optical devices such as this stand magnifier make print material accessible to individuals with low vision. *(Susan Islam)*

TELESCOPES

Telescopic devices are used for viewing distant objects, although some designed to be used by one eye only, can allow viewing of objects as close as 8 to 10 in away. There are many types of telescopes but the most common is the handheld monocular. Other types include binoculars, spectacle-mounted (full field, expanded field, wide angle, or bioptic), clip-on, headborne, behind-the-lens, and contact lens. Zimmerman (1996) provides more detail about the different types.

Monoculars (and binoculars) are most often used by adults to facilitate mobility (Hall et al., 1987), and bioptics are used to facilitate driving (Chapman, 1995; Vogel, 1991). Bioptics are explained in more detail later in this chapter. Mobility tasks include reading street signs, building addresses, or business signs. It is important that the team of professionals think in terms of clients' more global distance viewing tasks and not limit telescope prescription to use for quick spotting in mobility tasks only. Telescopes are also used for tasks of longer duration such as watching television or sporting events and viewing lectures or demonstrations.

Once the practitioner knows the client's distance vision goals, it is fairly easy to devise a training program based on them. The instructor needs to handle unrealistic goals as early in the intervention as possible. This involves working with the client to explain why those goals are not likely to be achieved and listening to the client's point of view as well. Whenever possible, alternative methods should be suggested to achieve goals that cannot realistically be achieved with telescope use. The following factors must be taken into consideration when selecting an appropriate telescopic device system:

➤ Type of mounting system

- Duration of targeted tasks: long-term vs. short-term.
- Client's operational skills with device.
- Client's preferences regarding device appearance.

➤ Choosing between a monocular or binocular telescope

- Client's visual limitations using eyes together.
- Client's preference for field of view and ease of use.
- Client's operational skills with device.

➤ Choosing final device magnification

- Distance of targeted tasks.
- Client's visual acuity with device.
- Client's preferences regarding image clarity, field of view, image illumination.

➤ Additional considerations

- Number of tasks for which the device can be used.
- Critical nature of task: There may only be one task for which a device can be used, but it may be crucial for the client to complete this task on a regular basis.
- Cost.

TELESCOPE USE FOR TELEVISION VIEWING. Training a client to use a telescope for TV viewing is a good example of training for viewing single, stationary targets. Many elderly adults with visual impairments want to watch TV more comfortably. They do not enjoy sitting close to the TV and would appreciate having a greater viewing distance. To provide them with the same or even a sharper image of the TV screen from a greater distance, magnification must be used.

Some people will not benefit from using telescopic devices for watching TV; they may prefer to sit close to view the TV. Many clients will think that use of a telescopic device will allow them to see TV as they did before their visual impairment. They need to be informed that the device will allow them to see TV more easily and clearly, but not as they used to. Clients also need to be informed that, even with a telescope, they may not be able to read print on the TV screen (Neve

& Jenniskens, 1994). Some people strongly prefer clarity over a wider field of view. They want to see things more clearly and will settle for seeing only a small portion of the screen at a time and moving their heads more to see the rest of the screen.

Cost is an important issue for most clients. The costs associated with particular devices should be clearly presented so that clients can consider cost factors in making decisions about devices.

It can be beneficial if the practitioner has a range of magnification that can be used. For example, the ophthalmologist or optometrist might recommend training the client with the telescopic devices that range from 2.5× to 4×. Even though the ophthalmologist or optometrist may have determined in the examination room that a certain power should be used, it is best to give the client the final say.

A number of different devices can be used for TV viewing, but more than 4× magnification is usually not helpful because too much field of view is lost with higher magnifications. That does not mean one needs to limit the magnification to 4×. It means that the field of view is disproportionately sacrificed for increased clarity, which is usually not worth the extra magnification. Going up to 6× or 8× magnification or more will greatly amplify the effect of small head and neck movements, which can make it more difficult for the person to view the television steadily. This often increases fatigue and shortens viewing time and pleasure. An alternative to increasing the magnification is decreasing the viewing distance (relative distance magnification), in addition to providing magnification. Using more than 4× power can be effective—as noted earlier, some clients insist on maximum clarity—but it should be at the client's insistence and with his or her understanding that the field of view decreases as power increases.

Since TV viewing is a long-term task, it is best for the client to use a head-borne device. His or her arm would get too tired if the telescopic device had to be held in order to see the TV. For other tasks, a handheld device may be more appropriate.

To ensure that the client understands how each device operates, it is necessary to spend adequate time familiarizing him or her with each device. It helps to point out (and perhaps demonstrate) how the device is worn, how to focus the telescope, and, if necessary, how to change the pupillary distance between the scopes on binocular devices.

Determining the client's visual acuity with the different telescopic devices is a good way to gain initial information from the client about the devices, paying attention to the following considerations:

➤ Allow the client enough time to focus each device properly and to get the clearest image through it.

➤ It is often helpful to instruct the client to focus one eye at a time by closing one eye.

➤ Sometimes the client's acuity in one eye will be much better than in the other eye. The eye with less acuity might interfere with the brain's interpretation of the images from the better eye. To prevent this from becoming irritating, one needs to block off visual input from the eye with poorer acuity as part of training with binoculars. This requires taping a dark piece of paper over the objective end of the telescopic lens or using an eye patch on the affected eye.

➤ Once both telescopic lenses have been focused, the focusing can be fine tuned with both eyes open.

Again, the cost of the device needs to be considered. The practitioner needs to determine if the client can afford the device and whether the benefits are worth the cost. It is more than likely that the better the acuity he or she can achieve, the better the chance that the client is going to prefer a device.

When the client's visual acuities have been determined, actually trying the task—in this case watching TV—with the device is a must. If the training is being done in a clinic or office, try to simulate the client's preferred viewing distance at home, so that the training session is close to the home situation. Even though the client might have a better acuity with a 4× device, that does not mean that the 4× will be the best for watching TV. The client might find the field of view too confining; he or she might want a larger field of view or a shorter viewing distance. For those reasons, it is best to let the client watch TV for a few minutes with more than one device. Allowing the client to make the choice is always best. It can be helpful to have the client view the TV at different distances using the different devices so that he or she makes the choice with consideration of magnification, field of view, and viewing distance. The practitioner may contribute to the decision, ultimately the client should choose which device allows him or her the most comfortable TV viewing.

When the client has used the device for the desired task for a specified period of time, ask him or her about any difficulties experienced with the device and provide assistance to address any reported problems.

TELESCOPE USE FOR MOBILITY. Binoculars and other telescopic devices can be used for O&M purposes, but monoculars are the most common choice. The training techniques described here were developed primarily for monoculars, although they can be used with any of the other devices.

The low vision evaluation report provides the range of magnification for devices to be used in training and should state the acuity that the client has achieved with each telescopic device. It is ideal if this acuity is close to the measurement achieved with the same devices outside the ideal conditions of the examination room. An acuity of 10/20 or better with the device is desired. A better value than 10/20 is an advantage; a worse value means that the client will have to be closer to signs in order to see them.

When beginning the training, it is best to begin with lower power and work up to higher powers, because higher powers result in smaller fields of view. When the specified range is 4× to 6×, for example, begin with the 4×.

Start by familiarizing the client with the components of the device and their operation. Show the device to the client, let the client handle it, point out the ocular and objective ends of the telescope (making sure the client knows which end goes closer to the eye), and how to focus. If necessary, demonstrate how to hold and then how to focus the device.

Next obtain the client's visual acuity with the device. Although this is done in the same manner as obtaining a measurement of visual acuity without the device, it provides an opportunity to introduce and reinforce the concept of eye-device-target alignment. That is, the device must be on a straight line between the eye and the target, or the client will not see anything through it.

Train the client in target localization by having him or her view the target first with the unaided eye, and then shifting to the device. Instruct the client to look at the target with the naked eye, keeping the vision on the target, slowly bringing the device up to the eye (never taking his or her vision off the target), until the device is at eye level and the client is looking through it. Using this method, the client usually achieves correct alignment quickly. Even though this procedure might seem difficult at first, it is actually easier than putting the device up to the eye and then looking for the target. Having the client repeat this alignment procedure with each line on a distance visual acuity test chart is a good way to reinforce the technique.

When the acuity with the lower power has been recorded, repeat the procedure with the other recommended telescopes. By this time the client has probably demonstrated efficiency in good alignment. If not, this efficiency needs to be stressed as he or she performs subsequent tasks.

The final choice of device should be the client's. Even though a better (or even much better) acuity might be achieved with a particular telescope, the client might not prefer it. Any number of factors can influence the choice: field of view restriction, size of the scope, manner in which the device focuses, or amount of light that comes through it. Two important ideas to stress for clients is that more power is not always better and that a bigger image is not always better.

Once the client has chosen a telescope, have him or her identify, at different distances, cards that have single letters or numbers on them. Make sure that the size of the letters or numbers is large enough for the client to see through the telescope. Varying the working distance is essential so that the client understands that refocusing at different distances is necessary to produce the clearest image for each target distance. Proceeding from single letters (or numbers) to two-, three-, and four-letter words, while varying the working distance, reinforces what has been taught. It should allow the client to understand clearly the nature and function of the scope.

Reading signs, seeing wall clocks, spotting room numbers, and other actual indoor tasks should be performed next. Performing these tasks at various distances is a good reinforcer.

When the client has achieved proficiency with indoor tasks, using the telescope for actual mobility tasks—reading street signs, business signs, and street addresses outdoors—is the final step. In some cases, the client will not be able to read a street sign from across a street and must be on the same corner as the sign to do so. Making sure the client has a realistic understanding of the limits of his or her vision with the telescope is important. If good communication (instruction and feedback) has been maintained, the client should not experience failure with the telescope. The client might not be able to do all that he or she wants to, but many tasks should be possible.

When the client has used the device for the desired task for a specified period of time, obtain feedback. Find out if the client is having any difficulties with the device and provide assistance to address any reported problems.

SPECIAL TRAINING CONSIDERATIONS. Some common problems and their solutions include the following:

➤ If the client has difficulty aligning the device, be certain that he or she is keeping the eye, the device, and the object of regard in line. Also make sure that the client is holding the device as close as possible to the eye or eyeglasses. Using a clip-on monocular might help.

➤ If the client has problems with alignment while sitting, resting the arms on a table or on the arms of a chair might help, as may bringing one or both elbows against the body.

➤ If the client is unsteady, suggest that he or she lean against a wall or a door jamb indoors and a tree, lamp post, parking meter, or building outdoors.

➤ If the client has difficulty locating sign poles across the street, he or she can use the crosswalk lines as a guide to trace across the street. Once he or she has located the curb across the street, scanning the area on top of and immediately behind the curb will allow him or her to locate the poles.

➤ If the client can locate the curb across the street but not any sign poles, he or she can use the crosswalk, as described previously.

➤ If the client has a central scotoma, remind him or her to use eccentric viewing.

➤ The client needs to know the range of focus of a telescope. Most telescopes can focus to very long distances. Binocular telescopes and many monocular telescopes have a range of focus that is limited so that the point of closest focus is well-beyond arm's length. Some monocular telescopes popular with users with low vision have a substantially wider range of focus, allowing the closest point of focus to be within arm's length.

MAGNIFIERS

The goal in using any type of magnifier is to read, write, or do other near vision tasks. Success depends on being able to see the print or symbol one is trying to decipher and to perform the task (e.g., reading or writing) with some degree of facility. As a general rule, reading 1M print is the goal. If the client can read print smaller than 1M, this is a bonus. The use of a reading stand or lap desk with any kind of magnifier will make its use easier. When clients have difficulty putting letters together to form words, reading training, as described earlier in this chapter, is needed before beginning any training with magnifiers for reading. As with telescopes, it is best if the practitioner has devices with a range of magnification for the client to try and from which he or she will make the final selection of a device.

HAND MAGNIFIERS. Most adults have had some experience with hand magnifiers, even if only through playing with them when they were younger. Most people, however, do not know the subtle techniques for their proper usage. In addition, most do not realize that the more powerful a magnifier is, the smaller the lens will be. Most want a bigger magnifier, erroneously thinking that it will magnify more, and do not realize that it will not be very powerful.

Smaller hand magnifiers are sometimes called pocket magnifiers and many people with low vision find them invaluable and carry them everywhere. Other hand magnifiers have a long handle and cannot easily fit in a pocket.

Hand magnifiers are available in powers from 4 to 40 diopters. They are often used for short-term reading tasks—generally less than 15 to 20 minutes—such as reading the return address on a letter, a telephone number, a credit card bill, or a price tag and other near vision tasks, but some clients will find them useful for long-term reading.

Some hand magnifiers have illumination built in and some do not. Providing additional lighting is a must. Let the client try different lighting arrangements before deciding upon his or her preferred lighting requirements. Issues to be addressed in determining optimal lighting arrangements can include the following:

➤ Bulb wattage

➤ Bulb type (incandescent, fluorescent, halogen, xenon, or a combination)

➤ Placement of the lamp

➤ Glare

➤ Light reflecting off the magnifier or page

➤ Distance of the lamp to the reading material

The practitioner needs to know the following training principles for hand magnifiers and convey them effectively to the client:

➤ The more power a handheld magnifier has, the closer it will need to be held to the material to be in focus. For example, a 32D magnifier will have to be held twice as close to the page as a 16D magnifier.

➤ It is usually best to begin by holding the magnifier flat against the material and moving it slowly away until the necessary magnification with the least distortion is obtained. This skill is sometimes called establishing the device-to-material distance. The device-to-material distance determines the amount of magnification. As this movement progresses, there is an increase in magnification, an increase in aberrations, and a decrease in the field of view. There is an upper limit to this distance: the point at which all images seen through the device will be blurry. When that happens, the device needs to be moved closer to the material.

➤ The eye-to-device distance is also important. As the eye-to-device distance is decreased, there is a decrease in aberrations and an increase in the field of view. The practitioner needs to be cognizant of both distances, to guide the client if he or she experiences difficulty using the device.

➤ When a person is wearing a bifocal spectacle correction, the eye-to-device distance and the power of the magnifier must be taken into account when determining which portion of the bifocal the person should use for viewing. In general, if the eye-to-device distance is greater than the focal length of the magnifier, the person should use the distance portion of his or her glasses to obtain more magnification. If the device-to-eye distance is less than the focal length of the magnifier, the person should view through the bifocal segment of his or her spectacles. (See Chap. 3 for a detailed discussion of spectacle corrections and optical device use.)

➤ The client needs to look directly into the middle of the magnifier and not off to the side. Looking to the side will increase the visibility of aberrations and decrease clarity. The client should hold the magnifier parallel to the material and maintain an effective device-to-material distance while moving the magnifier across the page. Maintaining an effective device-to-material distance is not easy: all people tend to shake a little as they move their hands. Cupping the body of the magnifier but not the lens in the palm of the hand and extending the fingers down to the page can help in holding a steady distance.

➤ Many clients, especially elderly clients who must use new body, head, and eye positions (Watson, 1996), may have difficulty with tracing and tracking skills involved in reading. These should be addressed before beginning training in the use of magnifiers. Many will have more difficulty with these skills with the introduction of magnifiers because magnifiers make the reading process more complicated. The section on reading training in this chapter provides methods for assisting clients.

➤ If eccentric viewing is needed, reinforce the proper angle while the client is looking through the magnifier.

As with telescopic devices, an optometrist or ophthalmologist often recommends a range of magnification or dioptric power. Manufacturers' magnification ratings are not always comparable, since methods for determining magnification are not consistent among different manufacturers (Bailey, Bullimore, Greer, & Mattingly, 1994). Determining the power of devices in diopters is comparable across manufacturers, however, so it is recommended that power in diopters be used when comparing devices for use with a particular client. (See Chap. 3 for a more complete discussion of methods for determining magnification.)

To determine which magnifier is best for a client, obtain a measurement of near vision acuity with the different devices recommended by the optometrist or ophthalmologist. In going through this process, the client gains experience handling and using each device and can compare their usefulness. The acuities that the optometrist or ophthalmologist obtained with the devices may differ, however, from that obtained outside of the examining room. Often there are differences between what works best while the client is in the examining room and what works best in the training program. Findings from the training program should form the benchmark, since the environment established in the training program can be made to replicate the client's working environment. After acuities have been obtained with the different devices, the client should choose which device is the best. The final choice might coincide with what the practitioner thinks, but it might not. A good practitioner will provide an opportunity for the client to try out magnifiers of different shapes and sizes, but all within the required range of magnification (Spitzberg & Goodrich, 1995). It might be necessary to let the client try the devices more than once.

Once the client has selected a magnifier, performing practical tasks will verify that the device allows the client to do what he or she requires. If the client wants to be able to look up numbers in the telephone directory, have a telephone book handy for that purpose. Having available menus, old bills, and receipts for reading can also instill confidence in a client's use of magnifiers and reinforce the correct way to use such devices.

Some clients will choose more than one handheld device, especially clients who have diverse needs related to their work. For example, a client may choose one handheld magnifier for reading the stock quotes in the newspaper at home and an additional, more portable, pocket magnifier for reading prices in a grocery store, because the print size being read is different.

When the client has used the device for the desired task for a specified period of time, obtain feedback to find out if he or she is having any difficulties with the device. Provide assistance to address any reported problems.

STAND MAGNIFIERS. Many adults may have seen stand magnifiers, but they are usually unaware of the best techniques for their use. As with hand magnifiers, clients may want a big magnifier, not realizing that a larger lens usually equals less power. Stand magnifiers come in a wide range of powers and are either illuminated or nonilluminated. Stand magnifiers are bigger and bulkier than pocket and hand magnifiers. For that reason, it is not as easy to carry them everywhere and it can be very difficult, if not impossible, to use one to write. However, they can be very useful for more protracted near vision tasks, particularly reading.

Stand magnifiers have a fixed focus and should be placed directly on the reading material. More magnification can be achieved by raising the magnifier away from the material, but doing so defeats the purpose of using it.

Since the magnifier is placed on the material and moved along, the client must be close enough to the magnifier to see the print through the lens. Some clients think they must be right on top of the magnifier; this is not always correct. Leaving an inch or two between the magnifier and the eye often gives better results.

It is difficult to use both eyes with stand magnifiers, so the better eye is usually used. In some cases, this will be the dominant eye, which might not be the eye with the best vision. If this is a deterrent to the client's successful use of the device, encourage him or her to use the better eye rather than the dominant one.

If a client has a near correction for lack of accommodation (reading glasses or bifocals), he or she should look through that correction when using the stand magnifier (see Chap. 3.). If eccentric viewing is needed, reinforce the proper angle while the client is looking through the magnifier.

As with hand magnifiers, a range of magnification or dioptric power should be recommended by the optometrist or ophthalmologist, including the actual devices to be used for trial purposes. However, the dioptric power rating of stand magnifiers is less predictive of the magnification effect of stand magnifiers compared to the predictive value of the dioptric power rating of handheld magnifiers (Bailey et al., 1994).

It is usually best to begin the training by obtaining an acuity with the different recommended magnifiers and letting the client choose a preferred magnifier after using each one. As with all other devices, the practitioner should never make the decision for the client but should guide him or her to a sound decision.

Keep in mind that the goal is to enable the client to complete meaningful tasks. If a client's goal is to keep track of his or her investments, the client will be disappointed if he or she can read articles in the newspaper but not the prices on the financial pages.

When the client has selected the best stand magnifier, he or she should use it in practical situations. If the client wants to read the newspaper, use a newspaper, not a large-print version. Many clients need to be encouraged to persist in reading with a stand magnifier. One reading session is usually not enough. Multiple sessions (usually about five) allow the client to gain proficiency in its use. This is usually marked by an increase in reading speed and duration (Goodrich, Mehr, & Darling, 1980; Goodrich et al., 2000a, 2000b).

A variety of graded reading materials are available. Clients' needs are best met when they read material of their ideal print size and interest level. If the client is given the newspaper sports pages to read, but does not like sports, the purpose is not being met. If at all possible, have the client bring reading material that he or she wants to read to training sessions. Reading this successfully shows the client that his or her critical reading desires are being met and motivates the client to continue.

When the client has used the device for the desired task for a specified period of time, obtain feedback to find out if the client is having any difficulties with the device. Provide assistance to address any reported problems.

SPECTACLE-MOUNTED MAGNIFIERS. Spectacle-mounted magnifiers, which have the lenses mounted in a spectacle frame, include aspherics, microscopic lenses, half eyes, and hyperoculars. Brilliant (1999) and Jose (1983) provide more detailed information about spectacle-mounted magnifiers.

As with the use of stand magnifiers, clients need encouragement to persist in reading with spectacle-mounted magnifiers. One reading session is usually not enough. Multiple reading sessions allow the client to note an increase in his or her reading speed and duration (Goodrich et al., 1980, 2000a, 2000b).

Using the correct amount of light is critical for success. Usually the light needs to come over the same shoulder as the eye that is being used: if the left eye is being used, the light needs to come over the left shoulder or from the left side. Allowing the client to have control of the placement of the lighting is usually beneficial. It is important to make sure that the light is not close to his or her head, and that the light does not cast shadows onto the reading material.

The initial trial with a spectacle-mounted magnifier should determine the client's preference using the acuity method described earlier. Once a selection has been made, and if no remedial training needs to be done, the client can use the magnifier in practical tasks.

When reading with spectacle-mounted magnifiers clients often feel that the reading distance is too close because it is much closer than when they had no visual impairment. This might be the only viable option for reading visually, however. They must hold the material at the focal distance, which is easily determined. Have the client start with the material against the nose and move it away until it comes into focus. That is more effective than holding the material at a normal reading distance and bringing it closer until it is in focus.

It is sometimes better to slide the reading material in front of the eye than to move the eye or the head to read across a line of print, especially when the person has to view eccentrically.

Make sure that the device allows the client to achieve success on tasks that are meaningful to his or her life. When the client has used the device for the desired task for a specified period of time, obtain feedback to find out if the client is having any difficulties with the device. Provide assistance to address any reported problems.

HEADBORNE MAGNIFIERS. Headborne magnifiers as defined here include clip-on loupes and headborne binocular loupes (Brilliant, 1999). These devices are typically used so that the client's hands are free for such activities as home repair, woodworking, hobbies, and other vocational and avocational pursuits.

With these devices, good lighting without shadows is vital. The focal point must be achieved or the client will see blurry images. Sometimes a client will see a double image due to the close focal point. If that happens, blocking off the lens for the eye with less acuity will usually prevent double vision. Patching the eye itself can also be successful. Acceptance by the client of the close working distance is vital for success. Training with headborne magnifiers requires the same techniques as described earlier for spectacle-mounted magnifiers. It is the client's choice as to which device works more effectively for him or her.

BIOPTIC TELESCOPES. A bioptic is a telescope mounted in the upper portion of a spectacle lens (called the carrier lens) in standard eyeglass frames. A person looks through the carrier lens the vast majority of time and through the telescope only a small percentage of time for short, spotting tasks. Bioptics are usually used for driving (Barron, 1991) but they can also expand the field of view in patients with visual field losses (Szlyk, et al., 1998, 2000). A client can use a bioptic telescope while driving to verify quickly the details of an object in the environment or for reading signs. Driving with a bioptic telescopic lens is not without controversy. Each state has its own laws governing driving while using these devices: the practitioner must check his or her state's department of motor vehicles for these requirements.

Bioptics may also be used for other purposes, such as card playing and hobbies. Telescopes may be mounted in the inferior portion of the carrier lens to allow the user to complete specific tasks. Lower mounts, however, pose significant mobility problems since the field of view is obstructed, and are relatively rare.

Using a bioptic telescope can pose a number of difficulties, including the following:

➤ Apparent (yet inaccurate) nearness of images or objects

➤ Small field of view

➤ Apparent speed with which objects come into and then leave the field of view (so-called jack-in-the-box effect)

➤ Inappropriateness of continually looking through the telescope due to its limited field of view

The bioptic telescope must be carefully prescribed by an ophthalmologist or optometrist. Training in the effective use of the bioptic system before the client uses it for driving can be done by a practitioner (Huss, 1998, 2000; Jose et al., 1983; Vogel, 1991). Using a bioptic telescope in conjunction with driving involves more than effective use of an optical device because driving involves the coordination of many complex skills. It is essential that a professional driving instructor who is experienced in working with drivers who use bioptic telescopes conduct the overall driver's training program.

Training a client to use a bioptic telescope is, like the other training regimens, a step-by-step process. Since the ultimate goal involves public safety, special care needs to be used to ensure good bioptic use. The concepts to convey to the client are use of the device for spotting, identifying, and scanning (described in the following sections). Even though these are different tasks, it is difficult to separate them when using a bioptic device for driving. While driving, a person does not have the time to think about which task is which. His or her functioning with the device should be so ingrained that he or she does it seamlessly, without conscious thought or delay.

Spotting is being able to view a target, through the telescope, without searching for it. Once the target is seen through the carrier lens, the client has to lower his or her head slightly, move the eye up to the telescope, look through the telescope, identify the target, and return to using the carrier lens. All this needs to be done in less than a second.

Identifying is taught in conjunction with spotting. A client needs to be able to identify targets quickly through the telescope in order to drive with a bioptic.

Scanning involves looking through the telescope at the environment (or, most likely, the traffic conditions) and obtaining information through the telescope that can not be gathered through the carrier lens. This also needs to be done very quickly. It is not easy, and it takes time to build good technique and confidence. The section on Scanning in this chapter provides good exercises for teaching this skill, which should begin once the client is able to use the telescope for spotting and identifying.

A good first step is to have the client display good skills and technique through the bioptic while riding as a passenger. Giving the client time and practice using the device in a car helps his or her confidence in using the scope. Once the client is proficient in the use of the bioptic in the training situations, professional driver's training is recommended.

Training in spotting can begin by having the client identify numbers or letters directly in front of him or her. The size should be such that the client needs to look through the telescope to make proper identification. A working distance of 10 to 15 feet is probably best. Getting the client used to dealing with distance is essential for good bioptic use. He or she should be instructed to look through the carrier at the number, lower the head and move the eye upward so the view is through the telescope, identify the number, lower the head, and resume looking through the carrier lens. This initial phase is so important that extra time should be spent on this. The instructor needs to emphasize that looking from carrier to telescope and back to carrier needs to take no more than 1 second to ensure safe driving.

When the client has mastered spotting objects directly ahead, the instructor can expand the activity a few degrees to the right and left of straight ahead. This sequence is continued, adding a few degrees each time the previous ones have been mastered. It is necessary to cover about a 60-degree (in diameter) visual field with these exercises; up and down directions need to be addressed in addition to left and right. (See Chap. 2 for a discussion of visual field).

If the client shows good spotting technique in a clinical setting, his or her success is likely to carry over to outdoor use. Outdoor training can be done first while the person is standing still and then while walking along a safe route. The instructor needs to emphasize to the client the distance that he or she needs to be from an object or sign in order to identify it through the telescope.

While the client is a passenger in a car, the instructor can emphasize again how far away he or she must be from signs or objects in order to identify them accurately through the telescope lens after he or she has spotted them through the carrier telescope. The client should not attempt to use the bioptic to identify targets until they are within or close to viewing range. Otherwise, he or she will need to make more than one attempt to identify the target, and this can be very dangerous while driving.

CLOSED-CIRCUIT TELEVISION MAGNIFICATION SYSTEMS. Closed-circuit television (CCTV) magnification systems (also known as video magnifiers) are an example of electronic magnification systems and are primarily used for reading and writing. Some models have recently become more versatile because they can focus at various distances. They can have black and white or color monitors; some units offer various color combinations for print and background.

Research with CCTVs indicates that training increases reading performance for most adult clients. Clients with central field losses may show improved reading speed and duration; clients with a peripheral field loss may gain reading duration but not necessarily reading speed (Goodrich et al., 2000a, 2000b). On average, seven training sessions are required to reach maximum reading speed, although some people reach their highest speed with fewer sessions (Goodrich, et al., 2000a, 200b). There appears to be little difference in reading speed and duration between use of CCTVs with an X-Y table (a table for placing the material to be viewed that has unrestricted, multidirectional movement) and the camera mounted on a stand compared to CCTVs that use a hand-scanned (mouselike) camera. However, clients may have definite preferences for one versus the other (Goodrich & Kirby, 2001), which may be influenced by the cost of the system. A summary of training guidelines is presented in the following sections (see Lund & Watson, 1997, for additional information).

Teaching someone to use a CCTV begins with familiarizing him or her with the monitor (TV screen), X-Y table, magnification, focus, contrast, polarity controls, and the on/off switch. The X-Y table most often has a lip at the back that allows the top edge of the reading material to be pushed against it. Making sure that the top edge is aligned with the table lip also ensures that the material will be presented straight across the screen and not uphill or downhill. The reading material should be placed in the middle of the table, with an equal amount of uncovered table to the left and right of the reading material.

For some clients, it is best to introduce the controls with the CCTV turned off because they might be distracted by the image on the screen when it is turned on. Some clients may need more than one explanation about the function of the various knobs, switches, and controls and the proper procedures for using them. Some units have an autofocus feature; the client touches a control and the camera does the focusing. Self-focusing units focus without input from the user when the magnification level is changed.

Reading material can be placed on the table either before or after the unit is turned on. Once the machine is on and the reading material is in place, the client moves the magnification knob or lever until the highest magnification level is attained. This often causes the image to be blurry or out of focus, and the client

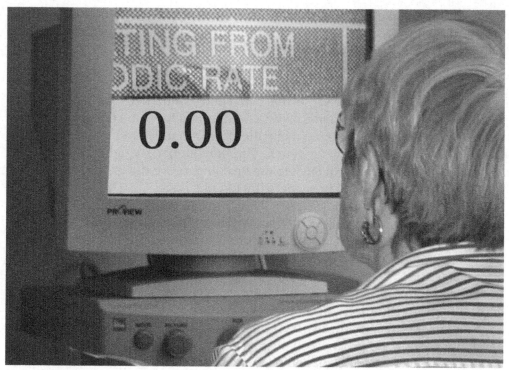

This client is learning to use a closed-circuit television system to read her monthly bills. *(Robert Barkaloff)*

must now turn the focus knob until the clearest picture is obtained. It is good practice to have the client use the controls to go from in focus to out of focus and then back into focus to obtain the clearest image. Focusing is done on the highest magnification since this results in an image that is in from the largest size to the smallest.

The next step is obtaining the desired magnification level. The goal is to use the smallest amount of magnification that allows the client to read comfortably. The client might be able to read an image that is 8 times larger than the actual print size on the CCTV but do so more comfortably using 12 times magnification. This indicates a preference for the larger magnification. Achieving the desired amount of magnification is obtained by moving the magnification control to that level. The magnification level for a client might change from day to day. One does not need to be concerned about this, although it is something to monitor. Reasons that magnification levels may change include variable vision due to diabetes, lack of sleep, or a hemorrhage in the eye. If significant changes persist, the client should be evaluated promptly by an ophthalmologist or optometrist, to determine any possible changes in visual status.

The positive or negative image control (polarity) can be introduced next and its use in conjunction with the various color combinations should also be explored. In order to make the best choice, the client needs to see positive (black on white) and negative (white on black) images, as well as the different colors of print and background available, which provide varying amounts of contrast and glare control. Clients may enjoy changing colors a few times within one reading session. For some clients, however, machines with color options may not be necessary.

After the controls have been set, the client can commence reading. The client can place one hand on each side of the X-Y table. It helps some clients if the practitioner initially moves the table while the client's hands are in contact with it, giving the client kinesthetic feedback. The practitioner should move the table across a line of print, move it back to the next line, move the table to read down the page, and move the table to get to the top of a page.

SRA Reading Laboratories (Parker, 2001) provides excellent reading material at different levels, which allow the instructor to begin reading training at each client's reading level. Each "laboratory" contains more than 100 stories of various lengths and complexity. The stories are divided into different reading levels from first grade to college, although none includes all levels. The print size varies from about 1.75M to 1M. Each story is printed on high-quality paper and includes comprehension questions, and other exercises in vocabulary and word study. Each series, sold separately, also has timed reading selections (usually only a few paragraphs long) and progress charts.

After the initial introduction and once the client understands the movements of the table, he or she should control it. Performance will improve as the client gains proficiency with the unit (Goodrich et al, 1980, 2000a, 2000b). However, expect the client initially to use more magnification than is eventually used and more magnification than would be prescribed for an optical device. Encourage eccentric viewing if the client requires it, and review all controls and operational procedures as often as needed.

Writing using a CCTV is practical and productive. It is generally best accomplished with a positive image (e.g., black print on a white background) and with magnification set at the lowest level at which the client can read the writing. Because handwriting is usually bigger than the printed word, clients will require less magnification than when reading printed material.

With handwriting, the action takes place on the X-Y table but is seen on the screen. Clients may need some practice to get used to this. It is sometimes best for the client to lock the X-Y table and move the paper across the stationary table while writing. It is important to remind clients that they must be able to see what they are writing: either the X-Y table or the paper must be moved to bring their handwriting into view.

Other tasks can be accomplished with the CCTV, including reading medicine bottles and filling an insulin syringe. Use of low magnification is recommended for these tasks. Despite some loss of detail, low magnification allows the client a broader view of what is on the screen. When the client has used the device for the desired task for a specified period of time, obtain feedback to find out if the client is having any difficulties with the device. Provide assistance to address any reported problems.

VISUAL FIELD ENHANCEMENT DEVICES

Visual field enhancement devices are used by clients who have small visual fields and, with the possible exception of spotting materials on desktops, almost exclusively used in conjunction with O&M activities. The purpose of a visual field enhancement device is to help the person with a small visual field be aware of more objects in the restricted visual field. It allows people to see obstacles that may be in their path that could not be seen without eye or head movements (Cohen, 1993).

Minifiers, or reverse telescopes, are the most common such devices. They do the opposite of magnifiers: They make images smaller (minification), thus providing the client with more information about what is ahead. Minfiers are to be used to gather information about the environment, but only when the client is standing still or sitting. The client must look through the device to become aware of any obstacles in his or her path. The objects seen will be smaller than normal or will appear farther away than they really are, but the client will have a good impression of them. The change in apparent size of, and distance to, the object when viewed though a minifier creates potential hazards. A tripping hazard or a drop-off may appear to be farther away than it is. If the person is walking while looking through the minifier, her or she may misjudge the distance and may trip or fall. For this reason, minifiers are recommended only as spotting devices.

Other visual field enhancement devices used to give clients information before they actually encounter objects include Fresnel prisms, mirrors (Bailey, 1982), high minus (concave) lenses, and amorphic lenses (Hoeft, 1992; Szlyk et al., 1998; Laderman, Szylyk, Kelsch & Seiple, 2000). A Fresnel prism is a plastic lens that can be pressed onto the back surface of an eyeglass lens (Brilliant, 1999). An amorphic lens is a reversed Galilean telescope that provides or creates minification (Brilliant, 1999). Fresnel prisms, mirrors, and amorphic lenses displace objects toward the functioning visual field and thus reduce the amount of eye movement a client needs to make in order to see those objects (Hoppe & Perlin, 1993). Reducing eye movement, while allowing the client to be more aware of such items, gives him or her access to more information more quickly, and thus should improve performance. Training for these devices involves an explanation of their uses and applications in everyday situations to determine if clients consider the devices useful.

A handheld reverse telescope is held close to the eye. The client looks through the device and sees compressed images, to which he or she must acclimate. Holding a reverse telescope farther from the eye defeats its purpose. It is also possible to have a reverse telescope put into an eyeglass frame through which the client can look.

High minus lenses and some minifiers are held 12 to 16 in away from the eye. Fresnel prisms are worn on glasses. Images seen through these devices are displaced instead of being compressed. The client is instructed to move the eye until the displaced image is seen. The amount of eye movement the client needs to make is less than if the device were not present.

CASE STUDIES

Low vision training is a crucial part of comprehensive low vision care that connects information concerning a person's visual abilities, medical and optical recommendations and prescriptions, and personal and family goals to a rehabilitation action plan. Instruction related to low vision, in its various forms, can lead to improved performance on tasks related to rehabilitation goals that serve to increase a person's independence and quality of life. Sometimes this instruction involves training in basic visual skills, and sometimes it can encourage clients to apply their visual skills in key tasks related to rehabilitation goals. It can involve the use of visual or nonvisual adaptations to ensure that desired tasks are performed successfully, albeit using alternative methods. Low vision training can also include the use of nonoptical, optical, or electronic devices that improve an individual's task performance. This training forms one part of the full array of rehabilitative services that may be required to address the expressed needs of adults with low vision.

The case studies that follow illustrate the process of providing comprehensive rehabilitation services for adults with low vision and the importance of tying instructional goals to tasks that have meaning in the client's life. These case studies were created from information about actual clients of the Southeastern Blind Rehabilitation Center (SBRC), an intensive in-patient facility, at the Veterans Affairs Medical Center in Birmingham, Alabama. This facility provides an extensive array of rehabilitation services to its clients, who are all veterans, including O&M, activities of daily living, written communication, manual skills, and computer access technology as well as low vision instruction. The veterans receive rehabilitation five days a week while attending classes seven hours per day. Provision of these types of comprehensive rehabilitation services covering a broad range of rehabilitation goals is the standard to which all rehabilitation programs for persons with low vision need to strive. As mentioned in Chapter 1, although a particular agency, program, clinic, or private office may not be able to provide all services needed by a client with low vision, practitioners can be part of a larger network of service providers, and clients can be referred to specialists within that network for the comprehensive low vision rehabilitation care they require.

Mr. Montoya

Mr. Montoya, a 38-year-old veteran, was admitted to SBRC with a diagnosis of optic nerve disease. He suddenly lost his vision in April 2000, but regained some in July 2000. Mr. Montoya received 36 hours of low vision assessment and training.

Mr. Montoya was employed as a welder and did a lot of artistic metal work before his vision loss. As a result of a functional vision assessment and interview, the following goals were established with Mr. Montoya: to do artistic metal work and welding; read; do woodworking; and access information from computer screens.

Mr. Montoya also received assessment and evaluation from specialists in O&M, rehabilitation teaching, manual skills, and computer access technology. A training program in each area was devised based on those evaluations and assessments.

Mr. Montoya's initial distance acuity without his glasses was OD 10/350, OS 10/300. His near acuity with his glasses was OD 0.07/4.00M OS 0.09/2.50M.

He had bilateral central scotomas with other areas of scotoma extending into the periphery. He stated that his visual field was like looking through swiss cheese. His best eccentric viewing position was looking temporally with each eye. He also stated that he was sensitive to light.

Mr. Montoya was examined by an optometrist who ordered new single vision eyeglasses for him. Improvement in visual acuity with this prescription was to 10/200 (OD) and 10/160 (OS). Training with optical devices was recommended, and it was successful. Mr. Montoya received training in the following areas: eccentric viewing (near and distance); use of telescopes, including aligning, spotting, scanning, and tracking; use of magnifiers, including tracing, tracking, and scanning; environmental adaptations for intermediate and near tasks; and use of electronic magnification devices.

As a result of training, Mr. Montoya met his goals and was able to resume his active artistic life. The following optical devices were issued to him and allowed him to meet those goals:

➤ Pocket magnifier (9× Eschenbach [32D]) for short-term reading tasks.

➤ Illuminated pocket magnifier (11× COIL [40D]) which he can use for short-term reading tasks, but which requires illumination in dim light.

➤ Spectacle-mounted telescopes (5.5× Beecher), OU, for watching TV at 8 to 10 ft.

➤ Handheld monocular (8×30) for spot checking at distance, such as O&M tasks.

➤ CCTV for most of his reading. He can read at 65 to 70 words/min with it for at least 40 min and can also use it to write.

➤ 8× (OS), aspheric allowed him to read gauges needed in order to continue to do his metalwork.

➤ Galilean reading telescope (3.5×) set for 16 in working distance, allowed him to do stained glass and blacksmith work.

➤ Smoke Solarshield sunglasses for outdoor use.

➤ NoIR U21 sunglasses for indoor use.

Mr. Montoya used the various optical devices in the other training areas and was able to ascertain the usefulness of each device. He could not meet his goal of welding because his vision did not allow him a comfortable working distance and enough working space. However, at the completion of his SBRC program, Mr. Montoya was functioning independently in his other personal and artistic endeavors.

Mr. Dillon

Mr. Dillon, a 59-year-old veteran, was admitted to SBRC with a diagnosis of diabetic retinopathy. He participated in the intensive rehabilitation program for five days a week, 7 hours a day. Mr. Dillon received 41 hours of functional vision assessment and training.

Mr. Dillon was a cabinet maker and was no longer able to do that type of work because of his vision loss. He was an avid reader and stated that reading was his main goal. Through the functional vision assessment and client interview, the following additional goals were set: to achieve glare control; pay his own bills; and learn skills and techniques to be able to live by himself.

Mr. Dillon also received assessment and evaluation from specialists in O&M, rehabilitation teaching, and manual skills. A training program in each area was devised based on those evaluations and assessments.

Mr. Dillon's initial distance acuity without his glasses was OD 10/160+, OS 10/160+. His near visual acuity without his glasses was OD 0.07/4.00M, OS 0.09/2.50M.

He had scattered scotomas and had undergone multiple laser treatments. He was examined by an optometrist who prescribed new eyeglasses, and training with optical devices was begun. However, during the training program, Mr. Dillon sustained another hemorrhage. Optical device training was halted, although he continued to attend his other rehabilitation classes. When he did resume functional vision training, new assessments were performed, the appropriateness of the optical devices already in use was reevaluated, and changes were made based on the new information.

At the end of his program he had received the following types of training: telescope training; spotting, scanning, and tracking for near and distance vision; environmental adaptations for near and distance vision; and electronic magnification device training. He also used the devices in his other rehabilitation classes. The following optical devices were issued to him and enabled him to meet his goals:

➤ Illuminated pocket magnifier (7× Coil [24D]) for short-term reading

➤ Handheld monocular (8 × 30) for mobility tasks

➤ Sport glasses (2.8×) for watching TV

➤ NoIR sunglasses for glare control indoors

➤ Grey/green Solarshield sunglasses for glare control outdoors

➤ CCTV for reading and writing: 35 min at 80 words/min

Mr. Dillon met his goals and was planning to find his own living quarters. He was most pleased to be reading again.

Mrs. Brooks

Mrs. Brooks, a 78-year-old veteran, was admitted to SBRC, with a diagnosis of age-related maculopathy. She received 39 hours of functional vision assessment and training.

Mrs. Brooks was retired. Before her vision loss she head been an accomplished seamstress and wanted to be able to continue sewing. She also enjoyed reading, cooking, and canning. As a result of her functional vision assessment and interview, the following goals were set: sewing; reading; participating in any training that would improve her visual functioning.

Mrs. Brooks also received assessment and training from specialists in O&M, rehabilitation teaching, and manual skills. A training program in each area was devised based on those evaluations and assessments.

Mrs. Brooks initial distance acuity without her glasses was OD 10/100, OS 10/100. With her glasses it was OD 10/100, OS 10/100. Her near acuity without her glasses was OD 0.20/3M, OS 0.21/3M. With her glasses it was OD 0.20/4M, OS 0.24/2.50M. She had bilateral central scotomas and, because of that, received eccentric viewing training. Her best eccentric viewing position was looking down. She also stated that she was sensitive to light.

Mrs. Brooks was examined by an optometrist, who prescribed new bifocals and new prescription sunglasses with a dark grey tint. There was no noted improvement in her visual acuity with the new prescription, but upon admission her glasses were a few years old and needed to be replaced. Training with optical devices was recommended, and it provided many benefits. Mrs. Brooks received training in the following areas: eccentric viewing (near and distance); use of telescopes, including aligning, spotting, tracking, and scanning; use of magnifiers, including tracing, tracking, and scanning; environmental adaptation for intermediate and near tasks; and electronic magnification devices.

As a result of training, Mrs. Brooks met her goals and was able to resume an active life. The following optical devices were issued to her and allowed her to meet her goals:

➤ Handheld monocular (7 × 25) for spot checking at distance, such as O&M tasks.

➤ Sports glasses (2.8×) for watching TV at 8 to 10 ft.

➤ Illuminated pocket magnifier (7× COIL [24D]) with which she can do short-term reading.

➤ Illuminated stand magnifier (6× Eschenbach [20D]) with which she can do long-term reading of mail and newspapers.

➤ Color CCTV with a flexible arm as Mrs. Brooks' main sewing and reading device. She can read for 50 min at 75 words/min with it and also write using it. In addition, she was taught to do hand sewing and needlepoint and to identify color swatches (for quilting) using the CCTV. The flex arm made these tasks easier and more efficient.

Mrs. Brooks used the various optical devices in her other training areas and was able to ascertain the usefulness of each device. Upon completing her SBRC program, she was functioning independently and her quality of life had improved significantly.

REFERENCES

Anstis S. M. (1974). A chart demonstrating variations in acuity with retinal position. *Vision Research, 14,* 589–592.

Bäckman, O. (1998). Reading proficiency following rehabilitation of visually impaired elderly patients. Vision 1996 International Conference on Low Vision Proceedings. Madrid, Spain: Organización Nactional de Ciegos Españoles: Book 2: 43–6.

Bäckman, O., & Inde, K. (1979). *Low vision training.* Malmo, Sweden: Liber Hermode.

Bailey, I. L. (1982). Mirrors for visual field defects. *Optometric Monthly, 73,* 202–206.

Bailey, I. L., Bullimore, M. A., Greer, R. B., & Mattingly, W. B. (1994). Low vision magnifiers—their optical parameters and methods for prescribing. *Optometry & Vision Science. 71,* 689–698.

Barron, C. (1991). Bioptic telescopic spectacles for motor vehicle driving. *Journal of the American Optometric Association. 62,* 37–41.

Brabyn, J. A., Haegerstrom-Portnoy, G., Schneck, M. E., & Lott, L. A. (2000). Visual impairments in elderly people under everyday viewing conditions. *Journal of Visual Impairment & Blindness, 94,* 741–755.

Brabyn, J., Schneck, M., Haegerstrom-Portnoy, G., & Lott, L. (2001). The Smith-Kettlewell Institute (SKI) longitudinal study of vision function and its impact among the elderly: An overview. *Optometry and Vision Science, 78*(5), 264–269.

Brilliant, R. L. (1999). *Essentials of low vision practice.* Boston: Butterworth-Heinemann.

Chapman, B. G. (1995). Driving with the bioptic. *Journal of Vision Rehabilitation, 9,* 19–22.

Chase, J. B. (2000). Technology and use of tools: Psychological and social factors. In B. Silverstone, M. A. Lang, B. P. Rosenthal, & E. E. Faye (Eds.), *The Lighthouse handbook on vision impairment and vision rehabilitation. Volume 2* (pp. 983–1002). New York, Oxford University Press.

Cohen, J. M. (1993). An overview of enhancement techniques for field loss. *Journal of the American Optometric Association, 64,* 60–70.

Cornelissen, F. W., Melis-Dankers B. J., de Booij, A., & Kooijman, A. C. (2000). Should we (only) use ecological tasks to assess optimal illumination levels? In C. Stuen, A. Arditi, A. Horowitz, M.A. Lang, B. Rosenthal, & K. Seidman (Eds.), *Vision rehabilitation: Assessment, intervention, and outcomes* (pp. 225–229). Lisse, Netherlands: Swets & Zeitlinger.

Crews, J. E. (2000). The evolution of public policies and services for older people who are visually impaired. In B. Silverstone, M. A. Lang, B. P. Rosenthal, & E. E. Faye (Eds.), *The Lighthouse handbook on vision impairment and vision rehabilitation. Volume 2* (pp. 1287–1300). New York, Oxford University Press.

Dargent-Molina, P., Favier, F. Grandjean, M. Baudoin, C., Schott, A. M., Hausherr, E., et al. (1996). Fall-related factors and risk of hip fracture: The EPIDOS prospective study. *The Lancet 348,* 145–149.

Defini, J., & Burack-Weiss, A. (2000). Psychosocial assessment of adults with vision impairments. In B. Silverstone, M. A. Lang, B. P. Rosenthal, & E. E. Faye. (Eds.), *The Lighthouse handbook on vision impairment and vision rehabilitation. Volume 2* (pp. 885–898). New York: Oxford University Press.

Duffy, M. A. (2002). *Making life more livable: Simple adaptations for living at home after vision loss.* New York: AFB Press.

Feinbloom, W. (1931). A case report on telescopic spectacles. *The 1931 Year Book of Optometry,* 440–452.

Fletcher, D. C., Schuchard, R. A., Livingstone, C. L., Crane, W. G., & Hu, S. Y. (1994). Scanning laser ophthalmoscope macular perimetry and applications for low vision rehabilitation clinicians. *Ophthalmology Clinics of North America, 7*(2), 257–265.

Freeman, P. B., & Jose, R.T. (1997). *The art and practice of low vision.* Boston: Butterworth-Heineman.

Goodrich, G. L., & Bailey, I.L. (2000). A history of the field of vision rehabilitation from the perspective of low vision. In B. Silverstone, M. A. Lang, B. P. Rosenthal, & E. E. Faye (Eds.), *The Lighthouse handbook on vision impairment and vision rehabilitation. Volume 2* (pp. 675–715). New York: Oxford University Press.

Goodrich, G. L., & Kirby, J. (2001). A comparison of patient reading performance and preference: Optical devices, handheld CCTV (Innoventions Magni-Cam), or stand-mounted CCTV (Optelec Clearview or TSI Genie). *Optometry, 72,* 519–528.

Goodrich, G. L., Kirby, J., Keswick, C., Oros, T., Wagstaff, P., Donald, B., Hazan, J., & Peters, L. (2000a). Reading, reading devices, and the low vision patient: Quantifying benefits of CCTV versus optical aids. In C. S. Stuen, A. Arditi, A. Horowitz, M. A. Lang, B. Rosenthal, & K. Seidman (Eds.), *Vision rehabilitation: Assessment, intervention, and outcomes* (pp. 333–337). Exton, PA: Swets & Zeitlinger.

Goodrich, G. L., Kirby, J. Keswick, C., Oros, T., Wagstaff, P., Donald, B., Hazan, J. & Peters, L. (2000b). Training the patient with low vision to read: Does it significantly improve function? In C.S. Stuen, A. Arditi, A. Horowitz, M. A. Lang, B. Rosenthal, & K. Seidman (Eds.), *Vision rehabilitation: Assessment, intervention, and outcomes* (pp. 230–236). Exton, PA: Swets & Zeitlinger.

Goodrich, G. L., Mehr, E.B., & Darling, N.C. (1980) Parameters in the use of CCTVs and optical aids. *American Journal of Optometry & Physiological Optics, 57*(12), 881–892.

Goodrich, G. L., & Quillman, R. D. (1977) Training eccentric viewing. *Journal of Visual Impairment & Blindness, 71,* 377–381.

Hall, A., Bailey, I. L., Kekelis, L. S., Raasch, T., & Goodrich, G. (1987). Retrospective survey to investigate use of distance magnifiers for travel. *Journal of Visual Impairment & Blindness, 81,* 418–423.

Hall, G. W., & Schultmeyer, M. (2002). The FUBI system for solar rating nonprescription eyewear. *Optometry, 73,* 407–417.

Hoeft, W. W. (1992). The amorphic lens. In B. Rosenthal & R. Cole (Eds.), *Problems in optometry: Patient and practice management in low vision.* Philadelphia: J.B. Lippincott.

Holcomb, J. G., & Goodrich, G.L. (1976). Eccentric viewing training. *Journal of the American Optometric Association, 47* (11), 1438–1443.

Hoppe, E., & Perlin, R. R. (1993). The effectivity of Fresnel prisms for visual field enhancement. *Journal of the American Optometric Association, 64,* 46–53.

Huss, C. P. (1988). Model approach—low vision driver's training and assessment. *Journal of Vision Rehabilitation, 2*(2), 31–44.

Huss, C. (2000). Training the low vision driver. In C. S. Stuen, A. Arditi, A. Horowitz, M. A. Lang, B. Rosenthal, & K. Seidman (Eds.), *Vision rehabilitation: Assessment, intervention, and outcomes* (pp. 268–270). Exton, PA: Swets & Zeitlinger.

Inde, K., & Bâckman, Ö. (1975). *Visual training with optical aids.* Malmo, Sweden: Hermods.

Jose, R. T. (1983). Treatment options. In R. T. Jose (Ed.), *Understanding low vision.* New York: American Foundation for the Blind.

Jose, R. T., Carter, K., Carter, C. (1983). A training program for clients considering the use of bioptic telescope for driving. *Journal of Visual Impairment & Blindness, 77,* 425–428.

Laderman, D. J., Szlyk, J. P., Kelsch, R. K. T., & Seiple, W. (2000). A curriculum for training patients with peripheral visual field loss to use bioptic amorphic lenses. *Journal of Rehabilitation Research and Development, 37*(5), 607–619.

Leonard, R. (2000). Vision impairment in working-age adults. In B. Silverstone, M. A. Lang, B. P. Rosenthal, & E. E. Faye. (Eds.), *The Lighthouse handbook on vision impairment and vision rehabilitation. Volume 2* (pp. 1201–1218). New York: Oxford University Press.

Leventhal, J., & Earl, C. (2000). Turning the printed word into speech: A review of Open Book Ruby Edition and Kurzweil 1000. *AccessWorld, 1,* 18–26.

Lott, L. A., Schneck, M. E., Haegerstrom-Poertnoy, G., Brabyn, J. A., Gildengorin, G. L., & West, C. G. (2001). Reading performance in older adults with good acuity. *Optometry and Vision Science, 78*(5), 316–324.

Ludt, R. (1997). Three types of glare: Low vision O&M assessment and remediation. *RE:view, 29,* 101–113.

Lund, R., & G. R. Watson, G.R. (1997). *The CCTV Book: Habilitation and rehabilitation with closed circuit television systems.* Lillesand, Norway: TERJES trykkeri as.

Mehr, E. B. & Freid, A. N. (1975). *Low vision care.* Chicago: The Professional Press.

Merriam, S. B., & Caffarella, R. S. (1999). *Learning in adulthood: A comprehensive guide.* San Francisco: Jossey-Bass.

Moore, J. E., & Wolffe, K. (1996). Employment considerations for adults with low vision. In A. L. Corn & A. J. Koenig, A.J. (Eds.), *Foundations of low vision: Clinical and functional perspectives* (pp. 340–362). New York: AFB Press.

Neve, J. J., & Jenniskens, A. J. W. (1994). In A. C. Kooijman, P. L. Looijestijn, J. A. Wellings, & G. J. VanderWildt (Eds.). *The legibility of TV-subtitles for the elderly and visually impaired. Low Vision: Research and New Developments in Rehabilitation* (pp. 243–250). Amsterdam: IOS Press.

Nilsson, U. L., Frennesson, C., & Nilsson, S.E.G. (1998). Location and stability of a newly established eccentric retinal locus suitable for reading, achieved through training of patients with a dense central scotoma. *Optometry and Vision Science, 75* (12), 873–878.

Parker, D. (2001). *SRA reading laboratories,* Columbus, OH: SRA/McGraw-Hill.

Quillman, R. D. (1980) *Low vision training manual.* Kalamazoo, MI: Western Michigan University.

Rosenbloom, A. A. (2000). Vision care for elderly individuals: Innovation and advancement in low vision services. In J. E. Crews & F. J. Whittington (Eds.), *Vision loss in an aging society* (pp. 85–107). New York: AFB Press.

Salive, M. E., Guralnik, J., Glynn, R. J., Christen, W., Wallace, R. B., & Ostfeld, A. M. (1994). Association of visual impairment with mobility and physical function. *Journal of the American Gerontological Society, 42,* 287–292.

Singer, H. W. (1999). Success with low vision patients: Realistic prognosis, reasonable goals. *Journal of Ophthalmic Nursing Technology 18,* 65–7.

Spitzberg, L. A., & Goodrich, G. L. (1995). New ergonomic stand magnifiers. *Journal of the American Optometric Association, 66,* 25–30.

Szlyk, J. P., Seiple, W., Laderman, D. J., Kelsch, R., Ho, K., & McMahon, T. (1998). Use of bioptic amorphic lenses to expand the visual field in patients with peripheral loss. *Optometry and Vision Science, 75*(7), 518–524.

Szlyk, J. P., Seiple, W., Laderman, D. J., Kelsch, R., Stelmack, J., & McMahon, T. (2000). Measuring the effectiveness of bioptic telescopes for patients with central field loss. *Journal of Rehabilitation Research & Development, 37*(1), 101–108.

Tuttle, D. W., & Tuttle, N. R. (1996). *Self-esteem and adjusting with blindness* (2nd ed.). Springfield, IL: Charles C. Thomas.

Vogel, G. L. (1991). Training the bioptic telescope wearer for driving. *Journal of the American Optometric Association, 62:* 288–293.

Warren, M. (1996). *Pre-reading and writing exercises for persons with macular scotomas.* Lenexa, KS: visABILITIES Rehab Services, Inc.

Watson, G. (1996). Older adults with low vision. In A. L. Corn & A. J. Koenig (Eds.), *Foundations of low vision: Clinical and functional perspectives* (pp. 363–394). New York: AFB Press.

Watson, G., Baldasare, J., & Whittaker, S. (1990). The validity and clinical uses of the Pepper Visual Skills for Reading Test. *Journal of Visual Impairment & Blindness, 84*(3), 119–123.

Watson, G., Whittaker, S., & Steciw, M. (1995). *Pepper Visual Skills for Reading Test* (2nd ed.). Lilburn, GA: Bear Consultants.

Watson, G. R., Quillman, R. D., Flax, M., & Gerritsen, B. (1999). The development of low vision therapist certification. *Journal of Visual Impairment & Blindness, 93,* 451–456.

Watson, G. R., Wright, V., & De l'Aune, W. (1992) The efficacy of comprehension training and reading practice for print readers with macular loss. *Journal of Visual Impairment & Blindness. 86*(1), 37–43.

Whittaker, S. G., & Lovie-Kitchin, J. (1993). Visual requirements for reading. *Optometry and Vision Science, 70,* 54–65.

Wolfe, K. E. (1996). Adults with low vision: Personal, social, and independent living needs. In A. L. Corn & A. J. Koenig (Eds.), *Foundations of low vision: Clinical and functional perspectives* (pp. 322–339). New York: AFB Press.

Wright, V., & Watson, G.R. (1995). *Learn to use your vision for reading workbook.* Lilburn, GA: Bear Consultants.

Zimmerman, G. J. (1996). Optics and low vision devices. In A. L. Corn & A. J. Koenig (Eds.), *Foundations of low vision: Clinical and functional perspectives* (pp. 340–362). New York: AFB Press.

Household Hints for People with Low Vision

General Hints

➤ Keep things orderly. Organization will help you to locate items more easily.

➤ Proper lighting is very important. Adjust the lighting according to the activity you are doing. Sometimes you will need more or less light than at other times. Use natural daylight when available.

➤ Color contrast will help make many tasks easier. Use light objects against dark backgrounds and dark objects against light backgrounds. Use the colors that you can see best.

Kitchen

➤ When pouring dark liquids (such as coffee), use a light-colored cup. Place the light-colored cup on dark-colored background.

➤ When pouring light-colored liquid (such as milk), use a dark-colored cup on a light background.

➤ To pour water use a dark-colored glass, not a transparent one.

➤ Use a frosted drinking glass or pour colored liquid into clear drinking glass before serving. This helps to locate the glass.

➤ Using trays is a helpful way to create a contrasting background on the kitchen counter. If you have a light-colored countertop and are pouring coffee into a light-colored cup, place the cup on a dark-colored tray to aid in locating the cup.

➤ Use a dark cutting board for light foods and a light cutting board for dark foods.

➤ Use brightly colored paint, or brightly colored vinyl or cloth tape on cupboards, cabinets, drawers, handles, to aid in locating them visually.

➤ Use a brightly colored paint or tape on the handles of kitchen equipment and utensils: pots, pans, measuring cups, etc.

➤ Use a pot with a colored interior (rather than aluminum). This makes it easier to see water boiling and various other foods.

➤ Stove and oven dials can also be marked with short strips of bright, contrasting tape, puff paint, or raised dots. Mark the oven dial at the temperature most frequently used, or use several contrasting colors for different temperatures.

➤ Use droppers when measuring liquids such as vanilla. Bend metal measuring spoons so that the handle is perpendicular to the spoon. The spoon can then be dipped into the item to be measured without fear of overpouring or spilling.

Compiled by Amanda Lueck, Angela Bau, and Helen Dornbusch for patients at the Low Vision Clinic, School of Optometry, University of California, Berkeley.

(continued on next page)

➤ Unless you absolutely need them, tape the back burners of your stove off. This will prevent you from reaching over a hot pan on a front burner.

➤ Use a timer. It will be easier than trying to check visually on items you are cooking.

➤ Color code recipe cards: one color for meat dishes, another for poultry, a third for desserts.

➤ Rewrite favorite recipes on index cards in large print with a black fiber-tip pen.

➤ Label groceries by rewriting the name of the item on light colored matte paper with a black fiber-tip pen. Secure the label to the item with a rubber band.

➤ Keep your kitchen organized: be the one in charge of putting groceries and other items away.

➤ Remember to completely close all kitchen cabinets, cupboards, and drawers.

Serving and Eating

➤ Use the contrast rule for setting the table: place light dishes on a dark tablecloth or placemat. Place dark dishes on a light contrasting tablecloth. Use a solid tablecloth or placemat only; patterns can be confusing.

➤ If proper lighting allows you to see the food on your plate, use it. Place a high-intensity lamp in position by your place setting to illuminate your plate.

➤ To aid a person in locating the position of different foods on a plate, use the clock system. The location of the food will correspond to the number position on the face of a clock. For example, chicken at the top of the plate would be at 12 o'clock, peas at the bottom of the plate would be at 6 o'clock, and so on.

➤ Use more solid textured foods to help guide hard to handle foods onto the eating utensil. For example, use potatoes or meat as a buffer against which you can gently push peas onto a fork. A roll or piece of bread will also work nicely.

Bathroom

➤ Use magnifying mirrors to help when shaving or applying makeup.

➤ A towel hung on the wall opposite the bathroom mirror, at the appropriate height, provides a contrasting background for the image of your head and hair. If you have light hair, use a dark towel; if you have dark hair, use a light towel.

➤ If glare in the bathroom is a problem for you, plastic or wood racks and accessories with a matte finish may cut down on the glare caused by items made of metal or glass.

➤ When choosing a shower curtain, clear plastic (with a design if desired) allows more light to be transmitted than an opaque solid color.

At Home

➤ Brightly colored vinyl or cloth tape provides color contrast to help locate the thermostat, electrical outlets, light switches, drawstrings on draperies, and other household items.

➤ For steps and stairs inside and outside of your home, mark the edge and riser of the steps with a contrasting adhesive, paint, or safety tape.

➤ Place colored tape around a wall socket so that it is not necessary to locate the socket with your hands.

➤ Use colored tape to mark the position of favorite stations on radio dials.

➤ When placing furniture in a conversational setting, consider the distance at which conversation would be most comfortable. Chairs placed too far apart may be just out of visual comfort distance for some persons with low vision.

➤ When white furniture is placed against or near a white wall, the edge of the furniture may be difficult to detect. Place a plant or brightly colored object at or near the edge to provide cues regarding edge and height of surface.

➤ Avoid bright patterns for such items as table cloths and furniture upholstery. They are often difficult to look at over a large area and small objects placed on or near them may be difficult to locate.

➤ Look for basic shapes and colors when identifying products in a supermarket. For example, two shelves of off-white jars with some blue indicates mayonnaise. A rectangle of red on containers in the same aisle indicates tomato catsup.

Recreational Activities

➤ When doing needlepoint or hooking rugs, place a dark cloth below the canvas. The strands of the canvas will stand out.

➤ When sorting two yarns or threads that differ slightly in color, compare each strand to a ball of one color. Against a solid background of color, it is easier to discriminate which strand is needed.

➤ When changing levels while hiking, measuring a level against oneself makes it easier to judge a height (e.g., the rock is up to my knee) if you have trouble with depth perception. When going down, being second in line is helpful so you can check the level of your feet against the person below (e.g., your feet are level with his or her knee).

➤ When playing sports or games choose balls and other objects that contrast the background (e.g., orange tennis balls and white or yellow ping pong balls). A stripe around a ball will give it a flicker effect and make it more visible. While some people prefer catching or hitting a ball that comes directly at them, others prefer to catch a "high fly" because the ball will be seen against the sky for a short time. Using a larger than average tennis racket may also be helpful and it does not detract from one's enjoyment of the game.

➤ When looking for friends in a movie theater, walk up to the screen and look back at the auditorium, letting the light from the screen illuminate the audience.

➤ Color televisions often permit people who have low vision to sit a little further from the screen; as with colored pictures, the detail is more easily seen than with black and white pictures.

(continued on next page)

➤ Leave a light on in the room while watching television. Although this is recommended for all viewers, it may be particularly helpful for some people who have low vision, such as those with nystagmus. The bright light of the TV in a darkened room appears to oscillate. A low level of ambient illumination in the room will reduce this effect.

➤ Photography is an enjoyable hobby that can also help maximize visual abilities. Taking a photograph and enlarging it may show facial features to a person who cannot see the features on the person, or it may be used to enlarge a variety of objects. Telephoto lenses, while larger than handheld monoculars, become, when turned toward the picture taker, instant (low power) monoculars as the viewer looks through the viewfinder.

➤ When enlarging music with large-print music paper (available from the American Printing House for the Blind; see Resources section) an ink pad and two pencil erasers save time to stamp out the notes. One pencil eraser is used as is, while the center of the other eraser is removed (with a cork borer or similar instrument). This second eraser is used for whole notes. These notes can be darkened as needed.

APPENDIX
GLOSSARY
RESOURCES
INDEX

Visual Consequences of Most Common Eye Conditions Associated with Visual Impairment

ROANNE FLOM

CONDITION	DESCRIPTION	STABILITY OF CONDITION	VISUAL ACUITY
Achromatopsia (rod monochromacy)	Normal rod photoreceptors in retina; few and abnormal cone photoreceptors; nystagmus	Stable	20/100 to 20/200
Albinism (includes ocular and oculocutaneous albinism)	Translucent irises, pale fundus, macular hypoplasia, nystagmus	Stable	20/60 to 20/400
Aniridia	Narrowed or absent iris	Cataract and glaucoma may develop	20/200 to 20/400
Coloboma	Notches or other defects involving the iris, lens, retina, choroid, and/or optic nerve	Usually stable; retinal complications may develop	20/20 to 20/400
Congenital cataract (with cataract removal)	Aphakia, deprivation amblyopia; nystagmus may or may not be present	Glaucoma may develop	20/40 to 20/400
Cortical visual impairment (cerebral visual impairment)	Dysfunction of posterior visual pathway (lateral geniculate to visual cortex), usually accompanied by other neurological disorders	Can improve at an early age; highly variable visual functioning	Varies
Delayed visual maturation	Brain dysfunction associated with varying causes	Improves by 8 months of age in most affected children	Varies

REFRACTIVE ERROR	PERIPHERAL VISUAL FIELDS	CONTRAST SENSITIVITY	PREFERRED TASK LIGHTING	SENSITIVITY TO AMBIENT LIGHTING	COLOR VISION	ACCOMMODATION
Astigmatism	Normal	Reduced	Dim	Very high	None, but can name some colors by brightness	Varies with age
Astigmatism	Normal	Normal	Dim to intermediate	High to very high	Normal	Varies with age
Astigmatism	Normal (unless advanced glaucoma present also)	Reduced	Dim to intermediate	High to very high	Normal	Reduced
Varies	Depends on retinal area involved; superior most common	Varies	Varies	Varies	Normal	Varies with age
High hyperopia	Normal (unless advanced glaucoma also)	Reduced	Varies	Moderate	Normal	Absent if cataract removed
Varies	Nearly always	Reduced	Varies	High in about 1/3 of cases	May prefer primary colors	Varies with age
Varies	Varies	Reduced	Varies	Varies	Varies	Varies with age

(continued on next page)

CONDITION	DESCRIPTION	STABILITY OF CONDITION	VISUAL ACUITY
Diabetic retinopathy	Abnormal retinal swelling and/or new blood vessel growth; glaucoma can develop	Laser treatment or surgery may stabilize	20/20 to NLP
Glaucoma	Optic nerve atrophy due to elevated intraocular pressure, insufficient blood flow, or other processes	Often stabilized or slowed with treatment	Reduced in advanced cases
Keratoconus	Thinning and distortion of cornea with possible scarring	Slowly progressive; may require surgery	20/20 to 20/60 with contact lenses
Macular degeneration (includes age-related, myopic, juvenile, Stargardt's disease, histoplasmosis, and toxoplasmosis)	Atrophy and/or scarring or retina at macula; abnormal new blood vessels can form	Usually progresses for several years	20/25 to 20/1000
Macular holes	Photoreceptor layers pulled away from center of macula	Stable; surgery may be possible in early stages	20/40 to 20/400
Marfans' syndrome	Connective tissue disorder causes crystalline lens to loosen; lens may dislocate partially or fully	Lens position may vary; glaucoma may develop	Near normal
Nystagmus (congenital)	Macular hypoplasia; nystagmus	Stable	20/20 to 20/120
Optic atrophy	Optic nerve atrophy; nystagmus may or may not be present	Usually stable	20/80 to 20/2000
Optic nerve hypoplasia	Congenitally small optic nerve; nystagmus may or may not be present	Stable	20/60 to 20/200
Retinal detachment	Photoreceptor layers of retina pulled away from underlying tissues	May recur	20/20 to NLP

REFRACTIVE ERROR	PERIPHERAL VISUAL FIELDS	CONTRAST SENSITIVITY	PREFERRED TASK LIGHTING	SENSITIVITY TO AMBIENT LIGHTING	COLOR VISION	ACCOMMODATION
Variable if sugar levels are dysregulated	Depends on retinal areas damaged	Reduced	Moderate	Moderate	Reduced	Reduced
Myopia more common	Mid- and then far peripheral; can be central	Reduced	Moderate	Moderate	Reduced	Varies with age
Contact lenses usually required	Normal	Reduced	Varies	Varies	Normal	Varies with age
Varies	Central scotomas	Reduced	Bright	High	Reduced	Varies with age
Varies	Small and central scotomas	Reduced	Moderate	Moderate	Normal	Varies with age
High myopia	Normal	Normal	Varies	Varies	Normal	Reduced
Varies	Normal	Normal	Normal	Normal	Normal	Varies with age
Varies	Varies	Reduced	Moderate	Moderate	Reduced	Varies with age
Varies	Varies	Reduced	Moderate	Mild to moderate	Reduced	Varies with age
Myopia more common	Varies	Varies	Varies	Varies	Varies	Varies with age

(continued on next page)

CONDITION	DESCRIPTION	STABILITY OF CONDITION	VISUAL ACUITY
Retinitis pigmentosa and Leber's amaurosis	Photoreceptor degeneration usually begins in midperiphery and extends outward and inward; nystagmus may or may not be present	Slowly progressive over decades	In advanced disease 20/40 to NLP; acuity loss may be early in some uncommon form of this condition
Retinoblastoma	Highly malignant hereditary eye tumor of early childhood mandates surgical eye removal	Surgical removal of eye mandated for survival	NLP
Retinopathy of prematurity	Incomplete retinal development and dragging of macula; nystagmus may or may not occur	Cataract and glaucoma may develop	20/20 to NLP
Stroke	Brain damage often limited to one hemisphere; nystagmus with oscillopsia may or may not occur	Stable after initial several months	20/20 to NLP
Trauma	Varies	Varies	20/20 to NLP
Venous occlusion (includes central retinal and branch vein occlusions	Blocked vein causes retinal damage	Blood and swelling may resolve early on; glaucoma may develop	20/20 to 20/400

NLP = no light perception.

REFRACTIVE ERROR	PERIPHERAL VISUAL FIELDS	CONTRAST SENSITIVITY	PREFERRED TASK LIGHTING	SENSITIVITY TO AMBIENT LIGHTING	COLOR VISION	ACCOMMODATION
Varies	Mid-peripheral, then tunnel vision, then complete field loss	Reduced	Moderate to bright	High	Reduced	Varies with age
Not applicable	Not applicable	Not applicable	Not applicable	Not applicable	Not applicable	Not applicable
Myopia	Varies	Reduced	Moderate	Moderate	Varies	Varies with age
Varies	Varies; hemianopsia, quadrant-anopsia, or complete field loss possible	Varies	Varies	Varies	Varies	Varies with age
Varies	Varies	Varies	Varies	Varies	Varies	Varies with nature of damage and age
Varies	Varies	Reduced	Moderate	Moderate	Reduced	Varies with age

Glossary

Absorptive lenses Eyeglasses with lenses tinted to absorb much of the sun's light and prevent it from entering the eye; sunglasses.

Accommodation The ability of the eye to maintain a clear focus as objects are moved closer to it by changing the shape of the lens.

Achromatopsia A congenital defect in or absence of cones, resulting in the inability to see color and reduced clear central vision.

Age-related macular degeneration A condition associated with vascular diseases such as arteriosclerosis and stroke, in which the central vision is gradually lost, decreasing in some people to 20/200 or less, but peripheral vision is usually retained. Also called age-related maculopathy.

Albinism, ocular Congenital absence of pigment in the iris and choroid, causing light sensitivity, nystagmus, and reduced visual acuity.

Albinism, oculocutaneous Congenital lack of pigment in the iris, choroid, hair, and skin resulting in reduced visual acuity, light sensitivity, and nystagmus.

Amblyopia Reduced vision without observable changes in the structure of the eye, caused by eyes that are not straight or by a difference in the refractive error in the two eyes, sometimes called "lazy eye." Not correctable with lenses, since the brain's suppression is the cause.

Amsler grid A graphlike card used to determine central visual field losses.

Angular magnification Increasing the apparent size of an object through the use of various lens systems, such as binoculars.

Aniridia A congenital malformation of the iris that can be accompanied by nystagmus, photophobia, reduced visual acuity, and often glaucoma.

Aphakia The absence of the lens, usually resulting from the removal of a cataract.

Arrangement test A type of color vision test that uses color caps to be arranged in a particular order by the individual being tested.

Assistive devices Optical, nonoptical, closed-circuit television, and computer-generated images that enable and/or encourage visual functioning.

Assistive technology Computer hardware and software used to make the environment and printed information accessible.

Astigmatism A refractive error caused by a spherocylindrical curvature of the cornea; correctable with a cylindrical lens.

Binocular vision Use of both eyes to form a fused image in the brain.

Compiled by Lori Cassels, California School for the Blind, Fremont.

Biobehavioral states A range of activity levels from sleep to alert or agitated. The ability to learn requires the maintenance of alert biobehavioral states.

Bioptic telescope A miniature telescope mounted on an eyeglass lens (called the carrier lens) and positioned above or below the direct line of sight when facing forward. It is used for momentary spotting of objects at a distance.

Blind spot See Scotoma.

Blink reflex A contraction of the eyelid muscles to close the lids that occurs spontaneously in response to sudden loud noises, bright lights, sneezing, or a perceived visual threat.

Cataracts A clouding of the lens, which may be congenital, traumatic, secondary to another visual impairment, or age related. When a cataract is surgically removed, an intraocular lens implant or contact lens or spectacle correction is necessary to provide the refractive function of the absent lens.

Central scotoma Area of diminished or absent vision that result in a blind spot in the center of the visual field.

Cerebral visual impairment See Cortical visual impairment.

Closed-circuit television system (CCTV) A device that provides electronic magnification by means of a video camera that projects the image onto a television monitor; also known as video magnifier.

Coloboma A congenital cleft in some portion of the eye, caused by the improper fusion of tissue during gestation; may affect the optic nerve, ciliary body, choroid, iris, lens, or eyelid.

Color vision The perception of color as a result of the stimulation of specialized cone receptors in the retina.

Concave lens A lens that spreads out light rays and is used to correct for myopia. Also called Minus lens. See also Spherical lens.

Cone dystrophy Hereditary degeneration of cones, resulting in decreased vision and a lack of color perception.

Cones Specialized photoreceptor cells in the retina, primarily concentrated in the macular area, that are responsible for sharp vision and color perception.

Confrontation visual field testing A method for making an approximate assessment of peripheral vision.

Contact lens A small plastic disc containing an optical correction that is worn directly on the cornea as a substitute for eyeglasses.

Contrast sensitivity The ability to detect small changes in brightness.

Convex lens A lens that bends light rays inward and is used to correct for hyperopia. Also called Plus lens. See also Spherical lens.

Cornea The transparent tissue at the front of the eye that is curved to provide most of the eye's refractive power.

Cortical visual impairment Visual impairment caused by change to the posterior visual pathways and/or the occipital lobe of the brain.

Depth of field The range of distances that an object can be from a lens and still appear to be in focus to the observer.

Depth perception Ability to determine relative spatial location of objects.

Diabetic retinopathy Range of retinal changes associated with long-standing diabetes. Stages include nonproliferative (early) and proliferative (when blood vessels grow abnormally and fibrous tissues form).

Diagnostic teaching The analysis of learning problems during lessons and targeted instruction to minimize or eliminate the problems.

Diopter The unit of measurement for the refractive power of a lens.

Eccentric fixation The use for visual fixation of a portion of the retina that is not specialized for sharp focus.

Eccentric viewing Looking to the side, above, below, or above an object of regard in order to place it in best focus. This often is necessary when there has been damage to the fovea.

Electronic magnification systems Machines that produce enlarged images, including closed-circuit televisions, computer systems, and low vision enhancement devices.

Emergent literacy The earliest phase in literacy learning, in which young children are actively engaged in experimenting with reading and writing and in gaining meaning from these activities.

Emmetropia The condition of a normal eye in which there is no refractive error.

Environmental adaptation or modification Change in the environment to maximize a person's ability to function.

Enlargement ratio The size of the image relative to the size of the object when viewed through a magnifier.

Esophoria The tendency of the eye to deviate inward.

Esotropia A form of strabismus in which one or both eyes deviate inward.

Exophoria The tendency of the eye to deviate outward.

Exotropia A form of strabismus in which one or both eyes deviate outward.

Field expansion systems A variety of optical devices for individuals with reduced visual fields, including prism lenses, mirror magnifiers, and reverse telescopes.

Figure-ground perception Ability to discriminate an object visually against its background.

Fixating Directing the eye so that the object of interest is imaged on the fovea or the preferred retinal locus.

Focal distance The distance between a lens and the point at which parallel light rays are brought to a focus.

Focal point The point at which parallel light rays are brought to a focus by a lens.

Following See Tracking.

Form constancy Ability to identify form regardless of size, orientation, or if embedded in other forms.

Fovea centralis An indentation in the center of the macula where the cones are concentrated, there are no blood vessels, and the clearest vision takes place.

Functional blindness Condition in which some useful vision may or may not be present but in which the individual uses tactile and auditory channels most effectively for learning.

Functional literacy The ability to apply reading and writing skills to practical tasks in everyday life.

Functional vision The ability to use vision in planning and performing a task.

Functional vision evaluation An evaluation of visual abilities as used in functional tasks, such as reading, tasks of daily living, vocational pursuits for older children and adults, and educational programming for students and most often conducted in the person's usual home, school, or work environment. Also known as functional vision assessment.

Glare Discomfort produced by too much light in the visual field.

Glaucoma An increase in intraocular pressure, associated with a buildup of aqueous fluid, which may cause damage to the nerves of the retina and the optic nerve and eventual visual field defects if left untreated.

Hemianopsia A defect in either half of the visual field. Also called hemianopia.

Hyperopia (farsightedness) A refractive error caused by an eyeball that is too short; corrected with a plus (convex) lens.

Hypertropia The upward deviation of one eye.

Hypotropia The downward deviation of one eye; the least common of the eye deviations classified as strabismus.

Independent living skills Skills for performing daily tasks and managing personal needs. Individuals with low vision often learn alternative or modified methods of performing these skills.

Individualized education program (IEP) A written plan of instruction for a student who receives special education services, developed by an educational team that includes the student and family.

Individualized family service plan (IFSP) A written plan developed by an educational team for the coordination of early intervention services for infants and toddlers with disabilities, with emphasis on family support, involvement, and implementation.

Individualized written rehabilitation program (IWRP) A contract between a person and a rehabilitation agency that describes the services needed to achieve that person's employment objective.

Interdisciplinary team Specialists who work individually with clients or students, but among whom there is communication.

Legal blindness A visual impairment in which distance visual acuity is 20/200 or less in the better eye with best correction or a visual field of 20 degrees diameter or less. Used as a criterion for determining eligibility for benefits or services in the United States.

Lens The transparent, biconvex structure within the eye that allows it to refract light rays, enabling them to focus on the retina; also, any transparent substance that can refract light in a predictable manner.

Light projection The ability to discern the source or direction of light, but not enough vision to identify objects, people, shapes, or movements.

Literacy The ability to read and write.

Literacy medium The method used by an individual to read and write.

Localizing Having an awareness of the location of an object of interest in the environment from visual, auditory, or kinesthetic cues so that a fixation can be directed toward it.

Low vision A vision loss severe enough to impede an individual's ability to learn or perform usual tasks of daily life, given that individual's level of maturity and cultural environment, but that still allows some functionally useful visual discrimination. Low vision cannot be corrected to normal by regular eyeglasses or contact lenses and covers a range from mild to severe vision loss but excludes complete loss of functional vision.

Low vision evaluation A comprehensive examination, performed by an optometrist or ophthalmologist, that investigates many of the same factors as in a basic eye examination, but also may involve the use of different techniques leading to more precise results for individuals with low vision.

Macula A small portion of the retina, with a concentration of cones for sharp central vision, that surrounds the fovea.

Macular degeneration Deterioration of central vision caused by a degeneration of the central retina.

Magnifier A device to increase the size of an image through the use of lenses or lens systems.

Michelson contrast The difference in luminance between the target and the background divided by the average of the luminances of the target and the background.

Microscope A high-power convex lens that magnifies near objects. Usually mounted into eyeglasses and prescribed for one eye only.

Minus lens See Concave lens.

Monochromatism Poor or no color perception; the presence of only one type of retinal cone (cone monochromatism) or the absence of all cone function (rod monochromatism).

Monocular telescope A telescope that can be used in the preferred eye.

Myopia (nearsightedness) A refractive error resulting from an eyeball that is too long; corrected with a concave (minus) lens.

Nonoptical devices Devices or modifications that do not involve lenses, used to make visual information more accessible to individuals with low vision, such as reading stands, trays, positioning and seating, modifications of illumination, and large print.

Null point Direction of gaze in which the oscillation of a person's nystagmus is reduced or eliminated due to eye position or direction of gaze.

Nystagmus An involuntary oscillation of the eyes, usually rhythmical and faster in one direction; may be horizontal or vertical.

Ocular motility Eye movement controlled by the extraocular muscles.

Oculomotor Relating to eye movements and muscular control.

Ophthalmologist A physician who specializes in refractive, medical, and surgical care of the eyes.

Optical device Any system of lenses that enhances visual function.

Optic nerve hypoplasia A congenitally small optic disk, usually surrounded by a light halo and representing a regression in growth during the prenatal period; may result in reduced visual acuity.

Optics The study of light, its ability to refract and reflect, and its behavior in lenses, prisms, mirrors, and the eye.

Optometrist A health care provider who specializes in refractive errors, prescribes eyeglasses or contact lenses, and diagnoses and manages conditions of the eye as regulated by state law.

Optotype Letter, number, or symbol used in tests of visual abilities.

Orientation and mobility (O&M) instructor A professional who specializes in teaching travel skills to persons with visual impairments.

Perimetry Methods to determine an eye's field of vision using objects that are moved from the nonseeing area to the seeing area (kinetic perimetry) or objects that are stationary but increased in intensity (static perimetry).

Perceptual span The amount of information that an individual can decode and store in short-term memory in one visual fixation.

Photophobia Light sensitivity to an uncomfortable degree; usually symptomatic of other ocular disorders or diseases.

Plano lens A lens that is parallel on both sides (has no refractive power).

Plus lens See Convex lens.

Polarity Ability of electronic magnification devices or computers to display the image in either positive or negative form; usual polarity is considered black on white; reversed polarity is white on black.

Preferred retinal locus (PRL) An alternative area of the retina used for best vision when the fovea is damaged.

Presbyopia A decrease in accommodative power (focusing at near) caused by the increasing inelasticity of the lens-ciliary muscle mechanism that occurs any time after age 40.

Pursuit movements Smooth, involuntary eye movements that keep the object of attention imaged on the fovea (or PRL) as the object is moving or as the head is turning or both. Pursuit movements occur when an object is moving, as in tracking or following, but also occur with head turns when looking at stationary objects.

Refractive error A condition correctable by eyeglasses or contact lenses such as myopia, hyperopia, and astigmatism, in which parallel light rays are not brought to a focus on the retina, thus creating a blurred retinal image.

Relative-distance magnification Increasing the size of an image on the retina by bringing the object to be viewed closer to the eyes.

Relative-size magnification Increasing the size of an image on the retina by increasing the size of an object to be viewed, such as large print.

Retina The inner sensory nerve layer next to the choroid that lines the posterior two-thirds of the eyeball, which reacts to light and transmits impulses to the brain.

Retinitis pigmentosa A group of progressive, often hereditary, retinal degenerative diseases characterized by decreasing peripheral vision; some cases progress to tunnel vision whereas others result in total blindness if the macula also becomes involved.

Retinoscopy A handheld light projected onto the pupil to measure the eye's refractive error by evaluating the behavior of the light reflected back from the retina.

Retinopathy of prematurity A series of retinal changes (formerly called retrolental fibroplasia) from mild to total retinal detachment, seen primarily in premature infants, that may be arrested at any stage. Believed to be connected to the immature blood vessels in the eye and their reaction to oxygen, but may be primarily the result of prematurity with very low birth weight. Functional vision in persons with this condition can range from near normal to total blindness.

Retrolental fibroplasia See Retinopathy of prematurity.

Rod monochromatism The absence of retinal cones or the presence of nonfunctional cones, resulting in the inability to differentiate color; characterized also by nystagmus, light sensitivity, and lowered visual acuity.

Rods Specialized retinal photoreceptor cells located primarily in the peripheral retina that are responsible for seeing form, shape, and movement and that function best in low levels of illumination.

Saccadic eye movement Rapid change in fixation from one point to another.

Scanning Making a series of fixations in order to inspect a large area visually.

Scotoma A blind spot in vision created by a dense and localized visual field defect.

Shape constancy The concept that objects remain the same shape, even though they may appear to change shape when viewed at different angles.

Shifting gaze Changing fixation to a new object of interest.

Size constancy The concept that objects remain the same size, even though they appear to change size when viewed from different distances.

Spectacles Eyeglasses that hold corrective lenses.

Spherical lens A lens whose shape is a segment of a sphere. A convex (plus) lens is thicker in the center and is used to correct hyperopia, a concave (minus) lens is used to correct myopia. Other types of spherical lenses are biconvex (when both surfaces curve outward), plano-convex (a single sided curve), biconcave (both surfaces curving inward), and planoconcave (when only one surface curves inward).

Stereopsis Fine depth perception resulting from the blending of the slightly different visual images received from each eye.

Strabismus An extrinsic muscle imbalance causing misalignment of the eyes; includes exotropia, esotropia, hypertropia, and hypotropia.

Tangent screen perimetry A flexible technique for examining visual fields with 30 degrees of fixation.

Teacher of students with visual impairments A specially trained and certified teacher who is qualified to teach special skills to students with visual impairments.

Telescope A lens system that makes small objects appear closer and larger.

Tracing Making a series of saccadic eye movements to shift fixation progressively along a line or a border.

Tracking Maintaining fixation on a moving object of interest using pursuit movements.

Transdisciplinary team Specialists working jointly to plan and implement assessment and instruction, often with designated professionals or family members as primary implementors of activities.

Typoscope Reading window or template made from card stock that allows a single word or line to be read.

Video magnifier See Closed-circuit television system

Visual ability Visual performance in real-world situations.

Visual acuity A measure of the ability to resolve fine detail.

Visual capacities Visual functions that are basic to the processing of visual stimuli, including visual acuity, visual field, contrast sensitivity, color, and response to light, as well as oculomotor functions used to control the receipt of visual information, including accommodation, convergence, saccadic eye movements, and pursuit eye movements.

Visual closure Identifying a form when only part of the form is presented.

Visual field The entire region of space off to all sides that is visible when steadily looking and facing straight ahead.

Visual functions Performance of the visual system in isolation and under standard measurement conditions; visual functions include visual acuity, visual fields, contrast sensitivity, color, response to light, oculomotor, control, accommodation, and so forth.

Visual impairment Any degree of vision loss that cannot be corrected to normal through eyeglasses or contact lenses that affects an individual's ability to perform the tasks of daily life, caused by a visual system that is not working properly or not formed correctly.

Visual memory The ability to remember a visual image or form after viewing.

Visual perception The process of attaching meaning to a visual image.

Visual acuity reserve A ratio of the size of the smallest print that can be read with best efficiency or comfort to the size of the smallest print that can be read at all at a given working distance.

Visual threshold The smallest size of print that can be read at all at a given working distance.

Weber contrast The contrast difference between the object and the background on which it sits.

Working distance The distance between the eye and an object of regard, such as a page being read.

Resources

This listing provides a starting place for readers to obtain additional information that can assist them in their work with people who have low vision and offers sources of products and evaluation tools. The national organizations listed here are primary sources of information, assistance, and referral for both professionals and consumers with low vision and their families. There is a separate section on sources for products, including optical and nonoptical devices and other supplies. A final section lists many of the commonly used assessment tools and instruments discussed throughout the book. A more comprehensive listing of organizations and services can be found in the *AFB Directory of Services for Blind and Visually Impaired Persons,* published by the American Foundation for the Blind, which can also be searched electronically at the AFB web site, www.afb.org.

NATIONAL ORGANIZATIONS

American Academy of Ophthalmology
655 Beach Street
San Francisco, CA 94109
(415) 561-8500
Fax: (415) 561-8533
www.aao.org
eyemd@aao.org

A national membership association of ophthalmologists offering programs for eye care physicians and other professionals. Offers print and electronic educational materials, including reference books, audio and videotapes, CD-ROMs, self-assessment programs, and an online education center. Represents eye care physicians and their patients before federal and state policymakers and with managed care organizations.

American Academy of Optometry
6110 Executive Boulevard, Suite 506
Rockville, MD 20852
(301) 984-1441
Fax: (301) 984-4737
www.aaopt.org
aaoptom@aol.com

A professional organization dedicated to maintaining and enhancing excellence in optometric practice by fostering research and the dissemination of knowledge in both basic and applied vision science.

American Association for Pediatric Ophthalmology and Strabismus
P.O. Box 193832
San Francisco, CA 94119
(415) 461-8505
www.aapos.org

A professional organization offering information on medical and surgical eye care of children and adults with strabismus for ophthalmologists, other health care providers, and the public; encourages research; and publishes the *Journal of AAPOS.*

American Association of the Deaf-Blind
814 Thayer Avenue
Silver Spring, MD 20910
(301) 588-8705
www.aadb.org
info@aadb.org

A consumer organization of deaf-blind persons and their families that conducts advocacy activities, conducts service programs, acts as a referral service, maintains a library of materials on deaf-blindness, and holds an annual convention.

American Council of the Blind
1155 15th Street, NW, Suite 1004
Washington, DC 20005
(202) 467-5081 or (800) 424-8666
Fax: (202) 467-5085
www.acb.org
info@acb.org

A national consumer organization that serves as national clearinghouse for information and promotes the effective participation of blind people in all aspects of society. Provides information and referral; legal assistance and representation; scholarships; leadership and legislative training; consumer advocate support; assistance in technological research; a speaker referral service; consultative and advisory services to individuals, organizations, and agencies; and assistance with developing programs.

American Foundation for the Blind
11 Penn Plaza, Suite 300
New York, NY 10001
(212) 502-7600 or (800) 232-5463;
    (212) 502-7662 (TDD/TTY)
Fax: (212) 502-7777
www.afb.org
afbinfo@afb.net

An information clearinghouse for people who are blind or visually impaired and their families, professionals, organizations, schools, and corporations. Conducts research and mounts program initiatives to improve services to visually impaired persons, including the National Literacy Center, the National Employment Center, National Aging Program, and National Education Program; provides information about the latest technology available for visually impaired persons through its Technology and Employment Center; advo-

cates for services and legislation; maintains the M.C. Migel Library and Information Center and the Helen Keller Archives; provides information and referral services; produces videos and publishes books, pamphlets, the *Directory of Services for Blind and Visually Impaired Persons in the United States and Canada*, the *Journal of Visual Impairment & Blindness*, and *AccessWorld: Technology and People with Visual Impairments*.

American Optometric Association
243 North Lindbergh Boulevard
St. Louis, MO 63141
(314) 991-4100 or (800) 365-2319
Fax: (314) 991-4101
www.aoanet.org

A federation of state, student, and armed forces optometric associations working to provide the public with quality vision and eye care. Sets professional standards, helping its members conduct patient care efficiently and effectively; lobbies government and other organizations on behalf of the optometric profession; and provides research and education leadership.

American Printing House for the Blind
1839 Frankfort Avenue
Louisville, KY 40206
(502) 895-2405 or (800) 223-1839
Fax: (502) 899-2274
www.aph.org
info@aph.org

The official supplier of textbooks and educational aids for visually impaired students under federal appropriations. Promotes the independence of blind and visually impaired persons by providing specialized materials, products, and services needed for education and life. Publishes braille, large-print, recorded, CD-ROM, and tactile graphic publications; manufactures a wide assortment of educational and daily living products; modifies and develops computer-access equipment and software; maintains an educational research and development program concerned with educational methods and educational aids; and provides a reference-catalog service for volunteer-produced textbooks in all media for students who are visually impaired and for information about other sources of related materials.

Association for Education and Rehabilitation of the Blind and Visually Impaired
4600 Duke Street, Suite 430
Alexandria, VA 22304
(703) 823-9690 or (877) 492-2708
Fax: (703) 823-9695
www.aerbvi.org
aer@aerbvi.org

Membership organization for professionals who work in all phases of education and rehabilitation with visually impaired persons of all ages on the local, regional, national, and international levels. Seeks to develop and promote professional excellence through such support services as continuing education, publications, information dissemination, lobbying and advocacy, and conferences and workshops. Publishes *RE:view*, a quarterly journal for professionals working in the field of blindness, and the newsletter *AER Report* and disseminates brochures and videotapes.

Canadian Council of the Blind
396 Cooper Street, Suite 401
Ottawa, ON K2P 2H7
Canada
(613) 567-0311 or (877) 304-0968
Fax: (613) 567-2728
www.ccbnational.net
ccb@ccbnational.net

A national self-help consumer organization of persons who are blind, deaf-blind, and visually impaired.

Canadian National Institute for the Blind
1931 Bayview Avenue
Toronto, Ontario M4G 3E8
Canada

(416) 486-2500
www.cnib.ca

Fosters the integration of persons who are blind and visually impaired into the mainstream of Canadian life and promotes programs for the prevention of blindness.

Council for Exceptional Children
1110 North Glebe Road, Suite 300
Arlington, VA 22201-5704
(703) 620-3660 or (888) 221-6830;
    (703) 264-9446 (TTD/TTY)
Fax: (703) 264-9494
www.cec.sped.org
service@ced.sped.org

A professional organization for teachers, school administrators, practitioners, and others serving infants, children, and youths who require special services. Publishes periodicals, books, and other materials on teaching exceptional children; advocates for appropriate government policies; provides professionals development; disseminates information on effective instructional strategies; and holds an annual conference. The Division on Visual Impairments focuses on the education of children who are visually impaired and the concerns of professionals who work with them and publishes the *DVI Quarterly*.

Council of Citizens with Low Vision International
1155 15th Street, N.W., Suite 1004
Washington, DC 20005
(800) 733-2258
www.cclvi.org

An advocacy group providing information on low vision concerns. Publishes *Vision Access*, a quarterly journal by, for, and about people with low vision.

DB-LINK (The National Information Clearinghouse on Children Who Are Deaf-Blind)
345 North Monmouth Avenue
Monmouth, OR 97361

(800) 438-9376
www.tr.wou.edu/dblink

A federally funded clearinghouse providing information and copies of written materials related to infants, children, and youths who have both visual and hearing impairments. Publishes the newsletter *Deaf-Blind Perspectives.*

Lighthouse International
111 East 59th Street
New York, NY 10022
(212) 821-9200 or (800) 829-0500;
    (212) 821-9713 (TTY)
www.lighthouse.org

A national clearinghouse on vision impairment and vision rehabilitation. Provides vision rehabilitation services; conducts research and advocacy; trains professionals; engages in advocacy; and provides educational and professional products and adaptive devices through its catalogs.

Helen Keller National Center for Deaf-Blind Youths and Adults
111 Middle Neck Road
Sands Point, NY 11050
(516) 944-8900 (voice and TDD)
www.helenkeller.org/national/contact.htm

Provides services and technical assistance to individuals who are deaf-blind and their families and maintains a network of regional and affiliate agencies.

National Association for Parents of Children with Visual Impairments
P.O. Box 317
Watertown, MA 02272-0317
(617) 972-7444 or (800) 562-6265
Fax: (617) 972-7444
www.spedex.com/napvi/
napvi@perkins.org

Provides support to parents and families of children who are visually impaired; operates a national clearinghouse for information, education and referral; promotes public understanding of the needs and rights of children who are visually impaired; supports state and local parents' groups and workshops that education and train parents about available services, and their children's rights; and publishes the newsletter *Awareness* for parents.

National Association for Visually Handicapped (NAVH)
22 West 21st Street
New York, NY 10010
(212) 889-3141
Fax: (212) 727-2931
www.navh.org
staff@navh.org

3201 Balboa Street
San Francisco, CA 94121
(415) 221-3201
Fax: (415) 221-8754
www.navh.org
staffca@navh.org

An information clearinghouse and referral center for persons with low vision, their families, and the professionals who work with them; produces and distributes large-print reading materials; offers counseling; sells low vision devices; and publishes *In Focus* for children and *Seeing Clearly* for adults.

National Coalition on Deaf-Blindness
175 North Beacon Street
Waterton, MA 02472
(617) 972-7347
Fax: (617) 923-8076

Advocates on behalf of deaf-blind persons. Provides information to consumers and professionals.

National Federation of the Blind
1800 Johnson Street
Baltimore, MD 21230

(410) 659-9314
Fax: (410) 685-5653
www.nfb.org
nfb@nfb.org

A national consumer organization working to improve social and economic conditions of blind persons. Monitors legislation affecting blind people; assists in promoting needed services; provides evaluation of present programs and assistance in establishing new ones; grants scholarships to blind persons; and conducts a public education program. Publishes the *Braille Monitor* and *Future Reflections*.

National Library Service for the Blind and Physically Handicapped

Library of Congress
1291 Taylor Street, N.W.
Washington, DC 20542
(202) 707-5100 or (800) 424-8567;
    (202) 707-0744 (TDD/TTY)
Fax: (202) 707-0712
www.loc.gov/nls

A national program to distribute free reading materials in braille and on recorded disks and cassettes to persons who are visually impaired and physically disabled who cannot utilize ordinary printed materials.

National Organization for Albinism and Hypopigmentation

P.O. Box 959
East Hampstead, NH 03826-0959
(603) 887-2310
www.albinism.org
info@albinism.org

Offers information and support to people with albinism, their families, and the professionals who work with them. Sponsors workshops and conferences on albinism and publishes a newsletter, *NOAH News,* and information bulletins on topics specific to living with albinism.

Recording for the Blind and Dyslexic

20 Roszel Road
Princeton, NJ 08540
(609) 452-0606 or (800) 883-7201
www.rfbd.org
custserv@rfbd.org

Provider of recorded educational materials, such as textbooks and reference materials, to people who cannot effectively read standard print because of a visual, perceptual or other physical disability.

TASH
(formerly The Association for Persons with Severe Handicaps)

29 West Susquehanna Avenue, Suite 210
Baltimore, MD 21204
(410) 828-8274 or (800) 482-8274;
    (410) 828-1306 (TDD/TTY)
Fax: (410) 828-6706
www.tash.org
info@tash.org

Serves as an advocacy organization for people with disabilities, their family members, other advocates, and professionals striving for human dignity, civil rights, education, and independence for all individuals with disabilities. TASH holds an annual conference, publishes the *Journal of the Association for Persons with Severe Handicaps* and the *TASH Newsletter.*

MANUFACTURERS AND SUPPLIERS OF OPTICAL AND NONOPTICAL DEVICES AND SUPPLIES

The companies and organizations listed in this section are the sources for various products mentioned throughout this book. They represent a sampling of those that manufacture or distribute both optical and nonoptical devices, adaptive daily living products, and evaluation instruments useful for vision professionals and their clients.

Academic Therapy Publications
20 Commercial Boulevard
Novato, CA 94949

Publishes curricula and assessments, including the Motor-Free Visual Perception Test.

Ai Squared
P.O. Box 669
Manchester Center, VT 05255
(802) 362-3612
Fax: (802) 362-1670
www.aisquared.com
sales@aisquared.com or
    support@aisquared.com

Manufactures products to make computers accessible for people with low vision, including screen readers and ZoomText screen magnifiers.

AllHeart.com
431 Calle San Pablo
Camarillo, CA 93012
www.allheart.com

Distributes a variety of supplies for health care professionals, including a variety of penlights.

Amcon
40 N. Rock Hill Rd.
St. Louis, MO 63119
(314) 961-5758 or (800) 255-6161
www.amcon-labs.com

Manufactures and distributes a variety of optical and eye care products, such as vision tests, occluders, and penlights.

American Printing House for the Blind
1839 Frankfort Avenue
Louisville, KY 40206-0085
(502) 895-2405 or (800) 223-1839
www.aph.org
info@aph.org

Publishes braille, large-print, recorded, CD-ROM, and tactile graphic publications; manufactures a wide assortment of educational and daily living products; modifies and develops computer-access equipment and software; maintains an educational research and development program concerned with educational methods and educational aids; and provides a reference-catalog service for volunteer-produced textbooks in all media for students who are visually impaired and for information about other sources of related materials. See listing under National Organizations.

Bernell
4016 N. Home Street
Mishawaka, IN 46545
(574) 259-2070; (800) 348-2225
Fax: (574) 259-2102
www.bernell.com
amartin553@aol.com

Distributes a variety of low vision, vision therapy, and vision assessment products, including eye patches, cover paddles, and clip-on occluders.

Beecher Research Company
906 Morse Ave.
Schaumburg, IL 60193
(708) 893-0187 or (800) 934-8765

Corning Ophthalmics
HP-AB-02
Corning, New York 14831
(800) 821-2020
Fax: (607) 974-8107
www.corning.com/ophthalmic

Manufactures glare-control and tinted lenses

Designs for Vision
760 Koehler Avenue
Ronkonkoma, NY 11779
(631) 585-3300 or (800) 727-6407
Fax: (631) 585-3404
www.designsforvision.com
info@designsforvision.com

Manufactures optical low vision devices.

Donegan Optical Company
P.O. Box 14308
Lenexa, KS 66285-4308
(913) 492-2500
www.doneganoptical.com
info@doneganoptical.com

Manufactures optical low vision devices.

Eschenbach Optik of America
904 Ethan Allen Highway
Ridgefield, CT 06877
(203) 438-7471 or (800) 487-5389 (for eye care
    and rehabilitation professionals only);
(800) 396-3886 (for consumers)
www.eschenbach.com
info@eschenbach.com

Distributes low vision devices, including magnifiers, telescopes, sun filters, binoculars, and electronic reading devices (CCTVs).

Exceptional Teaching Aids
20102 Woodbine Avenue
Castro Valley, CA 94546
(510) 582-4859 or (800) 549-6999
Fax: (510) 582-5911
www.exceptionalteaching.com
ExTeaching@aol.com

Distributes products and teaching aids for individuals of all ages who are visually impaired or have other special needs and for those who serve this population.

Goodkin Border and Associates
1862 Veterans Memorial Highway
Austell, Georgia 30168
(770) 944-8226 or (800) 759-6275
Fax: (770) 944-0256
www.gbacorp.com/
Goodkin@bellsouth.net

Distributes a variety of products for people who are visually impaired, including optical, nonoptical, and electronic low vision devices, as well as braille products and software, screen reading systems, systems integration, and training.

Good-Lite Company
865 Muirfeld Drive
Hanover Park, IL 60130
(800) 362-3860
Fax: (888) 362-2576
www.good-lite.com

Distributes vision charts and accessories including Lea Tests.

GretagMacbeth
617 Little Britain Road
New Windsor, NY 12553-6148
(845) 565-7660; (800) 622-2384
Fax: (845) 565-0390
www.gretagmacbeth.com

Distributes the Farnsworth color vision test and manufactures a variety of daylight illumination products.

Haag-Streit UK
Edinburgh Way
Harlow
Essex, CM20 2TT
United Kingdom
44-0-1279-414969
www.haag-streit-uk.com

Manufactures ophthalmic instruments and vision testing equipment, including the Cambridge Low Contrast Gratings and the Pelli-Robson Contrast Sensitivity Chart.

Independent Living Aids
200 Robins Lane
Jericho, NY 11753
(516) 937-1848 or (800) 537-2118
www.independentliving.com
can-do@independentliving.com

Distributes a wide variety of adaptive products for individuals who are blind or visually impaired.

JBliss Imaging Systems
100 W. El Camino Real, Suite 68
Mountain View, CA 94040
(650) 940-4115 or (888) 452-5477
Fax: (650) 903-4136
www.jbliss.com
info@jbliss.com

Develops PC-based reading and magnifying systems.

Keeler Optical Company
456 Parkway
Broomall, PA 19008
(610) 353-4350 or (800) 523-5620
www.keelerusa.com
keeler@keelerusa.com

Distributes ophthalmic and other medical products.

Lighthouse Professional Products Catalog
938-K Andreason Drive
Escondido, CA 92929-1920
(800) 826-4200
Fax: (800) 368-4111
www.lighthouse.org/prodpub_procat.htm
professionalcatatlog@lighthouse.org

Distributes optical, adaptive, and vision testing products for vision-care and vision rehabilitation professionals. See also the listing for The Lighthouse International under National Organizations.

Lighting Specialities Company
735 Hastings Lane
Buffalo Grove, IL 60089-6906
(847) 215-2000 or (800) 214-4522

Low Vision Aids
10086 W. McNab Road
Tamarac, FL 33321
(954) 726-5670 or (800) 364-1608

LS&S Group
P.O. Box 673
Northbrook, IL 60065

(847) 498-9777 or (800) 468-4789;
(866) 317-8533 (TTY)
www.lssgroup.com
lssgrp@aol.com

Distributes a variety of adaptive daily living products for people who are visually impaired or hard of hearing.

Luzerne Optical
Low Vision Aids
180 North Wilkes-Barre Boulevard
P.O. Box 998
Wilkes-Barre, PA 18703-0998
(570) 822-3143 or (800) 233-9637
www.luzerneoptical.com
vision@luzerneoptical.com

Luxo Lamp Corporation
36 Midland Ave.
Port Chester, NY 10573
(800) 222-5869
www.luxous.com
office@luxous.com

Develops and manufactures a variety of lighting products.

MaxiAids
42 Executive Boulevard
P.O. Box 3209
Farmingdale, NY 11735
(631) 752-0738 or (800) 522-6294
www.maxiaids.com/Scripts/

Distributes adaptive products and products for independent living.

National Library Service for the Blind and Physically Handicapped
Library of Congress
1291 Taylor Street, N.W.
Washington, DC 20542
(202) 707-5100 or (800) 424-8567;
(202) 707-0744 (TDD/TTY)
Fax: (202) 707-0712
www.loc.gov/nls

Distributes free reading materials in braille and on recorded disks and cassettes to persons who are visually impaired and physically disabled who cannot utilize ordinary printed materials.

NoIR Medical Technologies
6155 Pontiac Trail
P.O. Box 159
South Lyon, MI 48178
(734) 769-5565 or (800) 521-9746
www.noir-medical.com

Manufactures tinted lenses and sunglasses for low vision applications.

Ocutech
109 Conner Drive, Suite 2105
Chapel Hill, NC 27514
(919) 967-6460 or (800) 326-6460
www.ocutech.com
info@ocutech.com

Develops optical low vision devices.

Optelec U.S.
6 Liberty Way
Westford, MA 01886
(978) 392-0707 or (800) 828-1056
www.optelec.com
info@optelec.com

Manufactures video magnifiers.

The Psychological Corporation
19500 Bulverde Road
San Antonio, TX 78259
(800) 872-1726
www.psychcorp.com

Publishes a wide variety of assessment and intervention products.

Psychological and Educational Publications
1477 Rollins Road
Burlingame, CA 94010

Publishes the Gardner Test of Visual-Motor Perceptual Skills.

Recording for the Blind and Dyslexic
20 Roszel Road
Princeton, NJ 08540
(609) 452-0606 or (800) 883-7201
www.rfbd.org
custserv@rfbd.org

Provides recorded educational materials, such as textbooks and reference materials, to people who cannot effectively read standard print because of a visual, perceptual, or other physical disability.

Richmond Products
1021 S. Rogers Circle #6
Boca Raton, FL 33487
(561) 994-2112
Fax: (561) 994-2235
www.richmondproducts.com
Richmndpro@aol.com

Distributes a variety of vision screen tests and ophthalmic accessories, including color blindness screening products, occluders, and daylight illuminators.

Selsi Company
194 Greenwood Ave.
Midland Park, NJ 07432
(201) 612-9200 or (800) 275-7357
www.selsioptics.com
info@selsioptics.com

Distributes optical products, including prism binoculars, telescopes, monoculars, readers, and magnifiers.

Stocking Company
620 Wheat Lane
Wood Dale, IL 60191
(630) 860-9700
www.stoeltingco.com

Publishes psychological and educational tests, including the Developmental Test of Visual Perception.

Swift Instruments
952 Dorchester Ave.
Boston, MA 02125
(800) 446-1116
www.swift-optics.com
info@swiftoptics.com

Produces teaching, medical, veterinary, and industrial microscopes.

S. Walters
30423 Canwood St., Suite 115
Agoura Hills, CA 91301
(818) 706-2202 or (800) 992-5837
www.walterslowvision.com
walterslv@cs.com

Produces optical low vision devices and CCTVs.

Telesensory
520 Almanor Ave.
Sunnyvale, CA 94086-3533
(408) 616-8700 or (800) 804-8004
www.telesensory.com
info@telesensory.com

Develops, manufactures, and markets electronic and computer-based low vision products, video magnification systems and speech output systems.

University of California School of Optometry
360 Minor Hall
Berkeley, CA 94720-2020
(510) 642-0229

Distributes Bailey-Lovie eye charts.

Vision Associates
2109 U.S. Hwy 90 West
Suite 170 #412
Lake City, FL 32055
(407) 352-1200
www.visionkits.com

Distributes a variety of vision tests and materials.

Vistech Consultants
P.O. Box 13553
Dayton, Ohio 45413-0553
(937) 454-1355
www.vistechconsultants.com

Manufactures the VCTS 6500 vision contrast test system.

EVALUATION TOOLS AND INSTRUMENTS

This section lists tools and instruments referred to in this book that may be used in a functional evaluation of vision. The descriptions of the instruments indicate their salient characteristics. Sources for the products are listed; contact information may be found in the previous section on Manufacturers and Suppliers of Optical and Nonoptical Devices and Supplies.

Distance Acuity Charts

Bailey-Lovie Chart
Uses letters; maintains constant proportional
   changes in letter size and spacing.
Source: University of California School of
      Optometry; Lighthouse Professional
      Products

Distance Test Chart for the Partially Sighted
Uses numbers; does not adhere to proportional
   changes from row to row; size changes are
   not constant; very large range of number
   sizes.
Source: Lighthouse Professional Products
      Catalog

ETDRS (Early Treatment of Diabetic Retinopathy Study) Chart
Uses letters; maintains constant proportional
   changes in letter size and spacing.
Source: Lighthouse Professional Products
      Catalog

Illiterate or Tumbling E
Uses only one symbol ("E") oriented in one of four directions. Useful for non-English speakers.
Source: Bernell

Lea Symbol Charts
Uses shapes (circle, square, house, and heart); maintains constant proportional changes in symbol size and spacing. For adults and children and non-English speakers.
Source: Good-Lite; Vision Associates

Bailey-Hall Cereal Test
Good for young children and students with multiple disabilities.
Source: Vision Associates

Near Acuity Charts

Bailey-Lovie Word Reading Chart
Uses unrelated words; maintains constant size and spacing progression. For adults.
Source: Lighthouse Professional Products Catalog; University of California School of Optometry

Illiterate or Tumbling E and Tumbling Hands
Uses only one symbol ("E" or a hand) oriented in one of four directions. Useful for non-English speakers.
Source: Bernell

Lea Symbol Chart
Available in crowded and uncrowded formats; uses shapes or numbers; maintains constant proportional changes in symbol size and spacing. For adults and children and non-English speakers.
Source: Good-Lite; Vision Associates

Tests for Assessing Reading Skills

MN Read
Uses sentences with second- and third-grade-level words; maintains constant size and spacing progression. For children and adults.
Source: Lighthouse Professional Products Catalog

Morgan Low Vision Reading Comprehension Assessment
Source: Lighthouse Professional Products Catalog

Pepper Visual Skills for Reading Test
Source: Lighthouse Professional Products Catalog

Contrast Sensitivity Charts

Bailey-Lovie High and Low Contrast Chart
Uses letters at a variable test distance; provides variable target size and constant contrast.
Source: Lighthouse Professional Products Catalog; University of California School of Optometry

Cambridge Low Contrast Gratings
Uses square wave gratings (stripes); provides constant target size and variable contrast. For children and adults.
Source: Haag-Streit UK

Hiding Heidi Low Contrast Test
Uses a face at variable test distance (usually very close); provides a constant target size and variable contrast. For children and adults.
Source: Good-Lite; Vision Associates

Mr. Happy
Uses a face at variable test distance (usually very close); provides a constant target size and variable contrast. For children and adults.

Source: Lighthouse Professional Products
Catalog; University of California
School of Optometry

Pelli-Robinson Contrast Sensitivity Chart
Uses letters at 1 m test distance; provides
constant target size and variable
contrast.
Source: Haag-Streit UK

VCTS 6500
Uses sine wave gratings (stripes) at 1 m
distance; provides variable target size and
variable contrast.
Source: Vistech Consultants

Color Vision Tests

Color Vision Testing Made Easy
Simplified Ishihara Plate test for younger
children; tests for red-green defects
only.
Source: Vision Associates

Dvorine Color Plates
Plate test; tests for red-green defects only.
Source: The Psychological Corporation;
Richmond Products

Farnsworth D-15
Arrangement test; tests for both red-green and
blue-yellow defects.
Source: GretagMacbeth; Richmond Products

L'Anthony Desaturated D-15
Arrangement test; tests for both red-green and
blue-yellow defects; more sensitive than the
Farnsworth D-15.
Source: Bernell; Richmond Products

Ishihara Plates
Plate test; tests for red-green defects only.
Source: Bernell; Richmond Products

Tests for Visual-Perceptual Skills

**Development Test of Visual Perception,
2nd ed.**
(D. D/ Hammill, N.A. Pearson, & J. K. Voress,
1993)
Revision of the Frostig Developmental Test of
Visual Perception; has motor and nonmotor
components. For ages 4–10 years.
Source: Stoelting Company

**Gardner Test of Visual-Motor
Perceptual Skills**
Nonmotor test of visual perception; does not
require writing or drawing.
Source: Psychological and Educational
Publications

Motor-Free Visual Perceptions Test—3
(R. P. Colarusso & D. D. Hammill)
Nonmotor test of visual perception; does not
require writing or drawing.
Source: Academic Therapy Publications

Index